# The World Health Report 2004

**changing** history

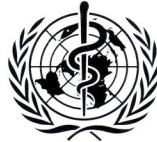

World Health Organization

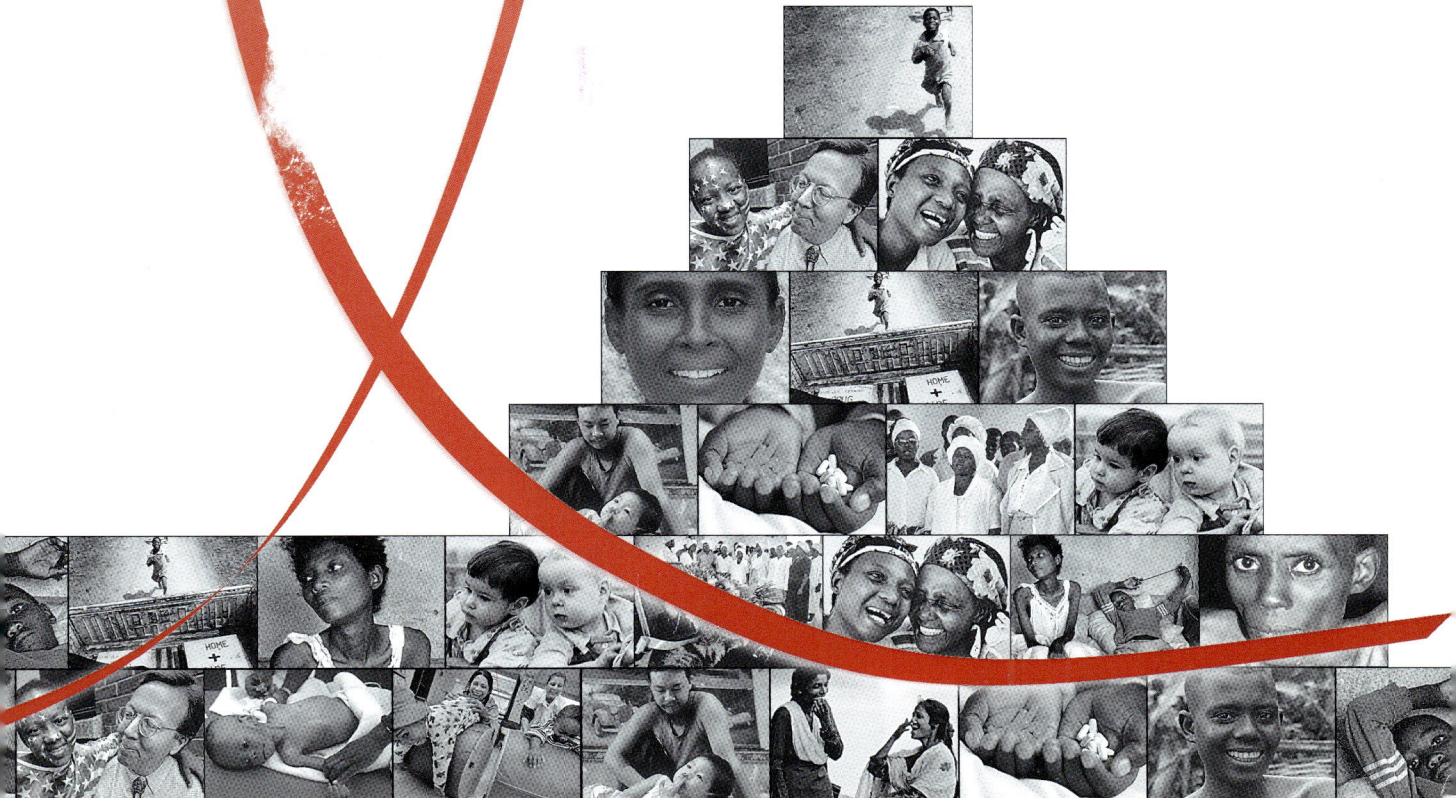

WHO Library Cataloguing-in-Publication Data

World Health Organization.
   The World health report : 2004 : changing history.

   1.World health - trends 2.HIV infections - therapy 3.Acquired immunodeficiency syndrome - therapy
   4.Acquired immunodeficiency syndrome - therapy 5.Anti-retroviral agents - supply and distribution
   6.Delivery of health care - organization and administration 7.World Health Organization I.Title
   II.Title: Changing history.

   ISBN 92 4 156265 X          (NLM Classification: WA 540.1)
   ISSN 1020-3311

Information concerning this publication can be obtained from:
World Health Report
World Health Organization
1211 Geneva 27, Switzerland
E-mail: whr@who.int

Copies of this publication can be ordered from: bookorders@who.int

This report was produced under the overall direction of Tim Evans (Assistant Director-General), Robert Beaglehole (Editor-in-Chief), Jim Kim (Special Adviser to the Director-General) and Paulo Teixeira (Director, HIV/AIDS). The principal authors were Robert Beaglehole, Alec Irwin and Thomson Prentice.

The other main contributors to chapters were: *Chapter One:* Ties Boerma, Jean-Paul Moatti, Alex de Waal and Tony Waddell. *Chapter Two:* Jhoney Barcarolo, Alex Capron, Charles Gilks, Alaka Singh and Marco Vitoria. *Chapter Three:* Hedwig Goede, Ian Grubb and Stephanie Nixon. *Chapter Four:* David Evans, Neelam Sekhri, Phyllida Travis and Mark Wheeler. *Chapter Five:* Don Berwick, Michel Kazatchkine and Yves Souteyrand.

Other contributors to the report were: Christopher Bailey, Michel Beusenberg, Boakye Boatin, Andrew Boulle, Guy Carrin, David Coetzee, François Dabis, Betina Durovni, Dominique Egger, Paula Fujiwara, Claudia Garcia-Moreno, Eric Goemaere, Peter Graaf, Raj Gupta, Kate Hankins, Kei Kawabata, Wayne Koff, Michael Lederman, Ying-Ru Lo, Naisiadet Mason, Kedar Mate, J.P. Narain, Carla Obermeyer, Amolo Okero, Catherine Orrell, Andreas Reis, Peter Reiss, Alan Stone, Tessa Tantorres, Kate Taylor, Roger Teck and David Walton.

Contributors to statistical tables were: Carla Abou-Zahr, Prerna Banati, Steve Begg, Christina Bernard, Ana Betran, Maureen Birmingham, Daniel Bleed, Monika Blössner, Anthony Burton, Laurent Chenet, Christopher Dye, Charu Garg, Peter Ghys, Patricia Hernández, Mehran Hosseini, Jose Hueb, Chandika Indikadahena, Mie Inoue, Peter Jackson, Doris Ma Fat, Colin Mathers, Sumi Mehta, John Miller, Bernard Nahlen, Mercedes de Onis, Richard Poe, Leonel Pontes, Jean-Pierre Poullier, Nathalie Proust, Eva Rehfuess, Kenji Shibuya, Karen Stanecki, Michel Thieren, Niels Tomijima, Nathalie Van de Maele, Catherine Watt and Hongyi Xu.

Valuable input was received from Assistant Directors-General, policy advisers to the Director-General at WHO headquarters, and many technical staff. Additional help and advice were kindly provided by Regional Directors and members of their staff.

The report was edited by Barbara Campanini and Leo Vita-Finzi. Translation coordination and other administrative and production support was provided by Shelagh Probst. The web site version and other electronic media were provided by Gael Kernen. The photographs and media kit were coordinated by Gary Walker. Proofreading was by Marie Fitzsimmons. The index was prepared by Kathleen Lyle.

Design: Reda Sadki
Layout: Steve Ewart, Sue Hobbs and Reda Sadki
Printing coordination: Keith Wynn
Printed in France
2004/15763 – Sadag – 20000

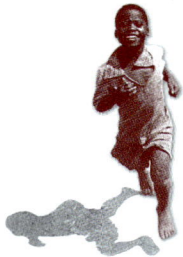

# contents

## Chapter 5

# message from the
# director-general

We are living in a time of unprecedented opportunities for health. In spite of many difficulties, technology has made important advances and international investment in health has at last begun to flow. Most of the increased funding is for the fight against HIV/AIDS. It brings a welcome and long overdue improvement in the prospects for controlling the worst global epidemic in several centuries. The responsibility of WHO and its partners in this effort is to ensure that the increased funding is used in such a way as to enable countries to fight HIV/AIDS and at the same time strengthen their health systems. HIV/AIDS control involves the full spectrum of economic, social and technical activities. A key role of WHO within this spectrum is to work with countries to build up the systems needed to provide treatment. Expanding the use of antiretroviral therapy will allow countries to support effective systems for delivering chronic care, thus extending their capacity to meet the long-term health needs of the population.

The initiative to make antiretroviral therapy available to 3 million people by the end of 2005 (known as "3 by 5") is aimed at accelerating this process. It provides new ways to pursue the objectives for which WHO has been working since it was founded 56 years ago. However, the stakes are high: rapid expansion of antiretroviral treatment is a large, complex and difficult undertaking. It certainly cannot by done by one agency working on its own. Partnerships are indispensable for a task of this magnitude. Making them work requires great commitment, goodwill and talent on all sides. The initiative draws its strength from many partners with large amounts of all these ingredients, and we expect much more. But I am well aware that we and our partners took a risk in embracing 3 by 5. What I strongly felt we needed was a time-limited, difficult goal that would change the way we work. This is the best way to challenge ourselves to make the contribution that we as WHO should be making to the global effort against HIV/AIDS. Future generations will judge our era in large part by our response to the AIDS pandemic. By tackling it decisively we will also be building health systems that can meet the health needs of today and tomorrow, and continue the advance to Health for All. This is an historic opportunity we cannot afford to miss.

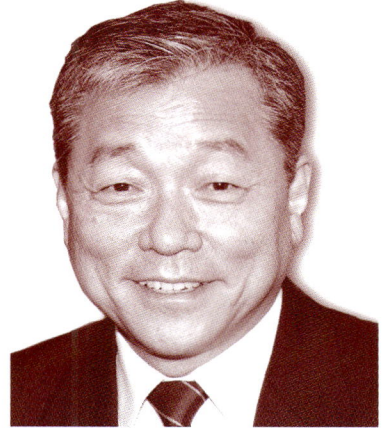

LEE Jong-wook
Director-General
World Health Organization
Geneva, May 2004

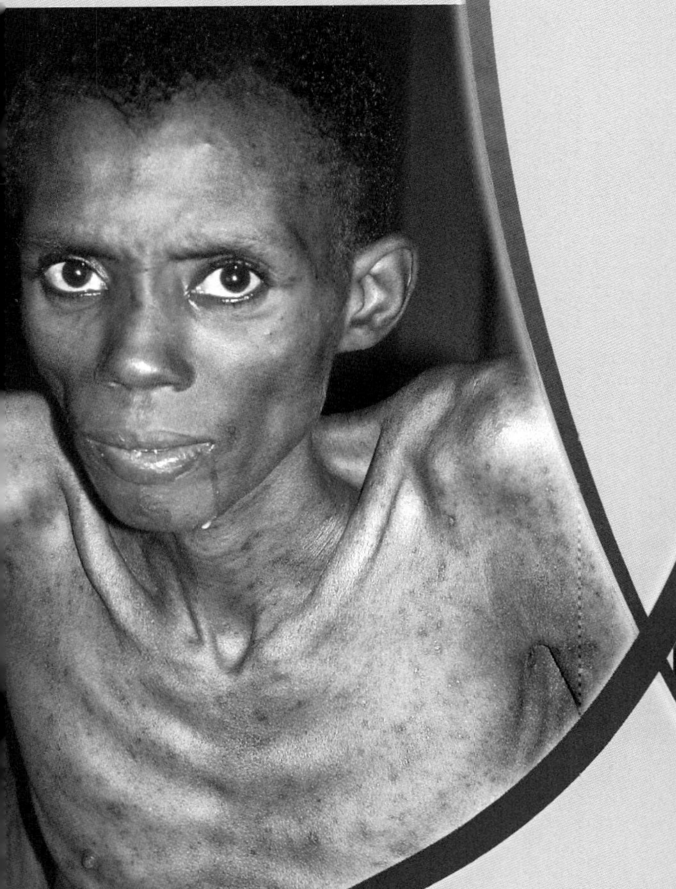

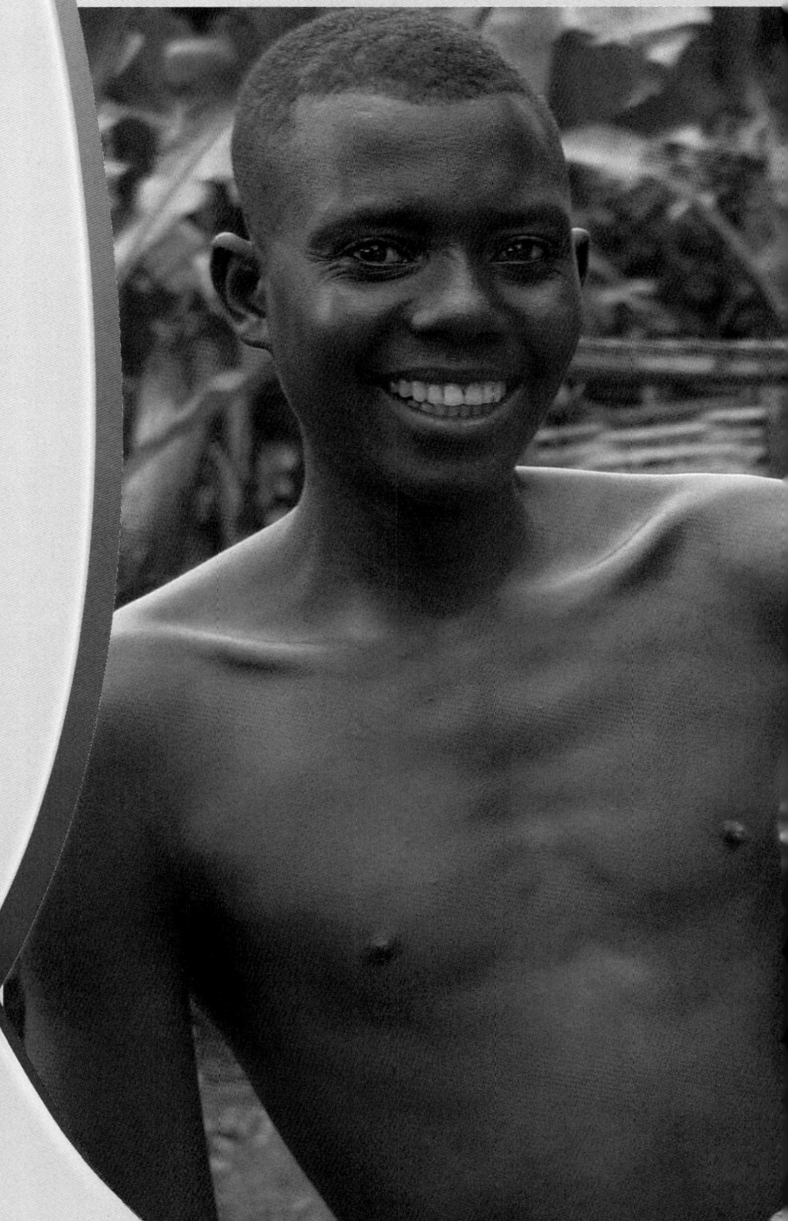

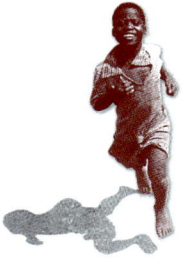

# overview

The two photographs on the opposite page show how the history of HIV/AIDS is changing. They are snapshots of the past and the present, a vivid example of how, today, innovative treatment programmes are not only saving lives but also helping to strengthen health systems on which to build a brighter future.

Joseph Jeune is a 26-year-old peasant farmer in Lascahobas, a small town in central Haiti. When the first picture was taken in March 2003, his parents had already bought his coffin. Suffering from the advanced stages of AIDS, Joseph Jeune probably had only weeks to live. The second picture, taken six months later, shows him 20 kg heavier and transformed after receiving treatment for HIV/AIDS and tuberculosis (TB) coinfection.

There are millions of people like Joseph Jeune around the world. For most of them, HIV/AIDS treatment is still beyond reach, but Joseph shows what can be achieved. He receives care at the small clinic in his home town. The clinic's HIV/AIDS and TB treatment programmes are part of a wider initiative to strengthen the health service infrastructure across much of Haiti's central plateau. The effort involves nongovernmental organizations, the public sector and communities, with major support from the Global Fund to Fight AIDS, Tuberculosis and Malaria. Using antiretroviral therapy as an entry point, the programme is building up primary health care in communities, for a total population of about 260 000 people. It does so through improved drug procurement and management, the expansion of HIV counselling and testing, increased salaries for local health care personnel, and the training of numerous community health care workers. Primary care clinics have been refurbished, restocked with essential medicines, and provided with new staff. They are receiving up to 10 times more patients for general medical care daily than before the project began.

*The World Health Report 2004* shows how projects like this can bring the medical treatment that saved Joseph Jeune to millions of other people in poor and middle-income countries and how, crucially, such efforts can drive improvements in health systems.

Effectively tackling HIV/AIDS is the world's most urgent public health challenge. Already, the disease has killed more than 20 million people. Today, an estimated 34–46 million others are living with HIV/AIDS. In 2003, 3 million people died and 5 million others became infected. Unknown a quarter of a century ago, HIV/AIDS is now the leading cause of death and lost years of productive life for adults aged 15–59 years worldwide.

A comprehensive HIV/AIDS strategy links prevention, treatment, care and support for people living with the virus. Until now, treatment has been the most neglected element in most developing countries. Yet among all possible HIV-related interventions it is treatment that can most effectively drive health systems strengthening, enabling poor countries to protect their people from a wide range of health threats. This report shows how international organizations, national governments, the private sector and communities can combine their strengths to expand access to HIV/AIDS treatment, reinforce HIV prevention and strengthen health systems in some of the countries where they are currently weakest, for the long-term benefit of all.

Almost 6 million people in developing countries will die in the near future if they do not receive treatment – but only about 400 000 of them were receiving it in 2003. In September 2003, WHO, the Joint United Nations Programme on HIV/AIDS (UNAIDS) and the Global Fund declared lack of access to AIDS treatment with antiretroviral medicines a global health emergency. In response, these organizations and their partners launched an effort to provide 3 million people in developing countries with antiretroviral therapy by the end of 2005 – the 3 by 5 initiative, one of the most ambitious public health projects ever conceived.

## A CHANCE TO CHANGE HISTORY

Advocacy by WHO and its partners for more global investment in health has begun to bear fruit. Official development assistance and other forms of global health investment are on the rise. Most of the increased spending is for HIV/AIDS. Along with the urgent need to tackle the pandemic, this fact now makes HIV/AIDS the key battleground for global public health. It also gives countries the chance to derive extra public health benefits from the new funds. The opportunity exists to invest these resources so as to save millions of threatened lives through treatment, reinforce comprehensive HIV/AIDS control and strengthen some of the world's most fragile health systems.

The objective of treating 3 million people in developing countries with antiretroviral drugs by the end of 2005 is a step on the way to the goal of universal access to antiretroviral therapy and HIV/AIDS care for all who need it. This goal far outreaches the capacities of any single organization. Through collaboration linking the skills of many partners, however, these aims can be achieved. The treatment initiative is important not only to tackle a grave health crisis, but also because it is building innovative mechanisms of collaboration in health, linking national governments, international organizations, the private sector, civil society groups and communities. Success in partnership on the initiative will accelerate other areas of global health work.

The initiative adapts lessons from HIV/AIDS programmes in developed countries and builds on the achievements of developing countries such as Botswana, Brazil, Senegal and Thailand in scaling up antiretroviral treatment. An increasing number of effective partnerships will mean that no country has to face the HIV/AIDS treatment challenge alone. UNAIDS has, for nearly a decade, kept HIV/AIDS at the forefront of global consciousness and spurred recognition that only an exceptional response can meet the challenge. Under its leadership, the entire United Nations system has embraced its responsibilities. The creation of the Global Fund has fostered partnership between governments, civil society, the private sector and affected communities. The World Bank has brought innovation, and is joined now by the European Union, bilateral initiatives such as the United States President's Emergency Plan for AIDS Relief, and the major contributions of individual governments and private foundations, including the Bill and Melinda Gates Foundation and the William J. Clinton Foundation. There have also been inventive new approaches to technical cooperation, such as hospital twinnings through the Ensemble pour une Solidarité

Thérapeutique Hospitalière en Réseau (ESTHER), initiated by the French government and now supported by Italy, Luxembourg, Spain and other partners.

Success in expanding HIV/AIDS treatment depends on the engagement of civil society. Without the mobilization of activist organizations and communities, the toll of HIV/AIDS over the past quarter-century would have been far heavier. The momentum for antiretroviral scale-up owes much to the sustained advocacy of treatment activists at local, national and global levels and to nongovernmental organizations such as Médecins Sans Frontières and Partners In Health-Zami Lasante, which demonstrated to the world the feasibility of delivering antiretroviral treatment in the poorest settings. This report shows WHO's commitment to work closely with national health authorities, the private sector, community-based organizations and others in delivering comprehensive HIV/AIDS programmes on the ground.

## WHY TREATMENT MUST BE SCALED UP

The long-term economic and social costs of HIV/AIDS have been seriously underestimated in many countries. More accurate projections now suggest that some countries in sub-Saharan Africa will face economic collapse unless they can bring their epidemics under control, mainly because HIV/AIDS weakens and kills adults like Joseph Jeune in their prime. Data in this report and the forthcoming UNAIDS/WHO *Global report* confirm that the social devastation of the epidemic continues to grow. Reinforced prevention is vital to safeguard future generations but, at the same time, antiretroviral treatment expansion is essential to protect the stability and security of communities, countries and regions and to strengthen the foundations of future development.

The fact that effective treatment exists but has not been made accessible to millions of people in urgent need is something that WHO must tackle, given its special responsibility within the UNAIDS family of cosponsors. WHO's Constitution charges the Organization to pursue the universal realization of the right to health: "the attainment by all peoples of the highest possible level of health". In the case of HIV/AIDS, for those in clinical need of treatment the realization of this right requires access to antiretrovirals.

## EXPANDING TREATMENT ACCESS

The report explains that the treatment initiative draws on the specific comparative strengths of multilateral, national and local actors and capitalizes on the motivating effect of a time-bound target.

Between the declaration of the global treatment emergency in September 2003 and the end of February 2004, more than 40 of the countries with the highest burden of HIV/AIDS expressed commitment to rapid treatment expansion and requested technical cooperation in designing and implementing scale-up programmes. WHO and its partners have worked closely with country health officials, treatment providers, community organizations and other stakeholders to revise treatment targets, design national treatment scale-up plans and launch implementation. In countries such as Kenya, the United Republic of Tanzania, and Zambia, WHO is linking with key bilateral partners to develop a target-focused, streamlined approach that will maximize efficiency under clear national leadership. Political commitment and national ownership of programmes are essential. The streamlined funding mechanisms developed by the Global Fund are enabling many countries to access funding and expand programmes more quickly.

As new funding flows in, technical and human resource capacities must be ready to ensure its effective use. Countries need technical cooperation to support implementation on the ground and have requested clear guidance on treatment delivery and programme management. WHO makes a fundamental contribution by providing such guidance.

An important task is to expand as rapidly as possible from small pilot projects to treatment programmes with national coverage, while maintaining quality of care in the face of serious resource constraints. For rapid expansion, noticing gaps in resources is the starting point for a plan to redesign care so that it is, from the outset, "scalable". The initiative takes a practical "engineering" or "system design" approach. The key is not to require that countries simply accumulate the usual resources for care – enough doctors, nurses, clinics, and so on – to reach the entire population; in many poor countries, that will just not work at present. Instead, the WHO strategy begins with clearly defined objectives, and then works to develop innovative system designs that can be expanded even when the usual medical resources are in very short supply. Such solutions will vary from country to country, but many factors are relatively constant, and many lessons can be shared. The strategy draws on solid evidence of the success of pioneering projects and some existing national programmes. Knowledge gained, systematically measured and reflected upon can be quickly reapplied and shared widely.

To help accelerate the initiative, WHO has developed a simplified set of antiretroviral drug regimens, testing and treatment guidelines that are consistent with the highest standards of quality of care. They have the added advantage of enabling much more effective use of nurses, clinical officers and community health workers to support treatment. While physicians supervise the clinical teams, day-to-day patient management and adherence support tasks can be safely and effectively delegated to other workers, including appropriately trained community health workers. In this way there is a better chance of delivering care quickly despite shortages of physicians, laboratories and other facilities. These simplified regimens are the critical element in ensuring that expansion of treatment in poor countries can be carried out equitably. WHO has also designed streamlined guidelines for training health workers in a wide range of skills related to the use of antiretroviral drugs, from HIV counselling and testing and recruitment of patients to treatment delivery, clinical management of patients and the monitoring of drug resistance.

WHO is now working on the ground with health officials, treatment providers and communities to overcome technical challenges; it is also serving as a coordination, communications and information-sharing hub to gather, analyse and disseminate data, and is feeding back the information so that it can be used rapidly to improve programme performance. This intensified collaboration on antiretroviral treatment scale-up is part of WHO's broad commitment to working closely with countries to meet their major health goals.

WHO, in partnership with UNICEF and the World Bank, has established the AIDS Medicines and Diagnostics Service as an operational arm to ensure that developing countries have access to quality antiretrovirals and diagnostic tools at the best prices. The service aims to help countries to buy, forecast and manage the supply and delivery of products necessary for the treatment and monitoring of HIV/AIDS.

As policy and technical support work at country level intensifies, WHO, UNAIDS and their partners will continue their global advocacy work to ensure that adequate resources flow to support countries. New resources available through the Global Fund and other partners will be critical to success. On request, WHO is providing countries with technical assistance in the preparation of applications to the Global Fund and other potential funders.

## TOWARDS HEALTH FOR ALL

The global HIV/AIDS treatment gap reflects wider patterns of inequality in health and is a test of the international community's commitment to tackle these inequalities. Beyond working to save millions of lives under immediate threat, WHO and its partners are confronting a broad range of health problems that afflict poor communities and keep them poor, viewing HIV/AIDS treatment expansion and the Millennium Development Goals as steps on the road to Health for All.

The treatment initiative will not end in 2005. Ahead lie the challenges of extending treatment to many more millions of people and maintaining it for the rest of their lives, while simultaneously building and sustaining the health infrastructures to make that huge task possible. The ultimate aim is nothing less than to reduce health inequalities by building up effective, equitable health systems for all.

## CHAPTER SUMMARIES

## Chapter 1. A global emergency: a combined response

This chapter describes the current epidemiological state of HIV/AIDS epidemics around the world and examines the daunting challenges that lie ahead. It shows that the world is far from ready for what is to come: it provides evidence that the social and economic consequences of unchecked HIV/AIDS epidemics will be catastrophic for many communities and countries.

Although it has seemed a familiar enemy for much of the last 20 years, the global HIV/AIDS pandemic is only now beginning to be seen for what it is: a unique threat to human society, whose impact will be felt by future generations. The most explosive growth of the pandemic occurred during the middle of the 1990s, especially in sub-Saharan Africa. Today, an estimated 34–46 million people are living with HIV/AIDS. Two-thirds of the total live in Africa, where about one in 12 adults is infected, and one-fifth in Asia. Globally, unprotected sexual intercourse between men and women is the predominant mode of transmission of the virus.

The chapter explains why WHO, along with its partners, believes an emergency global and comprehensive response is essential and must embrace prevention, treatment and long-term care. Prevention is essential to protect the many millions of young adults and children who are most at risk but who are not yet affected. Treatment is the difference between life and death for the millions of people who are HIV-positive but are currently denied access to antiretroviral medications. Long-term care is also essential. Almost 6 million people need treatment now – only about 400 000 received it in 2003. The chapter argues that a treatment gap of such dimensions is indefensible, and that narrowing it is a public health necessity.

Together, prevention, treatment and long-term care and support can reverse the seemingly inexorable progress of the HIV/AIDS epidemics, offering the worst-affected countries and populations their best hope of survival.

## Chapter 2. The treatment initiative

This chapter stresses the need for a comprehensive strategy that links prevention, treatment, research, and long-term care and support for people living with HIV/AIDS. But it points out that until now, treatment has been the most neglected component of this approach in much of the developing world. To accelerate prevention while limiting the social devastation now unfolding, rapid expansion of HIV/AIDS treatment with antiretroviral medicines in the countries hardest hit by the pandemic is needed immediately.

Despite mounting evidence that this treatment works in resource-poor settings, by late 2003 less than 7% of people in developing countries in urgent need were receiving it. The chapter examines public health arguments and economic and social arguments for scaling up antiretroviral therapy. It then presents WHO's strategy for working with countries and partners to reach the treatment target and provides an estimate of the global investment required. It explains the five pillars that support the strategy. These are: global leadership, strong partnership and advocacy; urgent, sustained country support; simplified, standardized tools for delivering antiretroviral therapy; effective, reliable supply of medicines and diagnostics; and rapid identification and reapplication of new knowledge and successes.

The opportunities and challenges facing selected countries are explored, highlighting the need to ensure that treatment scale-up reaches the poorest people. Finally, the chapter considers the wider importance of expanded treatment as a new way of working across the global health community for improved health outcomes and equity.

## Chapter 3. Community participation: advocacy and action

The participation of communities and civil society groups, particularly groups of people living with HIV/AIDS, is crucial to treatment scale-up and comprehensive HIV/AIDS control. This participation will include both advocacy and the involvement of community members in delivering services and support to patients. Community involvement is essential to prevention, treatment, care, support and research.

This chapter describes the background of community participation as a dimension of public health work and recalls key achievements of civil society HIV/AIDS activism. It then considers the roles that civil society groups and community members will play in scaling up antiretroviral therapy in resource-poor settings.

State leadership will be indispensable to successful scale-up, and civil society cannot replace the public sector. But a key task of effective government leadership will be creating partnerships with civil society organizations and mechanisms to make use of the skills available within communities. The commitment to community participation links the treatment strategy with the Health-for-All vision and an equity-based agenda in global public health. The values of human rights, health equity and social justice embraced by many civil society AIDS activist groups are closely related to WHO's constitutional objective: "the attainment by all peoples of the highest possible level of health". This chapter shows that these values provide a basis for ongoing collaboration and partnerships between communities, civil society groups, national governments and international organizations, including WHO.

Such collaboration will be crucial to future health progress. The role of the 3 by 5 initiative in catalysing innovative partnerships is part of how it is changing ways of thinking and working in global health. For example, communities educated and mobilized around HIV/AIDS control will be better able to take part in health promotion, disease control and treatment efforts regarding health problems related to other Millennium Development Goals: to combat malaria and other diseases, maternal and child mortality, and the growing burden of chronic adult diseases in low-income and middle-income countries.

## Chapter 4. Health systems: finding new strength

Health sector interventions against HIV/AIDS – especially the treatment initiative – are dependent on well-functioning health systems. In countries with a high burden of HIV/AIDS, systems are often degraded and dysfunctional because of a combination of underfunding and weak governance. HIV/AIDS places additional burdens on these weakened health systems.

The 3 by 5 initiative has the potential to strengthen health systems in a number of ways, by, for example, attracting resources to the health system in addition to those required for HIV/AIDS, stimulating investment in physical infrastructure, developing procurement and distribution systems of generic application, and fostering interaction with communities which can benefit a wide range of health interventions. It is important that any potentially adverse effects on the wider health system are anticipated and minimized.

The chapter continues with a consideration of the health systems context in resource-poor settings, taking note of the participation of both public and private providers. It then considers how health systems can be strengthened, so that they can implement the expanded treatment initiative while continuing to improve and expand many other health interventions. The conceptual framework of the four main functions of health systems is used: leadership, service delivery, resource provision, and financing. In the medium term, the financing gap will have to be closed mainly by external donors, because national governments and economies are incapable of generating much more than they do already, whereas donors, aware of their past pledges, can be enouraged to do more.

## Chapter 5. Sharing research and knowledge

This chapter records that, since scientists first identified the human immunodeficiency virus as the cause of AIDS in 1983, there have been many remarkable research achievements related to the disease and many people have benefited. Twenty years ago there was little effective treatment; today there is a range of antiretroviral drugs that dramatically improve patients' quality of life and chances of survival.

Despite significant advances, however, including the design and testing of more than 30 candidate HIV vaccines, it will be several more years at least before a safe and effective vaccine becomes widely available. In examining that continuing quest, the chapter also reviews research into other important areas of HIV/AIDS prevention, treatment and care.

There are four broad categories of challenges facing researchers.

- Prevention research – slowing down the growth and geographical expansion of the epidemic: a challenge for epidemiology and sociobehavioural aspects of prevention.
- Vaccine research – designing a safe and effective preventive vaccine, the best hope for the long-term prevention and control of HIV/AIDS.
- Treatment research – generating new antiretroviral drugs and designing new therapeutic strategies that would be active on "wild" and resistant strains of viruses, easy to take and better tolerated than currently available drugs: a challenge for basic and clinical research.
- Delivery system (operational) research – making care and antiretroviral treatment available to all of those who need it worldwide: a multidisciplinary undertaking.

The chapter examines important matters such as the prevention of HIV transmission from mother to child; the development and use of microbicides; the need to sustain long-term adherence to treatment; toxicities; drug resistance; joint approaches to HIV/AIDS and tuberculosis; economic issues; health policy analysis; equity issues; and international collaboration. The chapter leads on to the report's brief concluding section, which contains an optimistic view of the future. It emphasizes that a crucial moment has been reached in the history of HIV/AIDS, and that there is now an unprecedented opportunity to alter its course. Ahead lies the challenge of extending lifelong treatment to many more millions of people, while simultaneously building and sustaining the health infrastructures to make that huge task possible. The outcome can be better health for generations to come.

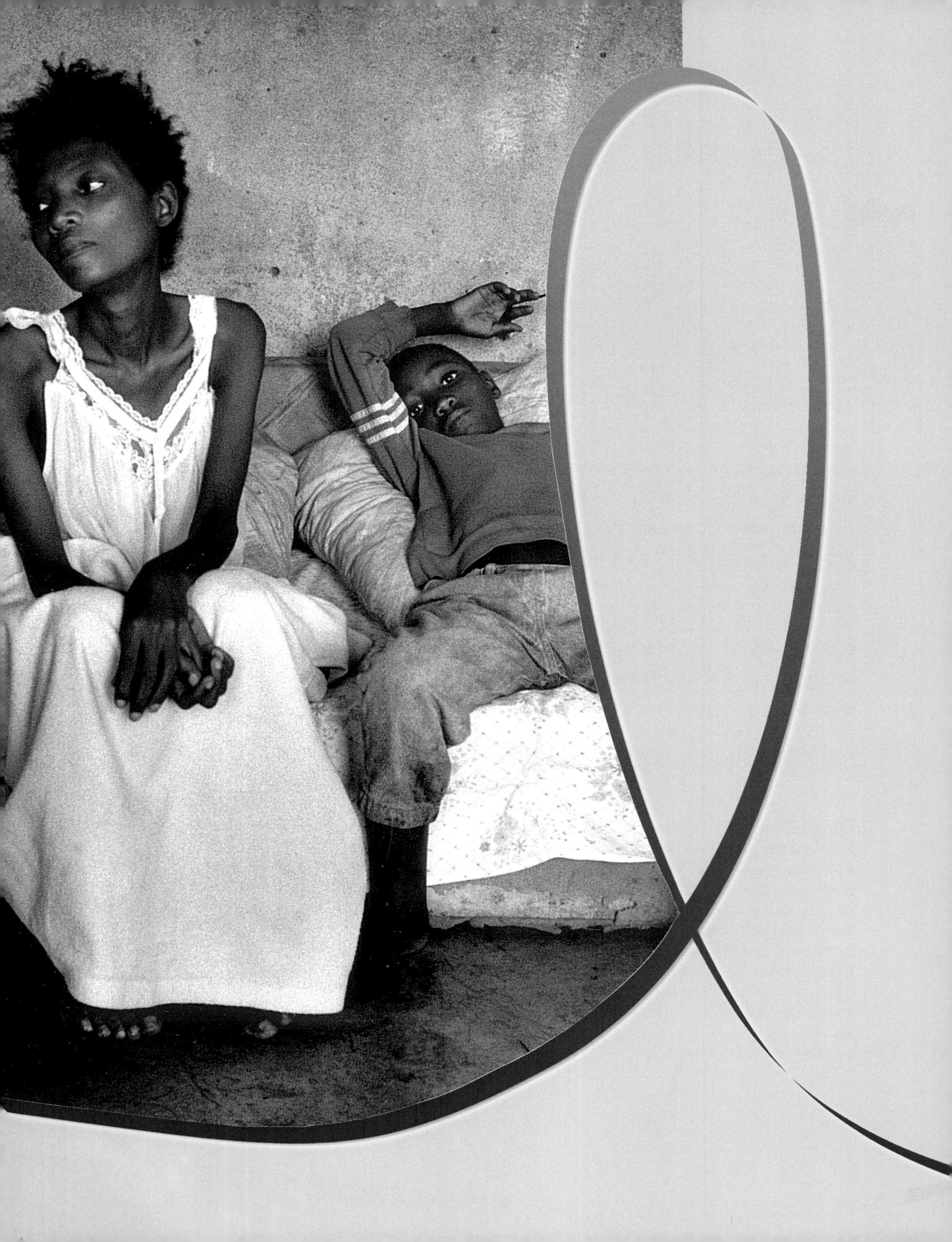

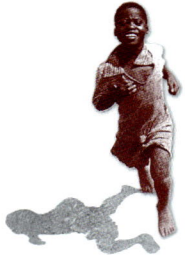

chapter one
# a global emergency:
# a combined response

**This chapter outlines the current state of the global HIV/AIDS pandemic and explains why an international response is needed. It describes some of the tragic social and economic consequences of the disease, including its destructive impact on health systems. The response must embrace prevention, support, treatment and long-term care. Together, these components can effectively combat the seemingly inexorable progress of HIV/AIDS epidemics, offering the worst-affected countries and populations their best hope of survival. Comprehensive action will accelerate progress towards all the Millennium Development Goals while offering an opportunity to help strengthen health systems.**

## THE GLOBAL SITUATION

Although it has seemed a familiar enemy for the last 20 years, HIV/AIDS is only now beginning to be seen for what it is: a unique threat to human society, whose impact will be felt for generations to come. Today, an estimated 34–46 million people are living with HIV/AIDS. Already, more than 20 million people have died from AIDS, 3 million in 2003 alone *(1)*. Four million children have been infected since the virus first appeared. Of the 5 million people who became infected with the virus in 2003, 700 000 were children, almost entirely as the result of transmission during pregnancy and childbirth, or from breastfeeding.

The most explosive growth of the epidemic occurred in the mid-1990s, especially in Africa (see Figure 1.1). In 2003, Africa was home to two-thirds of the world's people living with HIV/AIDS, but only 11% of the world's total population. Today, about one in 12 African adults is living with HIV/AIDS. One-fifth of the people infected with HIV live in Asia.

Globally, unprotected sexual intercourse between men and women is the predominant mode of transmission of the virus. In sub-Saharan Africa and the Caribbean, women are at least as likely as men to become infected.

Other important modes of transmission include unprotected penetrative sex between men, injecting drug use, and unsafe injections and blood transfusions. In many countries, including most countries in the Americas, Asia and Europe, HIV infection is mainly concentrated in populations engaging in high-risk behaviour, such as unprotected sex (particularly in the context of commercial sex work or between men) and sharing of drug injection

**Figure 1.1** Estimated number of adults infected with HIV, by WHO region, 1980–2003

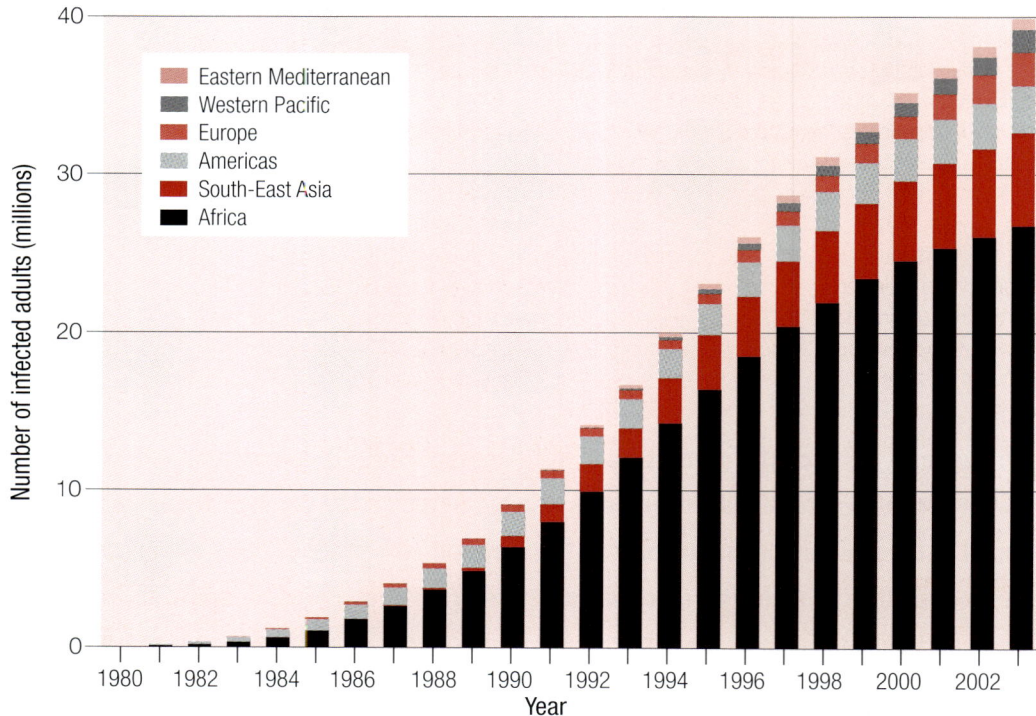

equipment. In such situations, however, there is a persistent threat that localized epidemics will spill over into the wider population. In some countries, rapid growth of the size of the vulnerable populations – as a result of civil unrest, a rise in poverty or other social and economic factors – triggers epidemic growth and wider spread of the virus.

The prolonged time lag between infection with HIV and the onset of full disease (on average 9–11 years in the absence of treatment) means that the numbers of HIV-associated tuberculosis cases, AIDS cases and deaths have only recently reached epidemic levels in many of the severely affected countries. Globally, the greatest mortality impact is on people between the ages of 20 and 40 years. Dramatic changes in life expectancy can be observed in the most affected parts of the world. The pandemic has reversed decades of gradual gains in life expectancy in sub-Saharan Africa *(2)*.

What does the global state of the pandemic mean in terms of progress towards the Millennium Development Goals? The eight goals, established following the historic Millennium Summit in New York in 2000, represent commitments by governments throughout the world to do more to reduce poverty and hunger and to tackle ill-health; specifically, to improve access to clean water and to reduce gender inequality, lack of education, and environmental degradation. This includes combating HIV/AIDS, and to have begun to reverse the spread of HIV by 2015. However, progress is not yet being made in many countries, and an unprecedented effort will be required in order for the worst-affected countries to make progress towards all of the Millennium Development Goals (see Box 1.1).

## The uneven spread of HIV

A brief analysis of the regional spread of the HIV/AIDS pandemic shows major differences between regions, within regions and within countries, which have important implications for prevention, care and support. The striking differences in the size of the epidemics in sub-Saharan Africa and other regions of the world have been well documented. While almost all countries in sub-Saharan Africa have been severely affected, widening variations are also emerging within the region, indicating that the consequences of the pandemic will vary substantially *(10)*.

The trends in HIV prevalence among pregnant women attending the same antenatal clinics since 1997 (see Figure 1.2) show that the epidemics in the countries of southern Africa are much larger than elsewhere in sub-Saharan Africa – and that the gaps appear to be widening. In eastern Africa HIV prevalence is now less than half that reported in southern Africa and there is evidence of a modest decline. In western Africa prevalence is now roughly one-fifth of that in southern Africa and no rapid growth is occurring. These striking differences are supported by data from population-based surveys and research studies (see Box 1.2). A range of socioeconomic, cultural, behavioural and biological factors are responsible, such as migration, male circumcision practices and the prevalence of herpes simplex virus type 2 infection *(12, 13)*.

In most countries in Asia the epidemics tend to be concentrated in drug injecting and commercial sex networks, although Cambodia, Myanmar, Thailand and six

## Box 1.1   The impact of HIV/AIDS on the Millennium Development Goals

HIV/AIDS epidemics are reducing the chances of achieving the Millennium Development Goals and targets for many heavily burdened countries, especially in sub-Saharan Africa.

The epidemics undermine poverty reduction efforts by sapping economic growth, thus hampering efforts to reach **Goal 1, to eradicate extreme poverty and hunger**. They have cut annual growth rates by 2–4% per year in Africa *(3)*. But the cumulative long-term macroeconomic effects may be much more devastating and could result in complete economic collapse in some high-burden countries.

Educational opportunities recede as HIV/AIDS cuts family incomes and forces people to spend money on medical care and funerals, thus affecting the chances of reaching **Goal 2, to achieve universal primary education**. For example, in Uganda, 80% of the children in HIV/AIDS-affected households in one village were removed from school because school fees could not be paid or the children's labour was needed *(4)*. In Zambia, the number of teachers killed by AIDS in 1998 was equivalent to two-thirds of the number of teachers trained in the same year *(5)*. Globally, HIV/AIDS is creating millions of orphans with even fewer educational opportunities.

In addition to killing millions of women, HIV/AIDS adds to the caregiving burdens of women and girls, reducing their chances of pursuing education and paid work, and hence undermining **Goal 3, to promote gender equity and empower women**. Girls are often required to care for their sick brothers and sisters at the expense of their own education. HIV-positive women face many forms of discrimination and psychological and physical abuse.

In the seven African countries with the highest adult HIV prevalence, AIDS has already produced a rise of more than 19% in infant mortality and a 36% rise in under-five mortality, thereby reducing many countries' chances of reaching **Goal 4, to reduce child mortality**. In Botswana, the under-five mortality rate will reach 104 deaths per 1000 live births by 2005. In the absence of HIV/AIDS, the rate would have been 45 deaths per 1000 *(6)*.

The disease reduces the chances of reaching **Goal 5, to reduce maternal mortality**. In Rakai, Uganda, maternal mortality was found to be 1687 per 100 000 live births among HIV-positive women and 310 per 100 000 live births among HIV-negative women *(7)*.

HIV infection also directly increases the risks of developing tuberculosis, and in HIV/AIDS-affected countries it is on the rise. In Malawi, for example, the incidence of tuberculosis doubled between 1986 and 1994, largely because people living with HIV/AIDS are seven times more likely to develop tuberculosis than those who are not infected with the virus *(8)*. In Uganda, HIV-infected women were more likely to develop malaria during pregnancy than HIV-negative women. The same study found that the mother-to-child HIV transmission rates were 40% among women with placental malaria compared with 15.4% for women without malaria *(9)*. Thus the pandemic also adversely affects the chances of contending with malaria and other diseases, as part of **Goal 6, to combat HIV/AIDS, malaria and other diseases**.

One target of **Goal 7, to ensure environmental stability**, is significant improvement in at least 100 million slum dwellers' lives by 2020. However, HIV/AIDS is likely to threaten many millions of them.

All goals depend on **Goal 8, to develop a global partnership for development**. This goal links donors, governments, civil society and the private sector. HIV/AIDS is undermining progress here, for example through its decimation of countries' skilled workforces. Providing access to essential medicines is a key target. Expanding HIV/AIDS treatment will be vital to progress.

**Figure 1.2**   HIV prevalence among pregnant women attending antenatal clinics in areas of sub-Saharan Africa, 1997–2002

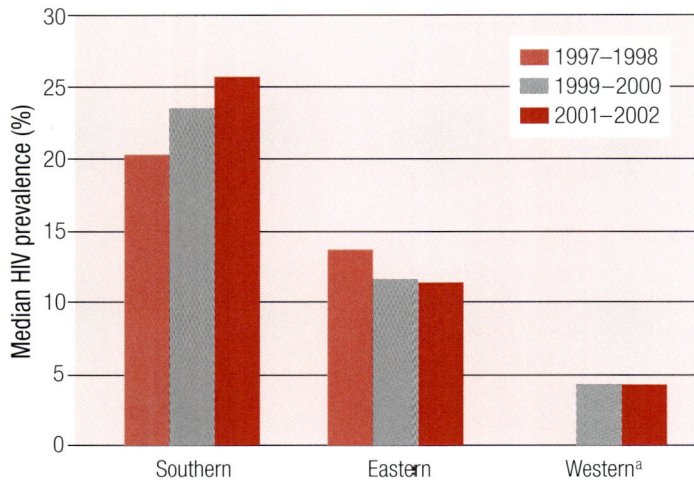

Median HIV prevalence (%)

Legend:
- 1997–1998
- 1999–2000
- 2001–2002

Southern   Eastern   Western[a]

[a] No estimate available for 1997–1998.

states in India have an estimated HIV prevalence among adults of more than 1%. The course of the epidemics in the two most populous countries in the world – China and India – will have a decisive influence on the global pandemic. In 2003 it was estimated that 840 000 people in China were living with HIV/AIDS, corresponding to 0.12% of the total adult population aged 15–49 years. About 70% of these infections are thought to have resulted from injecting drug use or faulty plasma-collection procedures; over 80% of all those infected are men. Official estimates in India for 2003 put the number of people infected at 3.8–4.6 million, with considerable variation between states; there has been a modest increase in recent years.

Countries in eastern Europe and central Asia are experiencing growing epidemics, driven by injecting drug use and to a lesser extent by unsafe sex among young people. In the Russian Federation, where national prevalence is estimated to be just under 1%, 80% of people living with HIV/AIDS are under 30 years of age. In western Europe, the estimated number of new infections greatly exceeds the number of deaths, largely as a result of the success of antiretroviral therapy in lowering death rates. There are, however, worrying signs of increased incidence of other sexually transmitted infections, such as syphilis and gonorrhoea, and reported increases in risk behaviours in several countries *(14, 15)*.

In the WHO Eastern Mediterranean Region it is estimated that there are around 750 000 people living with HIV/AIDS. Heterosexual sex is the main mode of transmission, accounting for nearly 55% of all reported cases. Injecting drug use has an increasing role in transmission and in the near future may become the driving force of the epidemics. A fivefold increase in infections among injecting drug users between 1999 and 2002 was recorded. In Sudan, the most affected country in the region, heterosexual sex is the predominant mode of spread.

In the Americas, the most affected area is the Caribbean, which has the second-highest prevalence in the world after sub-Saharan Africa: overall adult prevalence rates are 2–3%. In Latin America, an estimated 1.6 million people are now infected. Most countries here have concentrated epidemics, with injecting drug use and sex between men as the predominant modes of transmission. The predominant mode of transmission in the Caribbean is heterosexual sex, often associated with commercial sex work. In Central America, prevalence rates have been growing steadily and most countries there are facing a generalized epidemic. In the United States of America, 30 000–40 000 new infections occur every year, with African-Americans and Hispanics the most affected populations.

## Rises in mortality, reductions in life expectancy

In many countries there is evidence of a reversal of the declines in child mortality achieved during the 1990s, especially in those most severely affected by HIV/AIDS.

These reversals indicate the adverse impact of HIV/AIDS on the Millennium Development Goal of reducing child mortality. Once again, however, large variations between African countries in their HIV-prevalence trends and levels of child mortality not associated with HIV will mean very different impacts in different places. It has been estimated that HIV/AIDS was the primary cause of about 8% of deaths in under-fives in sub-Saharan Africa in 2001 *(16)*.

In the absence of vital registration and reliable cause-of-death information, evidence on the impact of HIV infection on child mortality is limited. It is known, however, that even before the introduction of antiretroviral therapy the progression of disease among children infected with HIV in Europe and the USA was considerably slower than that observed in Africa. In western and eastern Africa the median survival time is less than two years, compared with well over five years in developed countries *(17)*.

The most dramatic effect of the HIV/AIDS epidemic has been on adult mortality *(18)*. In the worst-affected countries of eastern and southern Africa, the probability of a 15-year-old dying before reaching 60 years of age has risen sharply – from 10–30% in the mid-1980s to 30–60% at the start of the new millennium. In community-based studies in eastern Africa, mortality among adults infected with HIV was 10–20 times higher than in non-infected individuals *(19)*. Overall, the greatest difference in mortality between infected and uninfected people is usually observed between the ages of 20 and 40 years. Women tend to die at an earlier age than men, reflecting the fact that the rates of HIV infection typically peak among women 5–10 years earlier than they do in men. The most reliable estimates of the median survival time following infection with HIV have come from the Masaka study in Uganda *(20)* where the figure was of the order of nine years – two years less than that observed in developed-country cohort studies even before the advent of effective treatment.

Vital registration systems, national censuses, demographic surveys and demographic surveillance systems have provided information on mortality trends *(18)*. Census and survey data from Kenya, Malawi and Zimbabwe have revealed steadily rising adult

## Box 1.2  HIV estimates and population-based surveys

Estimating accurately the number of people living with HIV/AIDS is important for purposes of advocacy, programme planning and evaluation. The estimates for countries with generalized epidemics are based on data generated by surveillance systems that focus on pregnant women attending sentinel antenatal clinics. For countries with concentrated epidemics, the estimates are based on data on HIV prevalence in both high-risk and wider populations.

Recently, several countries have conducted national population-based surveys that include HIV testing, and many more countries plan to do so in the near future. Demographic and health surveys have included HIV testing in the Dominican Republic, Kenya, Mali and Zambia. National surveys with HIV testing have also been conducted in Burundi, Niger, South Africa and Zimbabwe. HIV prevalence is generally lower in the population-based surveys than the existing estimates based on antenatal surveillance.

Nationally representative surveys have important advantages over antenatal surveillance, as they provide data on a wider sample of the population and especially on rural populations, which are often underrepresented in antenatal clinic surveillance systems. UNAIDS and WHO adjust data to correct for the underrepresentation of populations with lower prevalence, but this may not have been enough.

Population-based surveys vary in their methodologies, sampling approaches, biological sample collection methods, HIV testing strategies, and ways to deal with ethical issues and incentives for participation. Nonresponse rates at the household and individual levels complicate the interpretation of results. In particular, absence from the household is likely to be associated with higher HIV prevalence. In general, survey-based estimates can be expected to be somewhat lower than the true prevalence.

All estimates need to be critically appraised. A single method or data source will not usually provide the best estimate of HIV prevalence. The value of antenatal clinic-based surveillance lies primarily in the assessment of trends, and surveys conducted at 4–5-year intervals will help to improve estimates. High-quality population-based surveys can improve the assumptions that are used to estimate national levels of prevalence, for example assumptions related to rural adjustment and the computation of male prevalence. The results of population-based surveys point to the improvements needed in national HIV surveillance systems *(11)*.

mortality throughout the 1990s. In Kenya, the probability of dying between the ages of 15 and 60 years rose from 18% in the early 1990s to 48% by 2002 (see Annex Table 1). In Malawi the figure is now 63%; it was less than 30% in the early 1980s. In Zimbabwe, the 1997 probabilities of 50% for women and 65% for men have risen to an overall 80%. There is evidence that in Thailand and Trinidad and Tobago there have been increases in mortality, even though the prevalence of HIV infection is considerably lower in those countries than in most of Africa. In Thailand, for example, the crude mortality rate for those aged 15–49 years almost doubled from 2.8 to 5.4 per thousand between 1987 and 1996.

The advent of the HIV/AIDS pandemic has reversed the gains in life expectancy made in sub-Saharan Africa, which reached a peak of 49.2 years during the late 1980s and which is projected to drop to just under 46 years in the period 2000–2005 *(2)* (see Figure 1.3). This turnaround is most dramatic in those severely affected countries in southern Africa that had relatively high life expectancy prior to the appearance of HIV/AIDS. In Botswana, for example, life expectancy decreased from nearly 65 years in 1985–1990 to 40 years in 2000–2005; in South Africa it is expected to drop from over 60 years to below 50 years. The United Republic of Tanzania (whose epidemic is less than half the size of that in South Africa) is likely to have experienced a decline in life expectancy from 51 to 43 years in the last 15 years. In Nigeria (where the epidemic is about half the size of that in the United Republic of Tanzania) the gradual improvements that were being made have stalled.

Overall, life expectancy at birth in the African Region was 48 years in 2002; it would have been 54 years in the absence of HIV/AIDS. In the countries of southern Africa life expectancy would have been 56 years instead of 43 years (see Figure 1.4).

**Figure 1.3**   Trends in life expectancy in sub-Saharan Africa and selected countries, 1970–2010

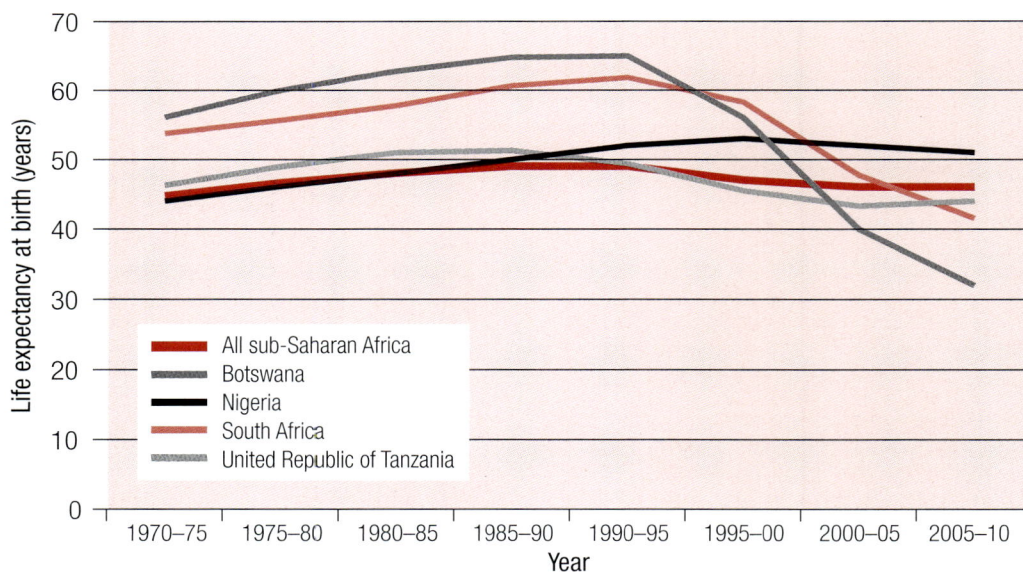

Source: *(21)*.

## THE DEADLY INTERACTION: HIV/AIDS AND OTHER DISEASES

The interaction of HIV/AIDS with other infectious diseases is an increasing public health concern. In sub-Saharan Africa, for example, malaria, bacterial infections and tuberculosis (TB) have been identified as the leading causes of HIV-related morbidity *(22)*. HIV infection increases both the incidence and severity of clinical malaria in adults *(23)*. In some parts of Africa, falciparum malaria and HIV infection represent the two most important health problems.

The pandemic has brought about devastating changes in the epidemiology of TB, especially in Africa where about one-third of the population is infected with TB but does not necessarily have the disease (it is dormant). However, by the end of 2000 around 17 million people in Africa and 4.5 million people in south-east Asia were infected with both TB and HIV *(24)*. A high proportion of these people can be expected to develop active TB unless they receive treatment *(25)*, because HIV, by weakening the immune system, greatly increases the likelihood of people becoming ill with TB.

In African countries with high rates of HIV infection, including those with well-organized control programmes, case-notification rates of TB have risen more than fourfold since the mid-1980s, reaching more than 200 cases per 100 000 population in 2002 *(25)*. In the USA, 16% of TB cases have been attributed to the virus.

In parts of Asia and eastern Europe, the number of people coinfected with multidrug-resistant TB and HIV is also likely to increase. In India, for example, where an estimated 1.7 million adults in 2000 were coinfected with TB and HIV, there is a multidrug resistance rate of up to 3% of previously untreated TB patients.

## THE AIDS TREATMENT GAP

The situation outlined above shows the devastating effects of the virus on the health of the world's people. But the effects are not evenly felt, and are often concentrated in the very places where treatment is least likely to be available. Overall, coverage with antiretroviral drugs is extremely low. In 2003, the estimated number of people worldwide needing treatment because they were in advanced stages of infection was nearly 6 million, although the numbers must be interpreted cautiously and the uncertainty range is large (4–8 million).

In 2003, about 400 000 people received treatment. Coverage is lowest in the African Region, where the burden is highest and only an estimated 100 000 people are receiving treatment: a coverage of 2%. Some 34 countries accounted for more than 90% of the number of adults in need of treatment in 2003. South Africa accounts for almost one in six people in need of treatment. Half of the global treatment needs are located in just seven countries: India and six countries in the WHO African Region.

**Figure 1.4** Life expectancy in Africa, with and without HIV/AIDS, 2002

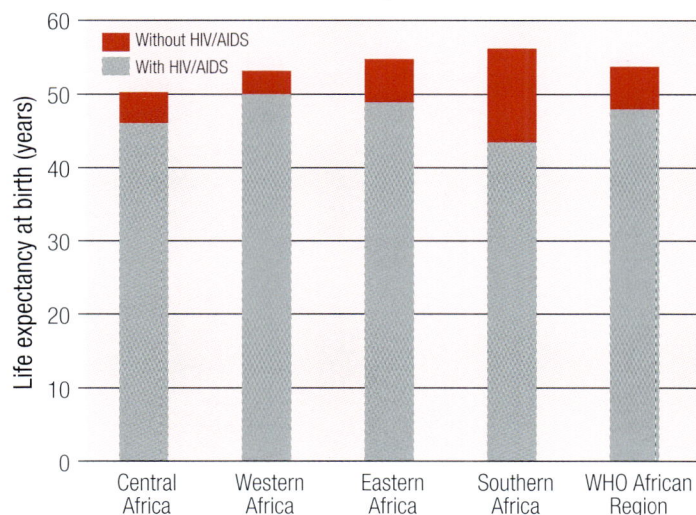

## THE HUMAN, SOCIAL AND ECONOMIC CONSEQUENCES

Epidemics of disease are like famines, wars and natural catastrophes in one major respect: they invariably bring further disasters in their wake. Globally, HIV/AIDS epidemics are already having a disastrous domino effect. Millions of children are orphaned, communities are destroyed, health services are overwhelmed, entire countries face hunger and economic ruin.

The disease affects the poor most severely: they are the most vulnerable to infection, and the poorest families are hardest hit by the suffering, illness and death caused by the disease. The effects include devastating financial hardships that lead in turn to further tragic consequences. The disease forces poor families deeper into poverty, and it also condemns households that were relatively wealthy to a similar fate.

Large-scale negative changes to patterns of economic and social behaviour are likely to result from the epidemic's impact on population structure and adult life expectancy *(26)*. Beyond the loss of income and the diversion of income to health expenditures, families resort to various "coping" strategies with negative long-term effects, including migration *(27)*, child labour, sale of assets and spending of savings. Families suffering from the illness or death of one or more of their members experience both the direct costs of medical and funeral expenditures and the indirect costs of the impact of the illness on productivity *(28, 29)*.

HIV/AIDS is changing the very structure of populations. There are increased dependency ratios in many African countries, for example, with smaller numbers of working-age adults on whom both children and elderly relatives depend; a situation that is becoming more severe.

The psychological effects on young people of seeing their immediate elders dying in huge numbers at such young ages, and consequent fears for their own future, are immense and will have profound effects on economic development. Moreover, as parents (most of them young adults) die prematurely, they fail to hand on assets and skills to their children. In this way, HIV/AIDS weakens the process through which human capital – people's experience, skill and knowledge – is accumulated and transmitted across generations *(30)*.

The crisis of children having lost either or both parents to HIV/AIDS has been afflicting Africa for a decade, and will get worse. Today there are about 14 million such children in the world of whom the vast majority are in Africa, but the projected total number will nearly double to 25 million by 2010 *(31, 32)*, a nation of children equal to the total population of Iraq. At that point, anywhere from 15% to 25% of the children in a dozen sub-Saharan countries will be orphans. Even in countries where HIV prevalence has stabilized or fallen, such as Uganda, the numbers of orphans will continue to rise as parents already infected continue to die from the disease. When orphans were relatively few, they could be cared for by extended families, but the numbers are now too great and many children end up living on the street.

### Women: unequally at risk

Women in many countries are already facing severe hardships resulting from inequality, discrimination and victimization, and HIV/AIDS often exacerbates the hardships. In fact, these very factors help explain why women suffer disproportionately from the disease. About 58% of all people living with HIV/AIDS in the WHO African Region are women. They are infected at younger ages than men by, on average, 6–8 years. Young women are often forced into unequal sexual relationships and are frequently unable to negotiate safer sex. The unequal losses of life among women resulting from this situation will create an imbalance in the adult population, with consequences that are unknown. One likely and ominous outcome, however, is that mature men will seek younger and younger women as partners, which in turn intensifies some of the risk factors for HIV spread.

## The underestimated economic threat

In many countries, the cumulative effects of the epidemics could have catastrophic consequences for long-term economic growth and seriously damage the prospects for poverty reduction. Until recently, most experts believed that a generalized HIV/AIDS epidemic at 10% adult prevalence would reduce economic growth by about 0.5% per year *(33)*. Several country-based studies have suggested that HIV/AIDS epidemics result in a reduction in gross domestic product (GDP) of around 1%, but recent economic studies and estimates suggest a much bleaker picture of current and future economic effects *(30, 34)*.

# A daughter's story

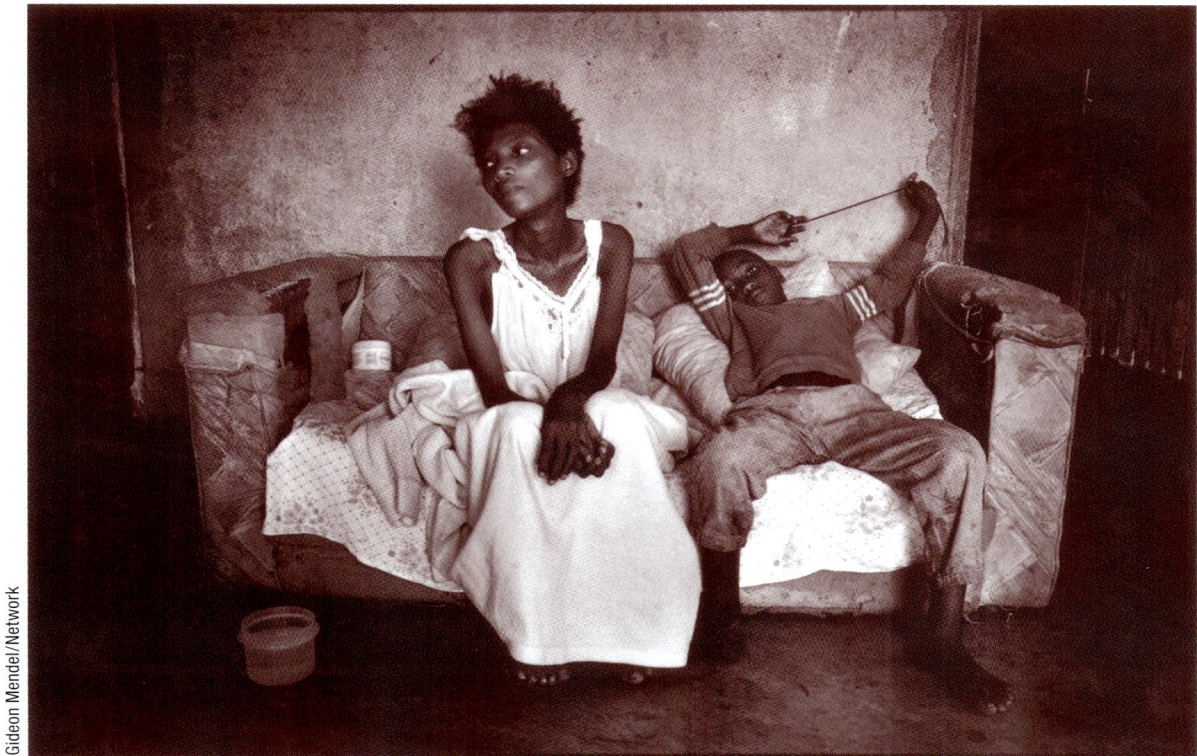

Gideon Mendel/Network

While being treated for tuberculosis at Ngwelezane Hospital, KwaZulu-Natal, South Africa, Samkelisiwe Mkhwanazi was diagnosed with HIV/AIDS. After leaving hospital she stayed for three months with a traditional healer and was treated with herbal medicines, but her condition did not improve.

Samkelisiwe, 30 years old, would normally be responsible for taking care of her child and her mother, Nesta, but now she has become dependent on her mother again. "I want to be with her until I die," she says. The entire family relies on Nesta, who must look after everyone, including Samkelisiwe's late sister's children (see Nesta's story in Chapter 5).

Samkelisiwe is just one of approximately 6 million people in developing countries who need urgent treatment with antiretroviral drugs. With health care systems that are unable to cope, most people living with HIV/AIDS must rely on their family or community for care.

Studies previously misinterpreted the effects of epidemics as being similar to those caused by one-off shocks, such as natural disasters or international economic downturns, which many economies can absorb and which are beyond the control of planners. Predictions have also frequently reflected assumptions that the worst-hit countries in Africa had an excess of labour, and suggested that a contraction in workforce numbers might lead to more efficient use of land and capital. The belief was that GDP per capita would actually increase if a fall in GDP were lower than the fall in population. Similarly, it had been thought that the destruction of the labour force and hence the reduction in labour supply caused by HIV/AIDS could result in an increase in the productivity of each remaining worker because each would have more land and capital with which to work. The result of these misinterpretations and assumptions was a widespread failure nationally and internationally to revise economic policies to take account of HIV/AIDS.

HIV/AIDS will have long-term and widespread effects that will last for generations, and which do not reveal themselves in many economic studies. Ill-health and premature death lead to wasted investment in human capital and globally reduce the incentives to invest in building for the future. An inadequate response to HIV/AIDS will allow the disease to continue to destroy education systems and other vital institutions, reduce human capital and the ability to transmit it, and contribute to a long-term decline in savings and investment. There will therefore be substantial benefits in responding to epidemics – even those of low prevalence.

## The threat of institutional collapse

The implications of reduced life expectancy in adults for societies heavily burdened by HIV/AIDS are becoming clear, though previous poor performance of institutions has sometimes obscured the specific impact of HIV/AIDS *(35)*. Institutional malfunctioning in Africa, for example, has been concealed by long-running inefficiency and low performance expectations. The survival and functioning of institutions in a number of southern African countries are now threatened. Incapacity is critical. Already there are major shortages of qualified personnel in key organizations. Posts are vacant or occupied on an "acting" capacity. Continuity of staff is low because of deaths and the reshuffles they occasion. Morale is equally low. Numerous studies and anecdotal evidence point to the slowing down and near paralysis of agricultural services, judiciaries, police forces, education systems and health services.

Many African businesses have also been severely affected by reduced labour supply, especially the loss of experienced workers in their most productive years, increased absenteeism, reduced profitability and loss of international competitiveness *(36)*. Threats to regional security caused by the epidemic are another example of indirect impacts that may negatively affect economic activities such as tourism *(37)* or inflows of foreign investment *(38)*.

Across southern and eastern Africa, the education sector is suffering as the loss of teachers exceeds those being trained *(39)*. This is not only a result of AIDS-related illness and death: some teachers are being hired by the private sector, which is also in need of skilled personnel, while others are migrating. The effects are masked by the fact that fewer children enrol in school because HIV/AIDS-affected families cannot afford school fees or need their children to work at home. The result will be lower educational achievement, with negative implications for efforts to reduce poverty, improve gender relations and decrease HIV transmission, and for the overall health of those who survive. The effort to enrol all children in school by 2015 (one of the Millennium

Development Goals) is being undermined with long-term negative consequences.

One of the many tragedies of HIV/AIDS is that it often strikes hardest where health systems are weakest, and deals a double blow. Systems that in any case cannot cope are weakened further by HIV/AIDS deaths and disability among large numbers of health personnel (see Chapter 4). In low-income countries which were already suffering from a lack of health care workers, health care systems are overburdened. In Côte d'Ivoire and Uganda, 50–80% of adult hospital beds are occupied by patients with HIV-related conditions. In Swaziland, the average length of stay in hospital is six days, but in 80% of cases increases to 30 days for patients with tuberculosis associated with HIV *(40)*.

The impact of HIV/AIDS on the health sector is often enormous. The severity and complexity of clinical opportunistic conditions are associated with high hospitalization rates, inpatient mortality and increasing treatment costs. In some sub-Saharan countries, the rate of general hospital bed occupation by AIDS patients is frequently higher than 50%. The introduction of antiretroviral therapy, however, has been shown to lead to a sharp reduction in HIV/AIDS-related mortality, morbidity and care expenditures, with substantial improvements in the quality of life of patients. Chapter 4 deals at length with the key issues linking HIV/AIDS, health systems and treatment expansion.

Given the daunting social and economic consequences of the spread of HIV, the need for effective and wide-ranging methods of prevention is as clear as it has been since the very first days of the epidemic in the 1980s. The next section looks at the current range of prevention and care strategies in play around the world.

## PREVENTION, CARE AND SUPPORT: STRATEGIES FOR CHANGE

HIV/AIDS may not be curable, but it is certainly preventable and treatable. It has been estimated that almost two-thirds of the new infections projected to occur during the period 2002–2010 can be prevented if the coverage of existing HIV prevention strategies is substantially increased *(41)*. Prevention efforts can and do work to halt the spread of the virus, and real advances in treatment hold out the hope of longer and better lives for those already infected. Scaling up treatment must become a way to support and strengthen prevention programmes. Careful integration of prevention and treatment services will ensure that those who test positive are linked to counselling and treatment, which can lead them to protect others from infection *(42)*. Furthermore,

## Box 1.3  Prevention and treatment in Brazil and the Bahamas

The Brazilian experience shows that scaling up antiretroviral treatment enhances, rather than impedes, prevention efforts if they are scaled up simultaneously. Since 1996 (the year Brazil's universal antiretroviral drug distribution programme began), sexual behaviour, and more recently HIV prevalence, have been monitored among nearly 30 000 male army conscripts. In 1999–2002, over 80% of the conscripts were sexually active and the proportion with multiple partners remained steady; but HIV prevalence among the men was low (0.08%) and condom use was high

and increasing. In 1999, 62% of men reported condom use at last sexual intercourse, and in 2000 and 2002, 70% did so. Condom use with a paid partner in the previous year increased from 69% in 1999 to 77% in 2002.

The impact of prevention interventions was also observed among injecting drug users. The most significant reduction in the index of sexual risk behaviour was found in this group *(43)*.

Similarly, in the Bahamas, the introduction of antiretroviral therapy has been accompanied by heightened prevention successes, in addition to significant reductions in deaths

(56% reduction in deaths from AIDS, including an 89% reduction in deaths among children). The success of prevention efforts is also evident from the fact that mother-to-child transmission of HIV was reduced from 28% to 3%; there was also a 44.4% reduction in new HIV cases, a 41% decline in HIV prevalence rate among patients being treated for sexually transmitted infections, and a 38% decline in HIV prevalence rate among pregnant women *(44)*.

people who might otherwise be afraid to undergo testing are more likely to seek services for sexually transmitted infections and HIV/AIDS when they have access to treatment (see Box 1.3).

## Preventing the sexual transmission of HIV

Prevention approaches can work in many populations, as long as they use evidence-based strategies, carefully tailored to the social and economic settings in which they are implemented and to the state of national HIV/AIDS epidemics. A comprehensive approach that supports social and individual rights, involves communities and is developed on the basis of their cultural values has been found to be effective when combined with the promotion of consistent condom use, voluntary testing and counselling for HIV, and delayed sexual initiation. Promotion of other strategies, such as abstinence and reduction in number of partners, also needs to be based on firm evidence.

## Box 1.4  Cambodia and Thailand – successes and challenges

HIV infection in Asia remains largely confined to those people at higher levels of risk – sex workers, injecting drug users, men who have sex with men – and their sexual partners. Those at elevated risk represent anywhere from 7% to 25% of the adult population, making severe epidemics a possibility in all the countries of the region.

However, the focused nature of risk means in turn that focused prevention efforts with high coverage can slow or reverse the course of the epidemics. By mounting intensive, well-funded and extensive efforts to reduce the risks in sex work, Cambodia and Thailand have changed the course of their epidemics. In both countries, the role of sex work in HIV

transmission was realized early on and major nationwide prevention efforts were mounted, working not only with brothel owners and sex workers, but also reaching out to the large client populations – almost 20% of adult males in the early 1990s. In response to these programmes, condom use between sex workers and clients rose to more than 90%, and the number of men visiting sex workers was halved.

Using this Asian Epidemic Model, the East-West Center and its collaborators have explored the impacts of these prevention efforts. Without aggressive prevention programmes, it is estimated that both countries would now be looking at expanding epidemics with 10–15%

of their adult populations living with HIV/AIDS, instead of the declining epidemics of 2–3% currently seen.

But as one avenue of HIV transmission is closed off, others appear. Programmes for injecting drug users, men who have sex with men, and sexually active young people have been weak and ineffective to date. The epidemic among injecting drug users in Thailand continues unabated, condom use among young people remains low at around 20%, and there are HIV levels of around 15% in men who have sex with men. If the two countries are to sustain their past successes, they must adapt responses to be as effective and aggressive with new evolving patterns of risk *(50, 51)*.

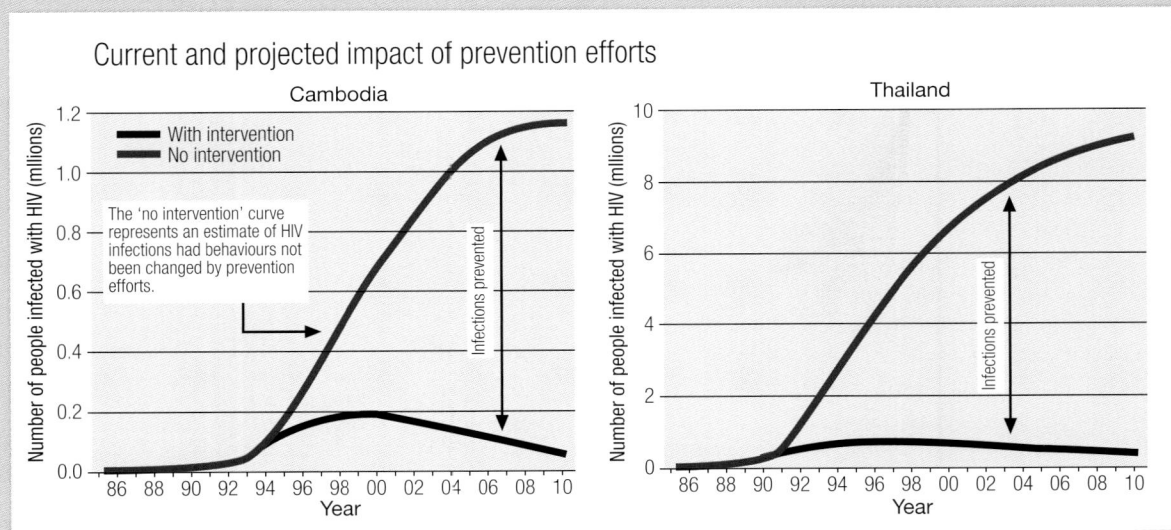

Current and projected impact of prevention efforts

Cambodia

Thailand

— With intervention
— No intervention

The 'no intervention' curve represents an estimate of HIV infections had behaviours not been changed by prevention efforts.

Number of people infected with HIV (millions)

Infections prevented

Year

Level of social and economic development, and cultural factors such as gender in-equality or access to education and health care, are all known to be obstacles to the successful implementation of prevention initiatives. Interventions that reduce the ef-fects of such obstacles – by implementing measures that allow girls to stay in school for longer, for example – can have a lasting impact on rates of HIV transmission. The promotion of human rights, combined with behavioural change programmes, also helps *(45, 46)*. Lessons learnt from various settings and communities show that the use of any chosen prevention measure requires that people not only have the proper knowledge but also the ability to apply it.

Consistent condom use demands a reliable distribution system to people who live in poverty or in difficult-to-reach areas *(47)*. Interventions that have targeted popula-tions at high risk such as men who have sex with men and female sex workers and their clients in Africa, Asia and Latin America are effective. In Abidjan (Côte d'Ivoire) and Cotonou (Benin), HIV prevalence among sex workers declined during the 1990s and the increased use of condoms contributed significantly to these declines *(48, 49)*; similar changes have been observed in sex workers in Cambodia and Thailand (see Box 1.4). Evidence from a South African mining community showed that interventions among those most at risk increased condom use and greatly reduced rates of sexu-ally transmitted infections – especially those most linked to HIV transmission – in the community *(52)*.

Effective prevention programmes aimed at young people can teach them responsible and safe sexual behaviour, according to some of the latest research. Recent findings from Uganda indicate that young people have changed their behaviour considerably over the last few years, and that HIV prevalence among them has dropped *(53)*.

## Breaking the link with other sexually transmitted infections

Sexually transmitted infections increase the risk of HIV transmission by at least two to five times *(49)*. They help drive the spread of HIV. If untreated, they not only increase the infectivity of HIV-positive individuals but also make those who are HIV negative more susceptible to infection. Early detection and treatment, and related efforts to reduce the prevalence of these infections, should therefore be an integral component of a comprehensive HIV prevention effort. The potential benefits are probably greatest in the early stages of a national HIV/AIDS epidemic when the virus spreads as a result of high rates of change of sexual partners, but evidence suggests that measures to control sexually transmitted infections have important effects even in more advanced epidemics.

## Preventing infection in infants and children

Every year an estimated 2.2 million pregnant women infected with HIV give birth, and about 700 000 neonates contract HIV from their mothers. HIV transmission from mother to child may occur during pregnancy, labour and delivery, or during breast-feeding. In the absence of any intervention, 14–25% of children born to HIV-infected mothers become infected in developed countries, 13–42% in other countries *(54)*. This disparity is mostly a result of different breastfeeding practices. It is estimated that 5–20% of infants born to HIV-infected women acquire infection through breast-feeding.

The most effective ways to prevent infection in infants and young children are to prevent HIV infection in women and to prevent unintended pregnancies among HIV-infected women. It is also possible, however, to prevent most cases of transmission from HIV-infected pregnant women to their infants. Antiretroviral prophylaxis in combination with other interventions such as elective caesarean section before onset of labour and rupture of membranes, and refraining from breastfeeding, have now almost entirely eliminated HIV infection in infants in the developed world, with transmission rates below 2%. In developing countries where breastfeeding is the norm, the risk of HIV transmission to the newborn child can be more than halved by short-course antiretroviral regimens, though this reduction is not sustained where feeding practices to reduce risk are not adopted.

To reduce the risk of postpartum transmission of HIV through breastfeeding, WHO currently recommends that when replacement feeding is acceptable, feasible, affordable, sustainable and safe, HIV-infected mothers avoid all breastfeeding. Otherwise, exclusive breastfeeding is recommended during the first months of life. To minimize the risk of postpartum transmission, breastfeeding should be discontinued as soon as is feasible, taking into account local circumstances, the individual woman's situation and the risks posed by using replacement feeding, including infections other than HIV and malnutrition.

Although progress is now being made in the delivery of these low-cost and relatively simple interventions on a large scale in the most-affected countries, it has been slower than anticipated. Women must be encouraged and helped to attend antenatal care

# Caring for HIV-positive infants in Moscow

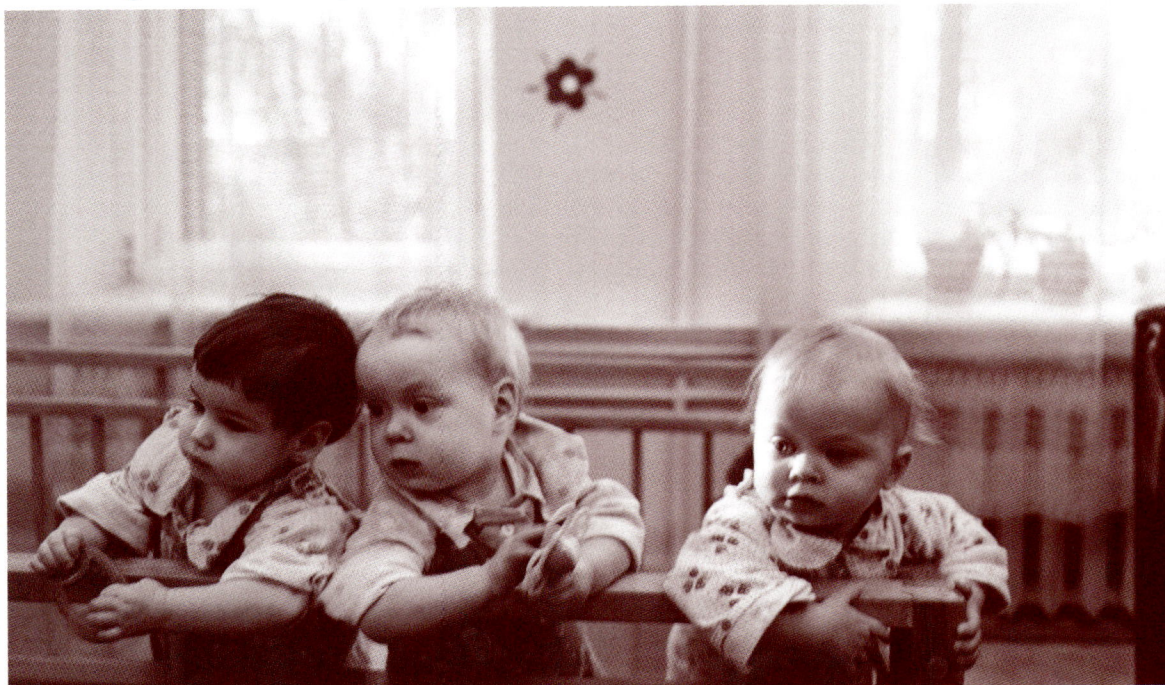

Ilse Frech/Lookat/Network

In eastern Europe and the former Soviet Union the number of HIV/AIDS cases has increased rapidly during the last decade. Unlike in most other regions, infection here is spread primarily though injecting drug use. Many women who become infected in this way transmit the virus to their babies. These three infants are being cared for at a small clinic in the Orechovo-Zoejevo Hospital, Moscow. The clinic provides a home for HIV-positive children whose mothers have died or are unable to look after them.

facilities, to accept counselling and testing, to return for test results and to adopt safer infant feeding practices, and must be given access to correctly administered antiretroviral drugs. Current challenges include achieving a rapid increase in acceptance of HIV testing and counselling, integrating prevention of infection in infants and young children into maternal and child health services, and extending the prevention of mother-to-child transmission to include HIV-related care, treatment and support for HIV-infected mothers, their infants and family.

## Injecting drug use – reducing the harm

There may be as many as 2–3 million past and current injecting drug users living with HIV/AIDS worldwide. There are HIV epidemics associated with such drug use in more than 110 countries. In the absence of harm-reduction activities, HIV prevalence among injecting drug users can rise to 40% or more within one to two years of the introduction of the virus into their communities. HIV transmission through the sharing of non-sterile injection equipment is augmented by sexual transmission among injecting drug users, and between them and their sex partners.

Injecting drug users should have access to services that help reduce the related risks of drug use and HIV infection. Drug treatment programmes should be accessible to those who want to stop using drugs or, through substitution therapy, to stop injecting. Harm reduction primarily aims to help injecting drug users to avoid the negative health consequences of injecting and to improve their health and social status. Interventions include projects that try to ensure that those who continue injecting have access to clean injection paraphernalia. One evaluation carried out in 99 cities showed a reduction in the risk of HIV transmission of 19% per year in cities with such projects (with no concomitant increase in drug use) compared with an 8% increase in cities without them *(55)*.

## Preventing transmission during health care

Improper blood-transfusion practices are another important route of parenteral HIV transmission. Policies and procedures are needed to minimize the risk of transmission through blood transfusion, including the creation of a national blood service, use of low-risk donors, eliminating unnecessary transfusions, and systematic screening of blood for transfusion.

Universal precautions in health care settings prevent the transmission of HIV and other bloodborne pathogens, and therefore increased access to safer technologies is needed. A review of published studies has shown that unsafe injections play a minor but significant role in HIV transmission in sub-Saharan Africa *(56)*. Irrespective of the exact contribution to the HIV/AIDS pandemic, unsafe injections are an unacceptable practice and efforts should be increased in all health care settings to reduce the exposure of patients and carers to bloodborne infections.

## Testing and counselling

The vast majority of people living with HIV/AIDS in low-income countries are unaware that they are infected. Testing is an essential means of identifying these people and beginning treatment, and for preventing infection in mothers and infants. It is also a critical component of a comprehensive strategy to prevent sexual transmission. Studies have shown that people who test positive for HIV tend to reduce risk behaviours *(57)*. Joint counselling and testing sessions with couples may increase condom use.

There is an urgent need to scale up access to counselling and testing, which should be offered as standard practice. An HIV test should always be performed with informed consent and appropriate confidentiality. Testing and counselling services must keep pace with the current new treatment and prevention opportunities. The onus will increase on national governments to provide high-quality testing and counselling services. Such services should become a routine part of health care, for example during attendance at antenatal clinics, or at tuberculosis and sexually transmitted infection diagnosis and treatment centres.

---

To accelerate prevention and care, while limiting the social devastation now unfolding, rapid expansion of HIV/AIDS treatment in the countries hardest hit by the pandemic is a public health necessity. Treatment with antiretroviral medicines is effective and is much cheaper than a few years ago; it saves lives and will help to prevent the social and economic disasters outlined in this chapter. The necessary response is described in the following chapter, which deals with the bold initiative to deliver treatment to 3 million people with HIV/AIDS by the end of 2005 and explains how this can help strengthen health systems.

# References

1. *AIDS epidemic update: December 2003*. Geneva, Joint United Nations Programme on HIV/AIDS and World Health Organization, 2003 (UNAIDS/03.39E).
2. *World population prospects: the 2002 revision*. New York, United Nations, 2003.
3. Dixon S, McDonald S, Roberts J. The impact of HIV and AIDS on Africa's economic development. *BMJ*, 2002, 324:232–234.
4. Topouzis D. *The socio-economic impact of HIV/AIDS on rural families with an emphasis on youth*. Rome, Food and Agriculture Organization, 1994.
5. *The progress of nations 2000*. New York, United Nations Children's Fund, 2000 (background paper).
6. *The impact of AIDS*. New York, United Nations, 2003 (United Nations Population Division, Department of Economic and Social Affairs).
7. Sewankambo NK, Gray RH, Ahmad S, Serwadda D, Wabwire-Mangen F, Nalugoda F et al. Mortality associated with HIV infection in rural Rakai district, Uganda. *AIDS*, 2000, 14:2391–2400.
8. Glynn JR, Warndorff DK , Fine PEM, Msiska GK, Munthali MM, Ponnighaus JM. The impact of HIV on morbidity and mortality from tuberculosis in sub-Saharan Africa: a study in rural Malawi and review of the literature. *Health Transition Review*, 1997, 7(Suppl. 2):75–87.
9. Brahmbhatta H, Kigozi G, Wabwire-Mangen F, Serwadda D, Sewankambo N, Lutalo T et al. The effects of placental malaria on mother-to-child HIV transmission in Rakai, Uganda. *AIDS*, 2003, 17:2539–2541.
10. *HIV/AIDS: epidemiological surveillance update for the WHO African Region 2002*. Harare, World Health Organization Regional Office for Africa, 2003.
11. *Reconciling survey and surveillance-based estimates. Report of Tropical Diseases Research Centre (Ndola, Zambia)/UNAIDS/WHO Technical Consultation, Lusaka, Zambia, 17–18 February 2003*. Geneva, World Health Organization, 2003 (http://www.who.int/hiv/strategic/mt170203/en/, accessed 14 February 2004).
12. Buve A, Carael M, Hayes R, Robinson NJ. Variations in HIV prevalence between urban areas in sub-Saharan Africa: do we understand them? *AIDS*, 1995, 9(Suppl. A): S103–S109.
13. Boerma JT, Nyamukapa C, Urassa M, Gregson S. Understanding the uneven spread of HIV within Africa: a comparative study of biologic, behavioral, and contextual factors in rural populations in Tanzania and Zimbabwe. *Sexually Transmitted Diseases*, 2003, 30:779–787.
14. Nicoll A, Hamers F. Are trends in HIV, gonorrhoea, and syphilis worsening in western Europe? *BMJ*, 2002, 324:1324–1327.
15. European Centre for the Epidemiological Monitoring of AIDS. *HIV/AIDS surveillance in Europe. End-year 2003, no.69*. Saint-Maurice, Institut de Veille Sanitaire, 2003 (http://www.eurohiv.org/reports/report_69/pdf/draft_rep69.pdf, accessed 3 February 2004).
16. Walker N, Schwartlander B, Bryce J. Meeting international goals in child survival and HIV/AIDS. *Lancet*, 2002, 360:284–289.
17. Newell M-L, Brahmbhatt H, Ghys P. Child mortality and HIV infection in Africa: a review. The impact of the AIDS epidemic on child mortality. *AIDS* (forthcoming).
18. Blacker J. The impact of AIDS on adult mortality: evidence from national and regional statistics. *AIDS* (forthcoming).
19. Porter K, Zaba B. The empirical evidence for the impact of HIV on adult mortality in the developing world: data from serological studies. *AIDS* (forthcoming).
20. Morgan D, Mahe C, Mayanja B, Okongo JM, Lubega R, Whitworth JA. HIV-1 infection in rural Africa: is there a difference in median time to AIDS and survival compared with that in industrialized countries? *AIDS*, 2002, 16:597–603.
21. United Nations Population Division. *World population prospects: the 2002 revision population database* (http://esa.un.org/unpp, accessed 18 February 2004).
22. Holmes CB, Losina E, Walensky RP, Yazdanpanah Y, Freedberg KA. Review of human immunodefiency virus type I-related opportunistic infections in sub-Saharan Africa. *Clinical Infectious Diseases*, 2003, 36:652–662.

23. Corbett EL, Steketee RW, ter Kuile FO, Latif A, Kamali A, Hayes RJ. HIV-1/AIDS and the control of other infectious diseases in Africa. *Lancet*, 2002, 359:2177–2187.

24. Corbett EL, Watt C, Walker N, Maher D, Williams BG, Raviglione MC et al. The growing burden of tuberculosis: global trends and interactions with the HIV epidemic. *Archives of Internal Medicine*, 2003, 163:1009–1021.

25. *Global tuberculosis control: surveillance, planning, financing.* Geneva, World Health Organization, 2004 (WHO/HTM/TB/2004.331, in press).

26. Barnett T, Whiteside A. *AIDS in the 21st century: disease and globalization.* London, Macmillan Palgrave, 2002.

27. Bronfman MN, Leyva R, Negroni MJ, Rueda CM. Mobile populations and HIV/AIDS in Central America and Mexico: research for action. *AIDS*, 2002, 16(Suppl. 3):S42–S49.

28. Mutangadura G, Mukurazita D, Jackson H. *A review of household and community responses to the HIV/AIDS epidemic in the rural areas of sub-Saharan Africa.* Geneva, Joint United Nations Programme on HIV/AIDS, 2000.

29. Over M. Coping with the impact of AIDS. *Finance and Development*, 1998, March:22–24.

30. Bell C, Devarajan S, Gersbach H. The long-run economic costs of AIDS: theory and application to South Africa. Washington, DC, World Bank, 2003.

31. *Orphans and other children affected by HIV/AIDS: a UNICEF fact sheet.* Paris, United Nations Children's Fund (http://www.unicef.org/aids/index_orphans.html, accessed 4 February 2004).

32. UNICEF/USAID/UNAIDS. *Children on the brink 2002. A joint report on orphan estimates and program strategies.* Washington, DC, The Synergy Project, 2002.

33. *Confronting AIDS: public priorities in a global epidemic.* Washington, DC, World Bank, 1999.

34. McPherson M, Goldsmith A. Africa: on the move? *SAIS Review*, 1998, 28:153–167.

35. Husain IZ, Badcock-Walters P. Economics of HIV/AIDS mitigation: responding to problems of systemic dysfunction and sectoral capacity. In: Forsythe S, ed. *State of the art: AIDS and economics.* Washington, DC, Policy Project, 2002:84–95.

36. Rosen S, Simon J, Vincent JR, MacLeod W, Fox M, Thea DM. AIDS is your business. *Harvard Business Review*, 2003, 81:80–87.

37. Forsythe S. HIV/AIDS and tourism. *AIDS Analysis Africa*, 1999, 9:4–6.

38. Hemrich G, Topouzis D. Multi-sectoral responses to HIV/AIDS: constraints and opportunities for technical co-operation. *Journal of International Development*, 2000, 12:85–99.

39. Grassly NC, Desai K, Pegurri E, Sikazwe A, Malambo I, Siamatowe C et al. The economic impact of HIV/AIDS on the education sector in Zambia. *AIDS*, 2003, 17:1039–1044.

40. *Accelerating access to HIV/AIDS care in Swaziland. A partnership between the Kingdom of Swaziland, the United Nations system, and the private sector.* Mbabane, Ministry of Health and Social Welfare, 2000 (Project document).

41. Stover J, Walker N, Garnett GP, Salomon JA, Stanecki KA, Ghys PD et al. Can we reverse the HIV/AIDS pandemic with an expanded response? *Lancet*, 2002, 360:73–77.

42. Global HIV Prevention Working Group. *Global mobilization for HIV prevention: a blueprint for action.* Menlo Park, CA, Kaiser Family Foundation, 2002 (http://www.kff.org/hivaids/200207-index.cfm, accessed 4 February 2004).

43. Coordenação Nacional de Dst e Aids [National Coordinating Office for STI and AIDS]. *Pesquisa entre os conscritos do Exército Brasileiro, 1996-2000: retratos do comportamento de risco do jovem brasileiro à infecção pelo HIV [Investigation among conscripts for the Brazilian army 1996-2000: portraits of behaviour involving risk of HIV infection among Brazilian youth].* Brasília, Ministério da Saúde, 2002 (in Portuguese).

44. Camara B, Lee R, Gatewood J, Wagner H-U, Cazal-Gamelsy R, Boisson E. *The Caribbean HIV/AIDS epidemic. Epidemiological status – success stories. A summary.* Port of Spain, Caribbean Epidemiology Centre, 2003 (CAREC surveillance report, 2003, Vol. 23, Suppl. 1).

45. Sumartojo E. Structural factors in HIV prevention: concepts, examples, and implication for research. *AIDS*, 2000, 14(Suppl. 1):S3–S10.

46. Auerbach JD, Coates TJ. HIV prevention research: accomplishments and challenges for the third decade of AIDS. *American Journal of Public Health*, 2000, 90:1029–1032.

47. *The male condom.* Geneva, Joint United Nations Programme on HIV/AIDS, 2000 (UNAIDS technical update).

48. Ghys PD, Diallo MO, Ettiegne-Traore V, Satten GA, Anoma CK, Maurice C et al. Effect of interventions to control sexually transmitted disease on the incidence of HIV infection in female sex workers. *AIDS*, 2001, 15:1421–1431.

49. Alary M, Mukenge-Tshibaka L, Bernier F, Geraldo N, Lowndes CM, Meda H et al. Decline in the prevalence of HIV and sexually transmitted diseases among female sex workers in Cotonou, Benin, 1993–1999. *AIDS*, 2002, 16:463–470.

50. Thai Working Group on HIV/AIDS. Projections for HIV/AIDS in Thailand: 2000–2020. Bangkok, Ministry of Public Health, 2001 (Department of Communicable Disease Control).

51. Cambodia Working Group on HIV/AIDS. *Projections for HIV/AIDS in Cambodia: 2000–2010.* Phnom Penh, National Center for HIV/AIDS and STD, 2002.

52. Steen R, Vuylsteke B, DeCoito T, Ralepeli S, Fehler G, Conley J et al. Evidence of declining STD prevalence in a South African mining community following a core-group intervention. *Sexually Transmitted Diseases*, 2000, 27:1–8.

53. Mbulaiteye SM, Mahe C, Whitworth JA, Ruberantwari A, Nakiyingi JS, Ojwiya A et al. Declining HIV-1 incidence and associated prevalence over 10 years in a rural population in south-west Uganda: a cohort study. *Lancet*, 2002, 360:41–46.

54. The Working Group on Mother-to-Child Transmission of HIV. Rates of mother-to-child transmission of HIV-1 in Africa, America and Europe: results from 13 perinatal studies. *Journal of Acquired Immune Deficiency Syndromes and Human Retrovirology*, 1995, 8:506–510.

55. McDonald M, Law M, Kaldor J, Hales J, Dore GJ. Effectiveness of needle and syringe programmes for preventing HIV transmission. *International Journal of Drug Policy*, 2003, 14:353–357.

56. Schmid GP, Buvé A, Mugyenyi P, Garnett GP, Hayes RJ, Williams BG et al. Transmission of HIV-1 infection in sub-Saharan Africa and effect of elimination of unsafe injections. *Lancet*, 2004, 363:482–488.

57. The Voluntary HIV-2 Counselling and Testing Efficacy Study Group. Efficacy of voluntary HIV-1 counselling and testing in individuals and couples in Kenya, Tanzania and Trinidad: a randomised trial. *Lancet*, 2000, 356:103–112.

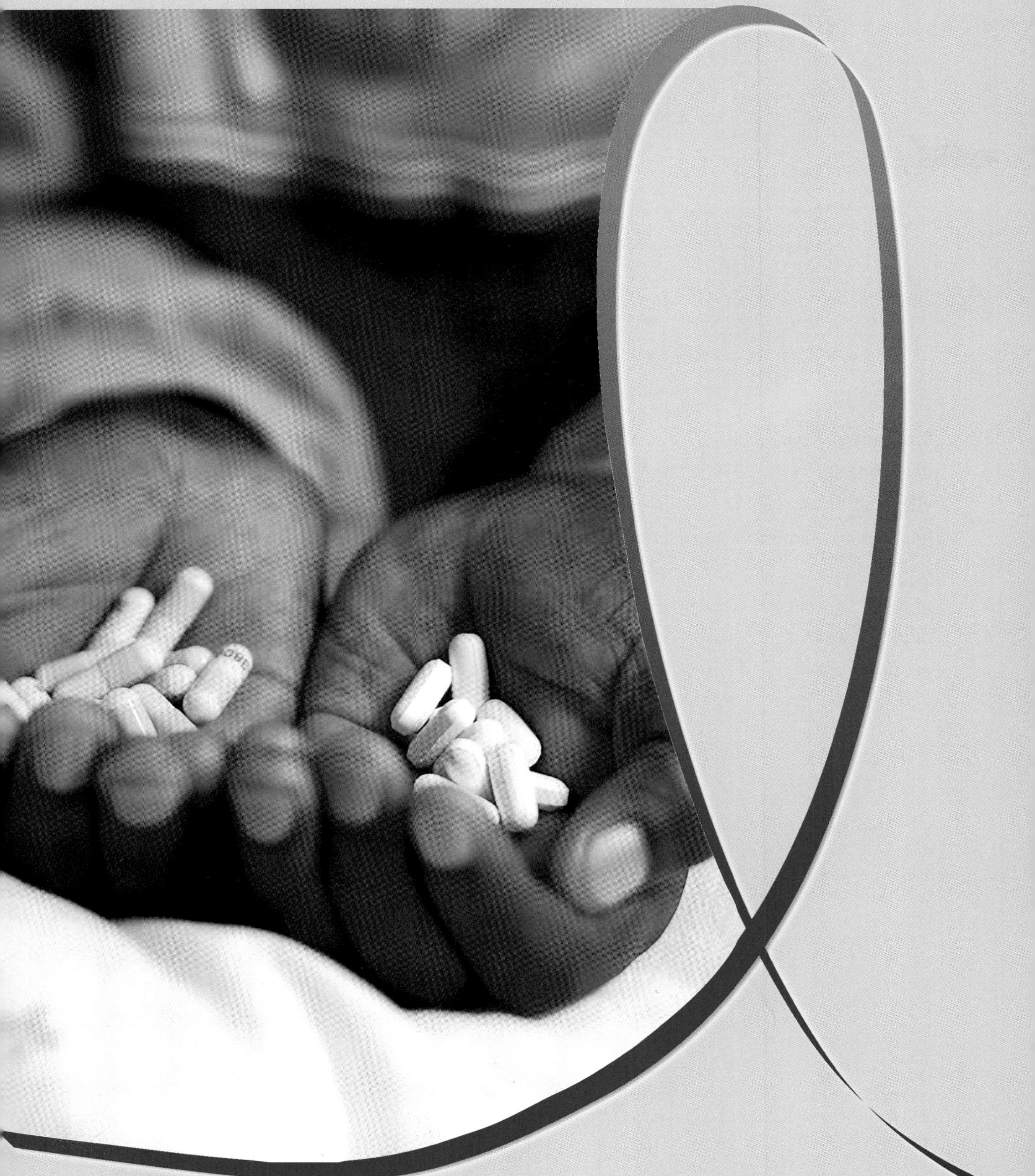

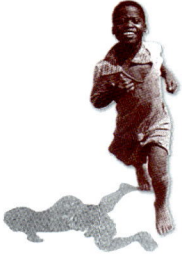

chapter two
# the treatment initiative

Chapter 1 showed the magnitude of the threat posed by HIV/AIDS. This chapter describes the magnitude of the task of responding to it and explains how WHO and its partners are supporting countries in one of the most ambitious endeavours in the history of public health. A comprehensive approach to HIV/AIDS links prevention, treatment and long-term care and support. In much of the developing world, however, treatment has until very recently been the most neglected component. It now needs to be rapidly expanded, along with accelerated prevention efforts, in the countries hardest hit by the pandemic.

Since 1996, more than 20 million people in the developing world have died of AIDS. If antiretroviral therapy had been rapidly deployed, most of these people would probably be alive today. Despite mounting political pressure and evidence that AIDS treatment works in resource-poor settings, by late 2003 less than 7% of people in developing countries in urgent need of antiretroviral drugs were receiving them (see Figure 2.1). In September 2003, LEE Jong-wook, Director-General of WHO, joined Peter Piot, Executive Director of UNAIDS, and Richard Feachem, Director of the Global Fund to Fight AIDS, Tuberculosis and Malaria, to declare the lack of access to antiretroviral therapy a global health emergency. In response, WHO, UNAIDS and a wide range of partners launched the "Treat 3 million by 2005" initiative – known as 3 by 5. Treating 3 million people by the end of 2005 is a necessary target on the way to the goal of universal access to antiretroviral therapy for everyone who needs it.

To reach this goal, major obstacles must be overcome. With few exceptions, HIV/AIDS has struck hardest in countries whose health systems were already weak. Many countries working to expand HIV/AIDS treatment face significant deficits in areas such as health sector human resources, HIV counselling and testing, drug procurement and supply management, health information systems, and laboratory capacity (including the ability to monitor drug resistance).

Delivering the results called for under 3 by 5 will challenge countries' capacities and test the will of the global health community. But it is an essential task whose implications go far beyond the immediate aim of saving millions of lives in the coming years. It may also be the key to saving some of the world's most fragile health

Figure 2.1 Estimated worldwide coverage with antiretroviral treatment, end 2003

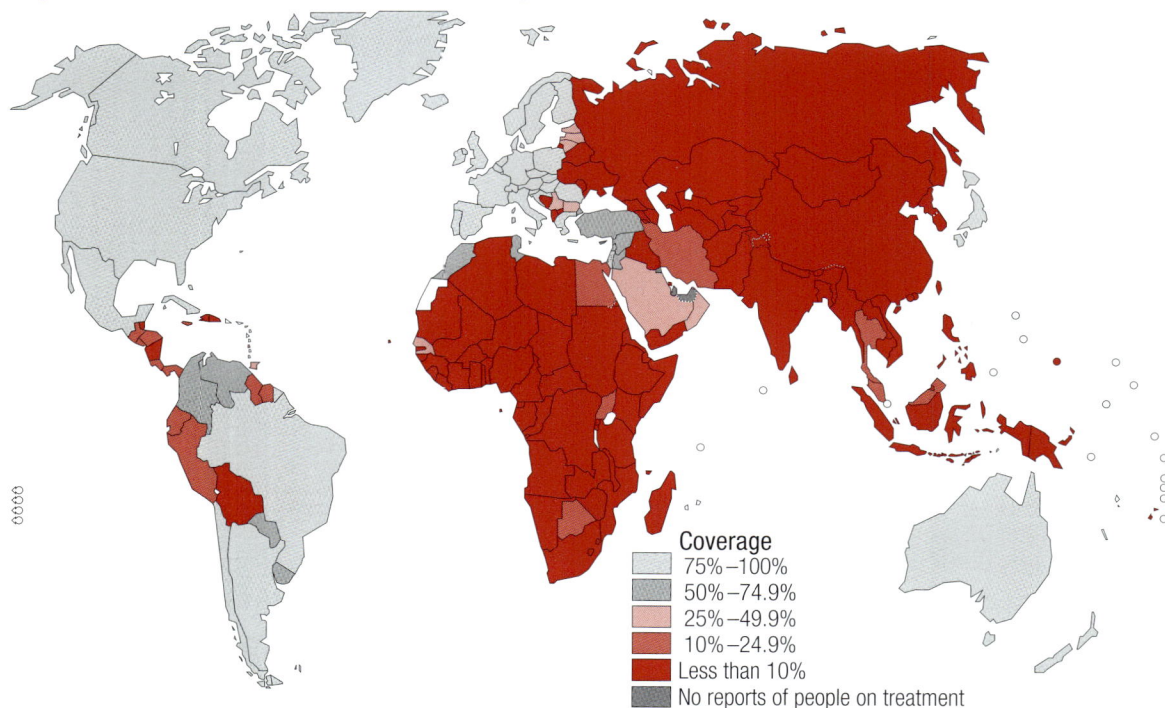

Coverage
- 75%–100%
- 50%–74.9%
- 25%–49.9%
- 10%–24.9%
- Less than 10%
- No reports of people on treatment

systems from further decline, and thereby offering whole societies a healthier future. Seen in this context, the 3 by 5 initiative is a vital opportunity to ensure that the new global resources flowing into HIV/AIDS are invested in ways that strengthen health systems for the long-term benefit of everyone.

This chapter examines public health, economic and social arguments for scaling up antiretroviral treatment in resource-poor settings. It then presents WHO's strategy for working with countries and partners, and provides an estimate of the global investment required. The opportunities and challenges facing countries are explored, highlighting the need to ensure that antiretroviral treatment reaches the poorest and most marginalized people. Finally, the chapter considers the wider importance of 3 by 5 as a new way of working across the global health community for improved health outcomes and equity.

WHO's commitment to support countries is guided by a broad assessment of resources and needs in global public health. Global investment in health has risen in recent years while many other sectors of international development assistance have stagnated, but the bulk of the new health investment is in HIV/AIDS. As the international agency charged with seeking the highest possible level of health for all people, WHO has the responsibility both to support expanded access to antiretroviral therapy and to work with countries and international partners to ensure that the new resources flowing into HIV/AIDS are invested so as to build sustainable health system capacities. Only an international public health agency can fulfil this technical cooperation and stewardship function. Health systems strengthening is the key both to sustainable provision of antiretroviral treatment and to reaching other public health objectives, including the health-related Millennium Development Goals and containment of the expanding epidemics of chronic diseases in the developing world.

## TREATMENT SCALE-UP: PUBLIC HEALTH ARGUMENTS

Two considerations stand out among the public health arguments for emergency treatment scale-up. First is the sharp reduction in HIV/AIDS-related morbidity and mortality associated with treatment. This has been documented in high-income countries, in Brazil's national treatment programme (see Box 2.1) and in pioneering projects in resource-poor settings *(1–3)*. Second is the synergistic effect that treatment can have on prevention efforts. The availability of treatment can enhance prevention in several ways:

- *Increased demand for voluntary counselling and testing*: providing opportunities for voluntary counselling and testing is crucial to effective prevention. As many as 9 out of 10 HIV-infected people in sub-Saharan Africa do not know their serostatus; and when treatment is unavailable, people may see little reason to find out. But the availability of treatment has been shown in numerous settings to increase voluntary counselling and testing – for example, it rose by 300% at a clinic in Haiti after antiretroviral therapy was introduced *(4)*.
- *Enhanced opportunities for secondary prevention*: coming to health centres for treatment offers patients the chance to receive information about prevention behaviours. The value of this approach is reflected in HIV-prevention strategies recently designed by the United States Centers for Disease Control and Prevention to target people known to be infected *(5)*.
- *Lower risk of transmission*: treatment lowers the likelihood of sexual transmission of HIV in the case of unprotected sexual intercourse. It must be recognized, however, that the longer life expectancy of patients on treatment will probably lead to an increase in sexual relations between people of different serostatus.

## Box 2.1  Checking the spread of HIV/AIDS in Brazil

Brazil is one of the few countries that has successfully checked the spread of HIV/AIDS. The country's first HIV/AIDS Programme was established in the State of São Paulo in 1983 when only four cases of HIV/AIDS had been reported. Since then the Brazilian response has evolved rapidly, influenced in particular by the structure and role of the public health system. By December 2002, almost 260 000 cases had been reported to the Ministry of Health, with approximately 145 000 deaths. Brazil's prevalence in the year 2000, which the World Bank had estimated in 1992 would reach 1.2%, was in fact 0.6%.

Brazil was the first developing country to implement a large-scale universal antiretroviral distribution programme. Initiated in the early 1990s with the distribution of AZT, the programme was signed into federal law in 1996. The programme now provides free drugs

for opportunistic infections to about 130 000 people – a coverage of almost all those people living with HIV/AIDS in the country.

As a result, morbidity and mortality rates have fallen by 50–70%. From 1996 to 2002, more than 60 000 HIV/AIDS cases, 90 000 deaths and 358 000 HIV/AIDS-related hospital admissions were averted, and the savings in outpatient and hospital costs have outweighed the costs of implementation by more than US\$ 200 million in four years. These results demonstrate the feasibility of antiretroviral therapy even in a resource-poor setting, where the ideal infrastructure is often lacking. Among the factors which have contributed to the Brazilian success are: the concerted early government response; the strong and effective participation of civil society; multisectoral mobilization; a balanced prevention and treatment approach; and the advocacy of human rights.

Although the prevalence of drug resistance has increased as access to antiretroviral therapy has expanded, Brazil's rate of resistance is substantially lower than that found in many developed countries. In 2001, 6.6% of new infections involved drug-resistant strains, a rate that is roughly one-third to one-half of that reported in North America and parts of western Europe. The low level of primary resistance is a result of well-planned actions by the Ministry of Health, in which the distribution of antiretrovirals was accompanied by guarantees of long-term treatment in health facilities, continuous training of health care workers, use of standardized guidelines, and the involvement of nongovernmental organizations in promoting adherence. The distribution of free antiretrovirals in itself prevented the problems associated with black-market or substandard regimens.

There is little evidence from developing countries of how treatment availability affects risk behaviours. Planning and careful measurement are needed to make treatment and prevention efforts work effectively together. As treatment is scaled up, programmes will continuously have to measure the impact on prevention and be able to adapt and respond promptly to any weakening of preventive behaviours.

## TREATMENT SCALE-UP: ECONOMIC AND SOCIAL ARGUMENTS

Economic and social analyses provide a clear rationale for emergency action on treatment scale-up. While a number of early studies suggested that the use of antiretroviral drugs was not cost-effective in poor countries, more recent analyses have indicated the contrary *(6)*. *The World Health Report 2002* suggested that some types of treatment would be cost-effective even in resource-poor settings *(7)*. Since then, prices of the drugs have fallen by more than 50%. Meanwhile, protocols developed for the 3 by 5 initiative should help make them even more cost-effective, particularly in countries where people with opportunistic infections are hospitalized. The use of antiretrovirals should reduce these infections for several years at least. This should in turn help cut health costs specific to HIV/AIDS, as has been documented in Brazil *(8)*.

As Chapter 1 showed, many early studies seriously underestimated the cumulative economic and social damage of HIV/AIDS in high-burden countries. Antiretroviral treatment can help stem the loss of human capital and productivity if it restores the health of millions of people and enables them to earn an income, raise their children and contribute to society. Under Brazil's universal access antiretroviral treatment programme, the average survival time of people with AIDS seeking care at government

## Box 2.2  Ensuring the supply of medicines to the developing world

The AIDS Medicines and Diagnostics Service is the access and supply arm of the 3 by 5 initiative. It aims to ensure that developing countries have access to high-quality antiretroviral medicines and diagnostic tools at the best prices, by helping them to buy, forecast and manage supply and delivery. The service builds on years of work by UNAIDS, WHO, the United Nations Children's Fund, the World Bank, the Global Fund to Fight AIDS, Tuberculosis and Malaria, and the global health community to tackle the treatment gap, and operates with input from these partners.

The service is available to governments, nongovernmental organizations, health insurance and employer-benefit schemes, and other not-for-profit supply channels. Current information on sources, prices, and the patent and regulatory status of high-quality antiretrovirals and diagnostics will be made available to buyers, particularly at country level, to help them make informed choices on procurement. WHO does not envisage buying medicines direct but will continue to purchase diagnostic tests as part of a bulk procurement scheme.

The AIDS Medicines and Diagnostics Ser-

vice will also provide information to manufacturers to enable them to forecast demand, thus ensuring that quantities produced reflect real needs at affordable prices.

Countries can access specific technical support services, including:

■ *Selection of core antiretroviral drugs and essential diagnostic tests* (advice on clinical guidelines; inclusion of products in the National Essential Medicines list).
■ *Patent status and licensing* (information on patent status; advice on options for legal importation of generic medicines).
■ *Registration and product specifications* (regulatory matters and registration status of antiretroviral drugs; strengthening capacity of drug regulatory agencies; quality and product specifications for procurement tenders and contracts).
■ *Prequalification of antiretroviral drugs and diagnostics* (advice on products that meet WHO standards for quality, safety and efficacy; operational standards for evaluating supply agencies and quality control laboratories).
■ *Market intelligence* (information on sources

and prices of antiretrovirals, other AIDS-related medicines and diagnostics; price indicators for raw materials for local production).
■ *Procurement* (global guidance and training programmes on procurement; access to the WHO/UNAIDS diagnostics buyers group technical support; access to procedures to obtain economies of scale through international rate contracts).
■ *Import taxes and margins* (tariffs, taxes and margins in other countries; technical and political support in efforts to reduce them).
■ *Supply management and monitoring* (guidance and training programmes in supply management and monitoring; consultant support in improving national supply systems; technical support in preparing estimates of quantities).
■ *Local production and quality assurance* (guidance on Good Manufacturing Practices standards; training courses on Quality Assurance and Good Manufacturing Practices; technical support to the national drug regulatory agency).

facilities has risen from less than six months to at least five years *(9)*. Patients' quality of life has also improved significantly: they go on working, sustaining their families, educating their children and interacting with their friends.

## THE 3 BY 5 STRATEGY

Countries are driving the process of treatment scale-up, supported by WHO, UNAIDS, the Global Fund to Fight AIDS, Tuberculosis and Malaria, the United States President's Emergency Plan for AIDS Relief, and other partners. On 1 December 2003, WHO published its global strategy, outlining how the Organization will contribute to the 3 by 5 target *(10)*. The strategy outlines key areas of activity in a framework of five pillars.

## Pillar One:
### Global leadership, strong partnership and advocacy

WHO is working closely with UNAIDS, the World Bank, and other multilateral organizations and international partners to ensure that the effort is integrated into the broader global development agenda. International resources committed to 3 by 5 should be additional to the support for countries' efforts to achieve targets such as the Millennium

# A haven for HIV-positive children

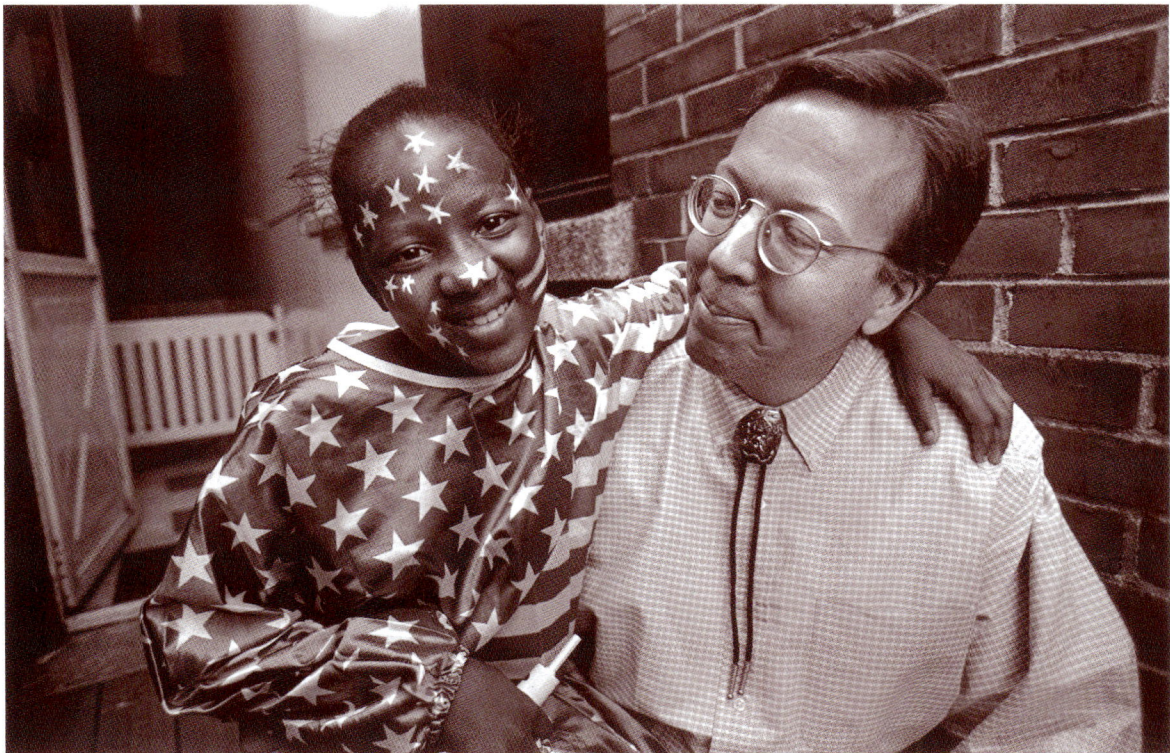

*Eugene Richards/Network*

At the Incarnation Children's Center in New York, USA, a girl called May shows her fancy dress costume to Dr Steve Nicholas. May comes from two generations of people with HIV/AIDS and is one of the children who, along with their families, receive care designed to minimize the effect of HIV/AIDS on their quality of life.

Founded in 1988, the Center meets the challenges of paediatric HIV/AIDS with a model of community-based care combining expertise and support, which takes children away from hospital wards. Since 1992, the Center has also operated an outpatient clinic for HIV-positive children living in the community.

Development Goals. WHO advocates for pro-equity approaches that promote gender equity and responsiveness to the needs of vulnerable groups.

### Pillar Two:
### Urgent, sustained country support

WHO is providing essential policy advice and tools, and will cooperate with countries at every stage of the design and implementation of national plans.

### Pillar Three:
### Simplified, standardized tools for delivering antiretroviral therapy

Rapidly scaling up antiretroviral therapy requires user-friendly guidelines and tools to help health workers identify and enrol people living with HIV/AIDS, deliver therapy and monitor results, including drug resistance. WHO is developing these tools.

### Pillar Four:
### Effective, reliable supply of medicines and diagnostics

The AIDS Medicines and Diagnostics Service has been established to help coordinate the many ongoing efforts to improve access to HIV/AIDS medicines. It provides a range of support services tailored to country needs (see Box 2.2).

### Pillar Five:
### Rapid identification and reapplication of new knowledge and successes

WHO is documenting experiences and lessons from successful national antiretroviral therapy programmes and pilot projects in resource-limited areas and is coordinating an agenda for operational research relevant to the needs of antiretroviral therapy programmes (see Chapter 5).

## PARTNERSHIPS: VITAL FOR SUCCESS

The 3 by 5 initiative will only succeed if it is supported by the many partners engaged in expanding treatment availability throughout the developing world. The initiative is above all a call for partnership – one whose strength lies in the different skills and comparative advantages of numerous organizations and communities (see Box 5.2).

The alliances and partnerships necessary for success involve national and local governments, civil society, bilateral donors, multilateral organizations, foundations, the private sector (including employers and pharmaceutical companies), trade unions, traditional authorities, faith-based organizations, nongovernmental organizations (international and national) and community-based organizations. People living with HIV/AIDS and the activist community are indispensable partners at all levels of WHO's activities. The full potential of the initiative will only be realized if it is linked to the work of the UNAIDS secretariat and other UNAIDS cosponsors.

Partnership and collaboration assume even greater importance as major programmes enter the implementation phase, including efforts financed by the Global Fund to Fight AIDS, Tuberculosis and Malaria and the World Bank's Multi-Country HIV/AIDS Program (see Boxes 2.3 and 2.4). At least US$ 4.5 billion has been committed by the Global Fund and the World Bank to the fight against HIV/AIDS. This figure is expected to rise substantially as the United States President's Emergency Plan for AIDS Relief takes off. However, the current lack of technical capacity in a large number of recipient countries is a major obstacle to the effective use of these resources. One of the greatest collective tasks will be to work with countries and recipients to ensure that the money achieves its intended results. Success depends on close collaboration between funders and technical agencies.

## DELIVERING TREATMENT: A PRACTICAL NEW APPROACH

Despite resource constraints and technical obstacles, health care planners and treatment providers are working in many settings to scale up treatment as rapidly as possible, expanding from small pilot projects to national programmes. To enable this to succeed, the 3 by 5 initiative incorporates a practical "engineering" or "system design" approach. The plan is to develop innovative system designs and treatment protocols that can be scaled up even when the usual medical resources are in very short supply. This depends on streamlining and simplification of programme logistics, delivery of treatment and monitoring. The simplified strategies should allow nurses or clinical officers to treat patients within a physician-supervised treatment team, with community health workers providing follow-up support and adherence monitoring. Pilot projects have shown that, with proper supervision and streamlined treatment models, community health workers can shoulder much of the daily burden of delivering and supporting treatment (see Chapter 3).

Reducing complexity is necessary in order to accelerate the roll-out of treatment in areas with weak health care systems and a severe shortage of trained health professionals. Simplification applies to drug regimens and biological monitoring procedures recommended in WHO guidelines. It also covers protocols for treatment delivery, patient monitoring and support, and drug procurement and supply management. Such simplification does not imply poorer outcomes for patients than would be the case in wealthier countries. Many aspects of delivery, programme logistics and monitoring can be streamlined while still providing patients with excellent care.

In its new streamlined treatment guidelines, WHO has cut the number of recommended first-line treatment regimens from 35 to four. All four regimens are widely used in high-income countries and are highly effective *(11)*. They use two different classes of antiretrovirals, reserving the protease inhibitor class for second-line therapy, and can be given to children, an important advantage for family therapy.

## Box 2.3  The Global Fund to Fight AIDS, Tuberculosis and Malaria

The Global Fund to Fight AIDS, Tuberculosis and Malaria attracts, manages and disburses resources through a new public–private partnership. It does so in order to make a sustainable and significant contribution to the reduction of infections, illness and death, and thus contribute to poverty reduction and the Millennium Development Goals.

The Global Fund relies on the knowledge of local experts for programme implementation. It finances proposals that reflect national ownership and are developed and implemented through multisectoral country partnerships among all relevant players within a country and across all sectors of society.

As a financing mechanism, the Global Fund works closely with other multilateral and bilateral organizations involved in health and development issues to ensure that newly funded programmes are coordinated with existing ones. The Global Fund actively seeks to complement the finance of other donors and to use its own grants to catalyse additional investments by donors and by recipients themselves. Since its inception in January 2002, it has designed and implemented systems for the technical review of grant proposals, efficient fund disbursement and the monitoring and evaluation of programme performance and financial accountability. In December 2002, the first grant agreement was signed and disbursement made. A year later, the Global Fund had awarded a total of US$ 2.1 billion over two years to 224 programmes in 121 countries and 3 territories.

Specific goals include increasing the supply of antiretroviral drugs and supporting voluntary counselling and testing services to prevent the spread of HIV. The Global Fund is also supporting orphans with medical services, education and community care; tripling the number of people treated for multidrug-resistant tuberculosis globally; delivering millions of combination drug treatments for resistant malaria; and financing millions of bednets to protect African families from transmission of malaria.

These four regimens do not require a cold chain, are widely available and cost less than regimens based on protease inhibitors. They use few pills, and the four combinations cover a variety of circumstances including tuberculosis coinfection and potential pregnancy. Other important advantages concern laboratory requirements and toxicity profile. Fixed-dose combinations are single pills containing all three antiretroviral drugs belonging to a triple therapy. Availability in a fixed-dose combination is an important criterion for preferred simplified first-line regimens. Weighing all these factors, the use of nevirapine-based regimens, particularly the d4T/3TC/NVP combination, is most suitable for initial therapy in resource-poor settings.

In addition to their logistic advantages, simplified treatment regimens, fixed-dose combinations and reduced pill count are much preferred by patients. They help ensure that patients adhere to treatment and that regimens work longer. Thus they can be expected to reduce the risks of drug resistance *(11)*.

Laboratory testing and diagnostic tools for monitoring the health of people living with HIV/AIDS must also be simplified and made more readily available to the poorest populations. Evidence shows that tests such as total lymphocyte count and haemoglobin colour-scale blood tests can be used where more sophisticated tests for viral load and CD4 cell count are not yet available. The simpler tests, combined with clinical evaluations by adequately trained health workers, can be effective in monitoring the progress of AIDS, the effectiveness of treatment and side-effects, even in settings with weak health infrastructure *(11–14)*.

Building on the simplified drug regimens, WHO has developed streamlined protocols for treatment delivery which aim to facilitate treatment scale-up, above all in the many areas where physician shortages are a major constraining factor. With simplified treatment models, it should become possible to decentralize antiretroviral delivery progressively to the health centre level; this is vital to reach the people most in need. Treatment can be initiated in facilities at all levels of the formal health care system, wherever the following are in place: HIV counselling and testing; personnel who are trained and certified to prescribe treatment and follow up patients clinically; an uninterrupted antiretroviral supply; and a secure, confidential patient record system. Rolling out treatment under this model will pose many complex challenges. It will require

## Box 2.4  Free antiretroviral therapy in Barbados

The Government of Barbados, with World Bank assistance (under its Multi-Country HIV/AIDS Prevention and Control Program for the Caribbean Region), has designed a multisectoral HIV/AIDS prevention and control project. The government has committed itself to universal and free provision of antiretroviral therapy for all citizens living with HIV/AIDS. The project has a total cost of US$ 23 million for strengthening prevention activities and scaling up antiretroviral treatment.

The scale-up of HIV/AIDS treatment and care includes:
■ a dedicated care and support outpatient facility, the Ladymeade Reference Unit, which was opened in early 2002 for voluntary counselling and testing and the provision of antiretroviral therapy;
■ the introduction of evidence-based treatment guidelines developed by WHO; they have proved to be easy to comply with, and adherence to the standard three-drug regimes has been very good;
■ provision of an expanded laboratory service to include Elisa testing, CD4, CD8, and viral load estimations;
■ a computerized HIV/AIDS case management, monitoring, evaluation and surveillance system.

The main outcomes achieved under the project so far include: an overall reduction in deaths of clinic-registered patients by approximately 56%; a total of 85% of patients with an adherence rate greater than 95%; hospital admissions for treatment of opportunistic infections among HIV/AIDS patients reduced by 42%; total hospital days reduced by 59.4%; average length of stay in hospital reduced by 30%; and a sixfold reduction in mother-to-child transmission, maintaining levels of less than 6% transmission over five years.

The Government of Barbados is committed to financing antiretroviral therapy beyond the life of the project and has allocated the funds required for further expansion of the number of patients receiving treatment.

high standards of operational research to help identify what works and what does not, and why, and to provide rapid feedback and dissemination of that knowledge.

Drug supply management is a significant challenge in many regions hit hard by HIV/ AIDS, but focusing on a small number of simplified drug regimens and using fixed-dose combinations should make it easier. Drugs are also a major part of the overall cost of 3 by 5 (see below), and minimizing these expenses is important to programme sustainability. WHO will work with countries and implementers to obtain the lowest possible prices on antiretrovirals of assured quality.

## Antiretroviral drug resistance: acting now to prevent a major problem

Although the benefits of antiretroviral drugs are universally recognized, there is concern that their widespread and inappropriate use could cause the virus to develop resistance to them, thus creating a major new public health problem. The question arises as to whether such resistance might be accelerated by treatment expansion.

Virus strains with reduced sensitivity to zidovudine, the first drug used to treat HIV infection, were first observed in 1989, three years after it was introduced. Subsequently, resistance to every currently licensed antiretroviral drug has been observed *(15)*.

WHO regards a surveillance system that enables monitoring of HIV drug resistance as an essential component of treatment scale-up. In this work, WHO and its partners are seeking the full support of the global HIV/AIDS scientific and public health community. WHO has established a coalition of 50 of the world's experts in policy, clinical management, and the science of HIV drug resistance (HIVResNet) to develop guidelines on how to conduct resistance surveillance in different settings and population groups.

Gathering reliable global data on the level of HIV drug resistance and its transmission has so far been extremely difficult. The prevalence of resistance in countries where antiretrovirals have been available for some years ranges from 5% to 27%. Recent data from 17 European countries showed that 10% of untreated patients carry drug-resistant virus. Very little data are available from the developing countries that will implement antiretroviral programmes, and much more information is required *(16)*.

The threat of increased levels of resistance cannot be an excuse for not delivering life-prolonging therapy: it has not been a reason to delay universal access in developed countries. Instead, monitoring HIV drug resistance and developing approaches to reduce its emergence and spread are required.

WHO and its partners have established the following objectives:

- to track HIV drug resistance and assess its geographical and temporal trend;
- to understand more completely the determinants of resistance, especially adherence to treatment and factors that undermine it;
- to identify ways to minimize its appearance, evolution and spread;
- to provide information to international and country-level policy-makers through a rapid and easily accessible dissemination system.

WHO has identified the need to give strong support to global surveillance of antiretroviral resistance. Since December 2003, WHO's *Guidelines for HIV drug resistance surveillance* have been available on the WHO web site *(17)*. These cover important aspects of a high-quality surveillance system such as sampling, data collection, laboratory testing, data management and analysis, quality control and ethical issues. The development and implementation of the HIV-resistance surveillance system will be primarily supported in high-burden countries where antiretrovirals are currently not widely available. Gathering data on HIV drug resistance prevalence in those areas will allow a baseline picture that can be compared with data obtained over time.

WHO and its partners are developing and implementing systems to measure HIV drug resistance in treatment-naïve people (those who have not taken antiretroviral medicines before) in 20 countries and to monitor HIV drug resistance among treated people in five countries. By 2005, 40 countries will have implemented surveillance systems and 15 countries will have monitoring systems.

## THE COSTS OF ACHIEVING 3 BY 5

The exact cost of reaching the 3 by 5 target will depend on how quickly care is scaled up in participating countries. It is likely to total at least US$ 5.5 billion by the end of 2005 in the set of high-burden countries that together account for 90% of the target *(18)*. This estimate assumes that 25% of the target is reached in 2004 and the remaining 75% the following year. It assumes that the prices of medicines remain at currently lowest available levels reported by the WHO Essential Drugs and Medicines Department (first-line treatment of US$ 304 per person per year). Total programme costs could be significantly reduced if drug prices for all countries approached those negotiated by the William J. Clinton Foundation for the 14 countries it supports (first-line treatment at less than US$ 140 per person per year).

Cost projections are based on the treatment regimens required for three different entry points: tuberculosis patients, antenatal clinics and health facilities. They include at the patient level:

■ counselling and condom distribution for the people tested as part of the programme;

■ antiretroviral drugs (first-line drugs for all people identified in late-stage disease and second-line drugs for treatment failures);

■ antiretroviral drugs to prevent mother-to-child transmission for women testing positive in antenatal care clinics and who are in early clinical stages of disease;

■ treatment and prophylaxis of opportunistic infections;

■ palliative care;

■ laboratory tests for toxicity for those showing signs of toxicity and switches of individual drugs in case of confirmed toxicity.

At the programme level, costs include training for doctors, nurses, clinical officers, community health workers and lay volunteers, supervision and monitoring, increasing the capacity of the medicines distribution and storage system, recruiting community health workers, universal precautions, and post-exposure prophylaxis. They also include purchasing an appropriate number of CD4 machines, automated

**Figure 2.2   Projected costs of the 3 by 5 initiative (total: US$ 5.5 billion), 2004–2005**

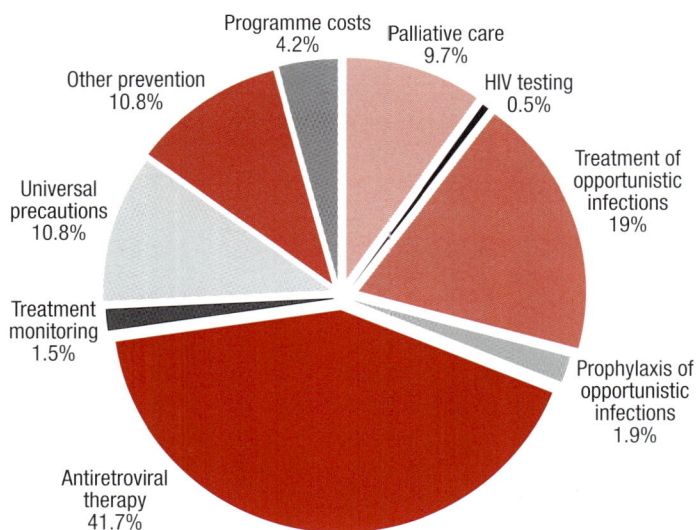

Programme costs 4.2%
Palliative care 9.7%
Other prevention 10.8%
HIV testing 0.5%
Universal precautions 10.8%
Treatment of opportunistic infections 19%
Treatment monitoring 1.5%
Prophylaxis of opportunistic infections 1.9%
Antiretroviral therapy 41.7%

# Handfuls of hope

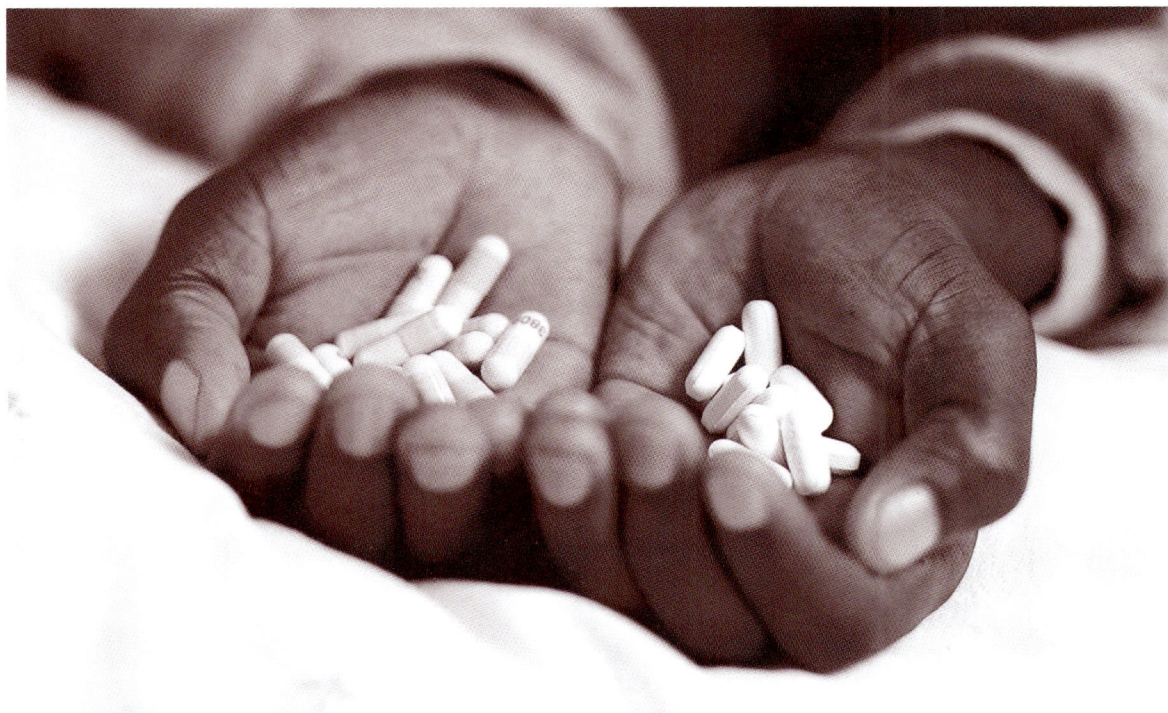

The AngloGold mining company in South Africa estimates the HIV/AIDS prevalence rate among its 44 000 workers to be between 25% and 30%. In July 2003 the company announced that it would offer anti-retroviral therapy to all its HIV-positive employees. The therapy is to be provided from 2004 onwards through the company's own privately funded non-profit medical service, the largest of its kind in the world. The service is conducting an implementation study to develop an un-derstanding of and solutions to the problems associated with treatment provision. The project is examining the operational requirements of pro-viding treatment, particularly with regard to supporting adherence to the drug regimen. It will include assessing what impact, if any, antiretroviral therapy has on patients' capacities to carry out their work, especially underground, as well as monitoring for drug sensitivity.

blood counters and blood chemistry machines in low-income countries, beginning in 2005.

Figure 2.2 shows the breakdown of estimated costs of 3 by 5 over the two-year period 2004–2005. Not surprisingly, antiretroviral drugs account for the greatest proportion, while treatment of opportunistic infections, palliative care and universal precautions are also major contributors.

These estimates include preventive activities required to support the 3 by 5 strat-egy directly. They also assume that other preventive interventions for HIV/AIDS will continue at the current rate. They do not include major changes to the health system infrastructure, which are not possible given the short time frame of 3 by 5. If other interventions are scaled up at the same time – perhaps for malaria and/or tuberculosis with financing from the Global Fund to Fight AIDS, Tuberculosis and Malaria – short-term constraints might be encountered in terms of shortages of personnel, health facilities or laboratory testing facilities. To achieve the Millennium Development Goals by 2015, including those related to HIV/AIDS, immediate investment in infrastructure and in health systems strengthening will be needed in many of the countries imple-menting 3 by 5. These issues are discussed further in Chapter 4.

The figure of US$ 5.5 billion concerns the countries with the highest burden from HIV/AIDS. Earlier, higher estimates have been superseded in other ways. For example, the model of care assumed in earlier calculations was more intensive in testing and staff time than that adopted by WHO to confront the AIDS treatment emergency. In addition, drug prices have fallen considerably.

## THE FRONT LINES: WORKING IN COUNTRIES

Countries are driving the rapid expansion of HIV/AIDS treatment under 3 by 5. Those countries already severely affected by HIV/AIDS and those with small but expanding epidemics have committed themselves to the emergency initiative.

Solving the emergency requires innovation backed by experience and expertise. It implies streamlining or suspending familiar but unsuitable procedures and devising effective new ones at short notice as events unfold. Key elements of the emergency response at country level include:

- adequate political and financial commitment to scaling up treatment;
- high-level national mechanisms for planning, coordinating and leading treatment efforts;
- ensuring continuous availability of drugs and diagnostics;
- moving quickly to build capacity in health services and communities;
- establishing appropriate systems for monitoring and evaluation and operational research as programmes are rolled out.

When a WHO 3 by 5 emergency mission is invited to a country, it can help stimulate work in all the above areas. Within days of the declaration of the global HIV/AIDS treatment emergency, the first WHO country mission was on the ground in Kenya. The mission began work with national health officials and political leaders, community and nongovernmental organization representatives, private-sector health care providers, international agencies, and other stakeholders to build consensus and catalyse action for rapid scale-up of treatment. Similar WHO emergency assessment teams have been sent out as countries request them. By mid-February 2004, 15 emergency planning missions had been completed and several more were planned in response to country requests.

Countries approach the 3 by 5 challenge from very different departure points, and with varying strengths and weaknesses. Yet important areas common to all have emerged. Announcements in late 2003 of national commitment to significant scale-up from China, India, Kenya, Malawi, South Africa, Zambia and others strengthened the growing, shared momentum. Now countries, communities and international partners are working to translate political commitments into action that saves lives. The following case-studies describe the range of situations countries face and some emerging common themes.

## China

More than 800 000 people in China are estimated to be living with HIV/AIDS. Injecting drug use has been the predominant mode of transmission, but heterosexual transmission related to sex work is on the increase. With new commitment from its political leaders, China has embraced the 3 by 5 initiative, which means aiming to provide treatment to 100 000 patients by the end of 2005.

Big problems must be tackled quickly. Epidemiological surveillance of HIV/AIDS needs further reinforcement. Implementation mechanisms for treatment are incomplete. Capacities need to be strengthened in many areas of work. Currently, despite provision of free antiretrovirals, patients must pay for HIV testing, symptomatic care, transportation costs and other expenses. These costs are serious obstacles to treatment access and adherence. Fortunately, China's strengths include a burgeoning domestic pharmaceutical industry which is now producing generic antiretroviral drugs. High-level commitment to intensified action on HIV/AIDS was underlined on World AIDS Day 2003, when Premier Wen Jiabao and Vice Premier Madam Wuyi visited people living with HIV/AIDS at Beijing's Youan Hospital.

## India

Official estimates in India for 2003 put the number of HIV-positive people at 3.8–4.6 million, with 600 000 in urgent need of treatment. India's national HIV prevalence rate is below 1%, but some regions and population groups are much more heavily affected. For example, more than 50% of commercial sex workers in the state of Goa and the city of Mumbai are HIV-positive. Efforts to scale up treatment will focus initially on six states – Andhra Pradesh, Karnataka, Maharashtra, Manipur, Nagaland, and Tamil Nadu – but there are immense difficulties. For example, the city of Mumbai alone has a larger population than Botswana and Zambia combined.

India's health system has significant strengths, including a large pool of skilled doctors and other health professionals. Training in HIV care is now part of all medical and nursing curricula, though few students yet receive adequate practical experience in clinical management. The country has numerous medical centres of excellence and an array of high-level research institutions. Without doubt, antiretroviral procurement and distribution will pose major challenges, but on the other hand successful models of drug supply management do exist, such as that in Delhi State *(19)*. India has a robust domestic pharmaceutical industry, which is also a major source of generic antiretrovirals (see Box 2.5).

## Box 2.5 How Asian drugs help African patients

The success of the 3 by 5 initiative relies on the availability of affordable and high-quality antiretroviral drugs. Some of the world's leading manufacturers of affordable generic antiretrovirals are found in the WHO South-East Asia Region: India and Thailand export to African countries such as Ethiopia, Kenya, Nigeria, Senegal and Zambia.

India in particular has emerged as a major manufacturer of affordable antiretroviral drugs. Several Indian pharmaceutical companies are taking the lead in pushing down global prices. The steep reduction in prices that has taken place in recent years was triggered by a breakthrough announcement that Indian generic drugs would be offered to patients in Africa for only US$ 350 per patient per year, through Médecins Sans Frontières. At that time, the price of the drugs provided by multinational companies ranged from US$ 10 000 to US$ 15 000 per patient per year. Thanks partly to the competition in generic drug production,

the price of antiretrovirals has dropped to one-thirtieth of its former level.

By December 2003, antiretroviral drugs manufactured by Indian pharmaceutical companies were available for as little as US$ 140 per patient per year, after a deal negotiated by the William J. Clinton Foundation. The Indian Government is working with the pharmaceutical companies to offer drugs to HIV/AIDS patients in India through a public–private partnership model at even lower prices. Low-cost drugs have already prequalified as "quality" drugs. Twelve antiretroviral drugs are presently in India's national essential drugs list. The fixed-dose combination lamuvidine+stavudine+nevirapine, manufactured generically in India, was also recently prequalified by WHO and is expected to simplify the treatment regimen, allowing patients to take only one tablet twice a day. Prequalification would allow the procurement of fixed-dose combinations from Indian

generic manufacturers by the United Nations for use worldwide.

However, some of the newer generic drugs will fall under patent protection from 2005, when the World Trade Organization Agreement on Trade-Related Aspects of Intellectual Property (TRIPS) takes effect in India. After this date, Indian generic manufacturers will have to wait until patents expire before they can begin production of new drugs, or the country may face trade sanctions. One option would be for the Indian pharmaceutical industry, as well as importers of generic drugs, to invoke the public health considerations of the Doha Declaration. It was agreed in a separate declaration at Doha that the TRIPS Agreement should not prevent members from taking measures to protect public health. Thus, the Doha Declaration will form a crucial element in expanding access to treatment.

On the eve of World AIDS Day in December 2003, as WHO released its 3 by 5 strategy, the Government of India announced a commitment to begin providing antiretroviral treatment free of charge to selected groups of patients in April 2004 and to place 100 000 people on treatment within a year. A WHO exploratory mission was invited to India within days of the government's announcement. WHO HIV/AIDS specialists are being deployed to each of the six high-burden states, with other initiatives aimed at supporting the country on issues such as clinical management, drug procurement, laboratory support and monitoring and evaluation.

By mid-February 2004, training of key staff in 16 institutions selected to initiate the treatment programme was advancing under the leadership of the National AIDS Control Organization. WHO worked with this organization on finalizing training curricula and materials, and a capacity-building plan.

### Kenya

About 1.8 million Kenyans are living with HIV/AIDS. Of the 280 000 Kenyans who urgently require antiretroviral therapy, about 11 000, or 4%, are currently on treatment. The majority of these patients are treated in the private sector or by nongovernmental and faith-based organizations.

Kenya has shown high-level political commitment to scaling up treatment and care, alongside prevention efforts. State health officials have set the following target: "Progressively deliver effective antiretroviral therapy, reaching 50% (140 000 patients) by 2005 and 75% (200 000 patients) by 2008, so as to increase the quality of life and survival by 10 years; reduce HIV-related hospital admissions by 60% and enhance significantly national prevention efforts". Major obstacles to this objective include a large financing gap, understaffed health facilities and high unemployment among trained health care workers. Treatment literacy – the understanding of what treatment is and how to manage it – is low. This is associated with very high levels of stigma among both health workers and the general population.

The government has declared HIV/AIDS a national disaster and is finalizing the legal provisions to enhance HIV/AIDS control, including provision of care and treatment on an emergency basis. Kenya has already made significant progress in preparation for institutionalization of care and treatment. The Ministry of Health has advanced plans for the phased opening of 30 comprehensive HIV/AIDS care centres, selected on the basis of geographical coverage, HIV prevalence, and the level of preparedness for antiretroviral treatment. Training of health care workers has begun. Legal barriers to the importation and local manufacture of generic antiretrovirals have been removed.

### Thailand

Around 100 000 people are currently in need of treatment in Thailand, but there are hopes that the country will reach the 3 by 5 objective of 50 000 patients by the end of 2005. Thailand has had a national, comprehensive HIV/AIDS control programme since the 1990s, integrating prevention, care and treatment (see Box 1.4).

By September 2003 the national antiretroviral treatment programme covered more than 13 000 patients. The government has allocated US$ 25 million to reach the 2004 target. The programme is continuing to strengthen infrastructures and capacity at management and service delivery level. Antiretroviral medicines will soon be covered by the universal health insurance plan. The biggest challenges are ensuring adherence and strengthening programme monitoring as well as drug resistance surveillance.

## Zambia

In Zambia, which has an adult HIV prevalence of 16%, about 1 million people are living with HIV/AIDS, and around 200 000 are in urgent need of antiretrovirals. The government has shown firm commitment to scaling up treatment, although progress has been slowed by limited resources and health system capacity. Only about 1000 patients were on antiretrovirals in the public sector at the end of 2003; an unknown number receive private-sector treatment. A national target of 100 000 people on treatment by the end of 2005 was adopted in 2003 after discussions between government health officials and a WHO delegation.

Obstacles to reaching this target are of similar scale and complexity to those encountered in many countries in sub-Saharan Africa. They include lack of funding to cover the projected costs of drugs, a significant health sector human resource shortage, weak laboratory capacity, weak monitoring and evaluation systems, and inadequate dissemination of information among stakeholders and communities. HIV/AIDS remains heavily stigmatized, limiting the number of people who seek testing and care in both the private and public sectors. Poverty and patients' inability to pay for medicines constitute major challenges for national treatment scale-up, given that 73% of Zambians are classified as poor *(20)*.

In his State of the Nation address to Parliament in January 2004, Zambian President Levy Mwanawasa affirmed commitment to 3 by 5. WHO has worked closely with health ministry officials in preparing an implementation plan, which includes an ambitious programme to train thousands of health workers, community workers and volunteers in aspects of treatment provision during 2004–2005. WHO is also providing policy and technical cooperation in Zambia's development of a proposal for funding from the Global Fund to Fight AIDS, Tuberculosis and Malaria. Funding from the United States President's Emergency Plan for AIDS Relief will further accelerate the national response.

## ETHICAL POLICIES FOR TREATMENT

The 3 by 5 initiative is an opportunity for countries not only to increase significantly access to antiretroviral therapy, but also to accelerate the drive to achieve Health for All. The principles of primary health care – health systems equity, greater community participation, and multisectoral approaches – are essential to the ethics of HIV treatment as well. Special attention must be paid to questions of fairness as programmes get under way, since more people need treatment than will receive it. Yet the risk that programmes will not be perfectly fair should not delay action. Making them transparent, accountable, and inclusive of all affected communities and stakeholders, and demonstrably taking account of people's views, not only makes it more likely that these programmes will be ethically defensible and sustainable in the long term but should help countries reach other important health goals as well.

A key challenge facing policy-makers is to decide whether there are any morally significant differences among people that would make it right to draw distinctions among them as recipients of treatment. For example, should a consciously "pro-poor" approach be followed on the basis that health systems often bypass their needs?

Among the issues to consider are the following:

■ To what extent should considerations of fairness constrain the usual objective of public health intervention, namely maximizing the benefits produced? The most efficient way to scale up treatment programmes may be to start with people already on waiting lists, or those already in the health system. If such lists now exist predominantly at elite hospitals with specialized clinics, then poor, rural, and otherwise marginalized or affected groups would be underrepresented. On the other hand, waiting until outreach programmes are able to serve such groups will result in a much smaller number of lives being saved in the first few years.

■ Should benefit be measured solely in terms of health effects? Some people have urged that antiretroviral therapy should be provided as a matter of priority to health workers on the assumption that if physicians and nurses are not saved, the health system will deteriorate further or collapse. Should the same apply to teachers, civil servants, police officers, soldiers, employees generally, family members, caregivers or others?

■ "Vertical" approaches to providing health care – such as setting up specialized HIV/AIDS clinics – may maximize the number of people treated in the short term, but are unlikely to be sustainable in many settings over the longer term, and could draw resources away from primary health care and the public system in general. This would disadvantage other groups of patients, especially the poorest and most vulnerable who are most dependent on such care. Likewise, the decision to start with existing waiting lists, which are predominantly at urban hospitals, may or may not affect the development of programmes for hard-to-reach groups.

■ Should people receiving antiretroviral therapy have to pay for it? The argument for making treatment free to users is often framed in medical and public health terms (charges will deter people from adhering to or continuing treatment, which could lead to drug resistance). An argument can also be made that a system in which fees are assessed based upon "ability to pay" is not only administratively burdensome but becomes a barrier that discourages poor people from getting care and undermines the ethical premise of solidarity that lies at the heart of Health for All.

■ For many countries, it is not clear how the long-term commitment to provide antiretroviral drugs will be sustained without support from donors. Such support is not guaranteed. Is the possibility that the drugs might be unavailable in the future a reason for not starting treatment, or would the failure to provide treatment for as long as possible be the greater wrong?

WHO and UNAIDS have taken the lead in developing guidance on these and other ethical aspects of policy through consultation with countries, implementers, advocates for the underserved, people living with HIV/AIDS and ethicists. Although WHO recognizes that Member States have legally binding obligations under the right to health, WHO's guidance will be framed as non-binding, policy-oriented, ethical principles. The guidance shows how a commitment to the principles of ethics, human rights, primary health care, and fair processes can assist in the resolution of the difficult choices that countries face.

## Making 3 by 5 work for the poor and marginalized

The AIDS treatment gap mirrors widening polarization in health and well-being between the world's haves and have-nots. The treatment initiative is an opportunity for the global community to unite in a bold effort to tackle health disparities through concrete, goal-driven action. Yet national authorities and implementers will face difficult political and ethical choices as they work to expand treatment.

Deep social and economic inequalities and disparities in access to health services characterize many areas in which 3 by 5 must work. HIV/AIDS treatment programmes alone cannot overcome these inequalities. However, programme planners and implementers, working with communities, can take steps to reduce the impact of existing inequalities on access, for example, by making it easier for women and children to receive treatment (see Box 2.6). Ensuring a fair chance for the poorest people in society, as well as for socially marginalized and stigmatized groups such as commercial sex workers and injecting drug users, will demand focused planning and ongoing vigilance in the design, financing and implementation of treatment programmes. The active involvement of groups representing poor and marginalized communities is crucial, as experience in the city of Rio de Janeiro, for example, has shown (see Box 2.7).

There are no simple answers to many of the ethical questions raised in connection with HIV treatment. WHO and UNAIDS have launched a consultative process on equitable access to HIV/AIDS treatment and care, involving many stakeholders. This will produce guidance for countries, treatment providers and communities. WHO and UNAIDS cannot impose uniform prescriptions, but can identify the relevant questions and procedural options.

The choices countries make on assigning priority for treatment may differ while respecting procedural fairness. Fundamental procedural requirements are that a clear, rule-governed mechanism be in place to determine priority in access and that this mechanism be designed and monitored through an inclusive, participatory process in which all stakeholder groups take part. Relevant stakeholders include people living with HIV/AIDS, health care workers, governments, medical associations, drug regulatory authorities, the private sector, donors, academic institutions and nongovernmental community-based and faith-based organizations. Involvement of communities is indispensable.

## Box 2.6  Ensuring equal access for women and men

In most countries, gender relations are characterized by an unequal balance of power between women and men, with women having fewer legal rights and less access to education, training, income-generating activities, property and health services. These factors affect their ability to protect themselves from HIV as well as their access to health knowledge, treatment and care. Ideally, health interventions will not only recognize and respond to the existing situation, but promote transformative approaches which challenge unequal gender roles and relations.

The following are crucial considerations in the design of treatment programmes.

**Access to information**. Providing information about the availability and benefits of antiretroviral treatment ("treatment literacy") is vital to generating and sustaining demand. The avenues (such as radio, drama and peer groups) used to reach people with information, and the messages given, may be different for women and men.

**Access to services**. Services need to tackle the gender-specific barriers that women face: economic, cultural, opportunity cost (distance, timing of services and waiting time may make the service inaccessible to women), stigma and discrimination, and quality of care. Involving people in the design of services can help identify these barriers, enhance the design of services and involve communities in providing support.

**Entry points for antiretroviral treatment**. While antenatal care is an obvious entry point for identifying women in need of treatment, it is necessary to go beyond this to reach out to women with HIV who are not pregnant, particularly young women.

**Barriers to testing and counselling**. The decision to seek testing is influenced by risk perception. Many married women who are monogamous and faithful may not feel themselves to be at risk. Women often fear the negative outcomes of testing.

**Barriers to disclosure**. Women's justifiable fears of the consequences of disclosure, such as violence and rejection, need to be tackled. These appear to be more common when a woman is tested before her partner. Couple counselling and testing, mediated disclosure by a trained counsellor, and education of communities and family members can all help to reduce stigma and discrimination against women who test positive. Women's right to confidentiality should be respected.

**Monitoring and follow-up**. Monitoring should be ongoing in order to identify who is being reached and who is not, and to make the necessary adjustments. Countries should be encouraged to set targets for women, based on local epidemiology.

**Training of providers**. Integrating gender considerations into treatment initiatives is an opportunity to focus on gender-based violence and other barriers.

## BEYOND 2005

The 3 by 5 initiative has set a time-bound target, which is useful for the purposes of motivating performance and measuring results. But the initiative will not end in 2005, partly because people will need to remain on treatment for the rest of their lives. Moroever, beyond the immediate target stands the goal of universal access. The target covers only half the global HIV/AIDS treatment gap. Another 3 million people will remain in urgent need of antiretroviral therapy. Eventually, almost all of the 40 million people now infected with HIV worldwide will require access to therapy. Progress achieved in scaling up access by 2005 must rapidly be extended to people who are still deprived.

The immediate target and the wider goal of universal coverage will challenge communities, countries and global institutions concerned with health. But the challenge must be faced. The expansion of treatment is no longer a question of if, but how. The use of antiretroviral medicines in developing countries will expand rapidly in the coming years. Many people with HIV/AIDS, even very poor people, will find ways to obtain medicines that promise to extend their lives. Will this take place efficiently through rational programmes able to set high standards for drug quality, patient care and support, treatment adherence and monitoring? Will principles of equity and fair access be respected? Or will the inevitable increase in the use of antiretrovirals in resource-poor settings take place in a piecemeal and anarchic way, with access largely determined by geography, social status and the ability to pay? Will this involve only limited support for treatment adherence and scant oversight of drug quality and resistance monitoring?

Without serious commitment to treatment access, the latter scenario is the more likely, and will inevitably result in the exclusion of large numbers of patients in need, poorer outcomes for numerous patients who do obtain some form of treatment, and rapid spread of resistance to drugs. Shared commitment to treatment access across

## Box 2.7  Reaching the poor in Rio de Janeiro

Rio de Janeiro is the second largest city in Brazil with 5.8 million inhabitants, including more than a million people living in the city's slums. The first HIV/AIDS case was registered there in 1982; since then, the municipal HIV/AIDS programme has been notified of 24 000 cases, an epidemic that is concentrated in the poorest neighbourhoods. Despite the large number of hospitals and clinics in the city, providing access to care has been very difficult. Since 1992, following the national government's example, a comprehensive package of prevention activities and care services has been implemented. Universal free access to triple antiretroviral treatment began in 1996.

To overcome the problem of lack of access to services, a continuously updated training programme of health care workers was launched. Today, staff at 51 health facilities, including university hospitals and primary care

units, provide antiretroviral drugs to more than 19 000 HIV/AIDS patients in all areas of the city. More than half of all patients are followed in primary care units where tuberculosis treatment, antenatal care and other health programmes are also in place.

At the same time as the training programme began, several projects directed at vulnerable populations were started by nongovernmental organizations in partnership with the municipal programme, and with financial support from the Ministry of Health. A total of 120 health units carry out prevention activities, including condom distribution, and nongovernmental organizations run more than 50 projects tackling the epidemic in specific populations.

A community health workers' programme has also been initiated and partnerships with community-based organizations have been established to disseminate prevention measures, bring those unaware of their infection to

where they can receive help, and reduce stigma. Training and support groups to promote adherence were started in clinics, with active contribution by nongovernmental organizations. So far, the evaluation of adherence and resistance in Brazil has shown results similar to those in developed countries.

Locally, partnership with civil society fosters the innovation required to tackle the epidemic. Political support at the local and national levels has been vital to the recognition of HIV/AIDS as a public health problem and hence the fast scale-up of activities through the entire health system. As a result of this multisectoral effort, AIDS-related deaths decreased by around 70% in Rio de Janeiro. A drop in hospital admissions and a rise in outpatient clinic visits demonstrate that there has been a widespread improvement in the treatment of AIDS-related illness (21–23).

the global health community can ensure that the process of expanding access to antiretroviral therapy unfolds quickly and fairly, maximizing benefits while limiting public health risks.

Such shared commitment will also strengthen partnerships that are vital to the future of global public health. Previous successful global campaigns – including smallpox eradication, the worldwide battle against tuberculosis, massive mobilization against polio and the response to SARS – provide important lessons for treatment scale-up. All of these efforts surmounted great obstacles and most ran into unforeseen difficulties. Yet none of them matches the HIV/AIDS treatment challenge in scope and complexity. The 3 by 5 initiative is catalysing new ways of working within WHO and across the global health community based on results-oriented teamwork among many partners, strong linkages between communities, national authorities and international institutions, and an overarching commitment to health equity.

Looking beyond 2005, WHO, UNAIDS and their partners will be developing a new strategic approach to maintain the gains of 3 by 5 and to extend them, using sustainable financing and delivery mechanisms, so that antiretroviral therapy becomes part of the primary health care package provided at every health centre and clinic. Mobilizing the resources and building the chronic care infrastructure needed to deliver lifelong treatment in primary care settings at the periphery will make lasting changes to health systems. As the next chapter explains, moving forward successfully in these directions will also depend on the close partnerships being forged between the formal health sector and many communities and groups, especially people living with HIV/AIDS.

# The story of Anna Vincent

Like Joseph Jeune (see Overview), 36-year-old Anna Vincent had been very ill before being brought to the Lascahobas clinic in central Haiti, where she was diagnosed with HIV/AIDS and tuberculosis. She was hospitalized for three weeks and put on antiretroviral therapy. Since then, Anna has recovered very well and gained over 16 kg in weight.

"Without antiretroviral therapy, I would not be here for my children. I would not be here at all. My family has always been there for me, but without treatment they could only arrange my funeral. Now I can create a future for my children," says Anna.

She plans to resume her seamstress classes and in the meantime has been awarded a grant by the Lascahobas clinic to become a market vendor. She can now be seen daily in the local market with a smile on her face.

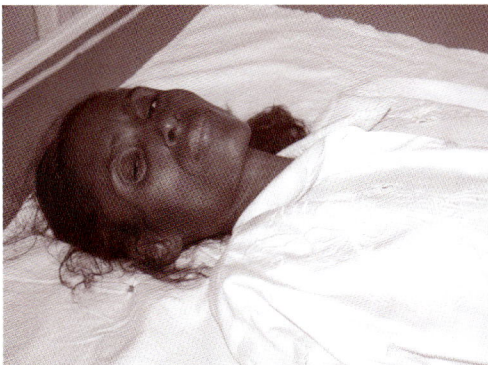

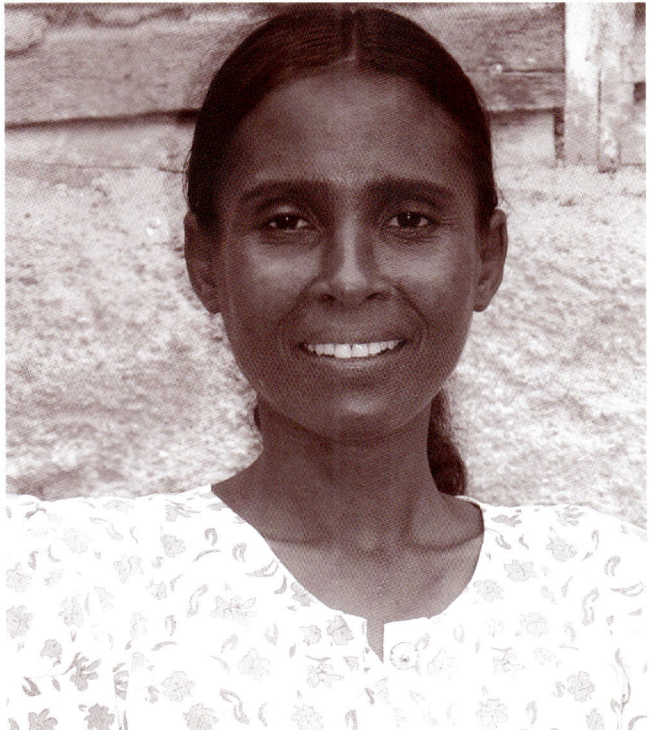

David Walton/Partners in Health

## References

1. *Access to antiretroviral treatment and care: the experience of the HIV Equity Initiative, Cange, Haiti*. Geneva, World Health Organization, 2003 (http://www.who.int/hiv/pub/prev_care/en/Haiti_E_Final2004.pdf, accessed 16 February 2004).

2. *Antiretroviral therapy in primary health care: experience of the Khayelitsha programme in South Africa*. Geneva, World Health Organization, 2003 (2. http://www.who.int/hiv/pub/prev_care/en/South_Africa_E.pdf, accessed 16 February 2004).

3. *Scaling up antiretroviral therapy: experience in Uganda*. Geneva, World Health Organization, 2003 (Perspectives and Practice in Antiretroviral Treatment Series; http://www.who.int/hiv/pub/prev_care/en/Uganda_E.pdf, accessed 16 February 2004).

4. Farmer P, Léandre F, Mukherjee JS, Gupta R, Tarter L, Yong Kim J. Community-based treatment of advanced HIV disease: introducing DOT-HAART (directly observed therapy with highly active antiretroviral therapy). *Bulletin of the World Health Organization*, 2001, 79:1145–1151.

5. Centers for Disease Control and Prevention. Advancing HIV prevention: new strategies for a changing epidemic – United States. *Morbidity and Mortality Weekly Report*, 2003, 52:329–332.

6. *The long-run economic costs of AIDS: theory and application to South Africa*. Washington, DC, World Bank, 2003.

7. *The world health report 2002 – Reducing risks, promoting healthy life*. Geneva, World Health Organization, 2002.

8. Teixeira PR, Antônio Vitória M, Barcarolo J. The Brazilian experience in providing universal access to antiretroviral therapy (http://www.iaen.org/files.cgi/11066_part_1_n2_Teixeira.pdf, accessed 16 February 2004).

9. Marins JR, Jamal LF, Chen SY, Barros MB, Hudes ES, Barbosa AA et al. Dramatic improvement in survival among Brazilian AIDS patients. *AIDS*, 2003, 17:1675–1682.

10. WHO/UNAIDS. *Treating 3 million by 2005: making it happen. The WHO strategy*. Geneva, World Health Organization, 2003.

11. *Scaling up antiretroviral therapy in resource-limited settings: treatment guidelines for a public health approach. 2003 revision*. Geneva, World Health Organization, 2003 (http://www.who.int/3by5/publications/en/ARVGuidelinesRevised2003.pdf, accessed 16 February 2004).

12. Badri M, Wood R. Usefulness of total lymphocyte count in monitoring highly active antiretroviral therapy in resource-limited settings. *AIDS*, 2003, 17:541–545.

13. Kumarasamy N, Mahajan AP, Flanigan TP, Hemalatha R, Mayer KH, Carpenter CC et al. Total lymphocyte count (TLC) is a useful tool for the timing of opportunistic infection prophylaxis in India and other resource-constrained countries. *Journal of Acquired Immune Deficiency Syndromes*, 2002, 31:378–383.

14. van der Ryst E, Kotze M, Joubert G, Steyn M, Pieters H, van der Westhuizen M et al. Correlation among total lymphocyte count, absolute CD4+ count, and CD4+ percentage in a group of HIV-1-infected South African patients. *Journal of Acquired Immune Deficiency Syndromes*, 1998, 19:238–244.

15. Stevens W, Kaye S, Corrah T. Antiretroviral therapy in Africa. *BMJ*, 2004, 328:280–282.

16. *How will the 3 by 5 initiative deal with HIV drugs resistance?* Geneva, World Health Organization, 2003 (WHO/HIV/2003.10; http://www.who.int/3by5/publications/briefs/en/drug_resistance.pdf, accessed 17 February 2004).

17. *Guidelines for surveillance of HIV drug resistance*. Geneva, World Health Organization (craft document for review; http://www.who.int/3by5/publications/documents/hivdrugsurveillance/en/, accessed 16 February 2004).

18. WHO/UNAIDS. *Estimated cost to reach the target of 3 million with access to antiretroviral therapy by 2005 ("3 by 5")*. Geneva, World Health Organization (http://www.who.int/3by5/publications/documents/en/cost_of_3by5.pdf, accessed 17 February 2004).

19. Chaudhury R, Bapna S. Effect of interventions on rational use of drugs. Paper presented at: Conference on the State of the Art and Future Directions, Chiang Mai, Thailand, 1–4 April 1997 (http://www.who.int/dap-icium/posters/4D1_TEXT.html, accessed 17 February 2004).

20. *Zambia poverty reduction strategy paper 2002–2004*. Lusaka, Ministry of Finance and National Planning, 2002.

21. Brindeiro RM, Diaz RS, Sabino EC, Morgado MG, Pires IL, Brigido L et al. Brazilian Network for HIV Drug Resistance Surveillance (HIV-BResNet): a survey of chronically infected individuals. *AIDS*, 2003, 17:1063–1069.

22. Szwarcwald CL, Bastos FI, Barcellos C, Esteves MAP, de Castilho EA. Dinâmica da epidemia de AIDS no Município do Rio de Janeiro, no período de 1988–1996: uma aplicação de análise estatística espaço-temporal [Spatial-temporal modelling: dynamics of the AIDS epidemic in the municipality of Rio de Janeiro, Brazil, 1988–1996]. *Cadernos de Saúde Pública*, 2001, 17:1123–1140.

23. Marins JR, Jamal LF, Chen SY, Barros MB, Hudes ES, Barbosa AA. Dramatic improvement in survival among adult Brazilian AIDS patients. *AIDS*, 2003, 17:1675–1682.

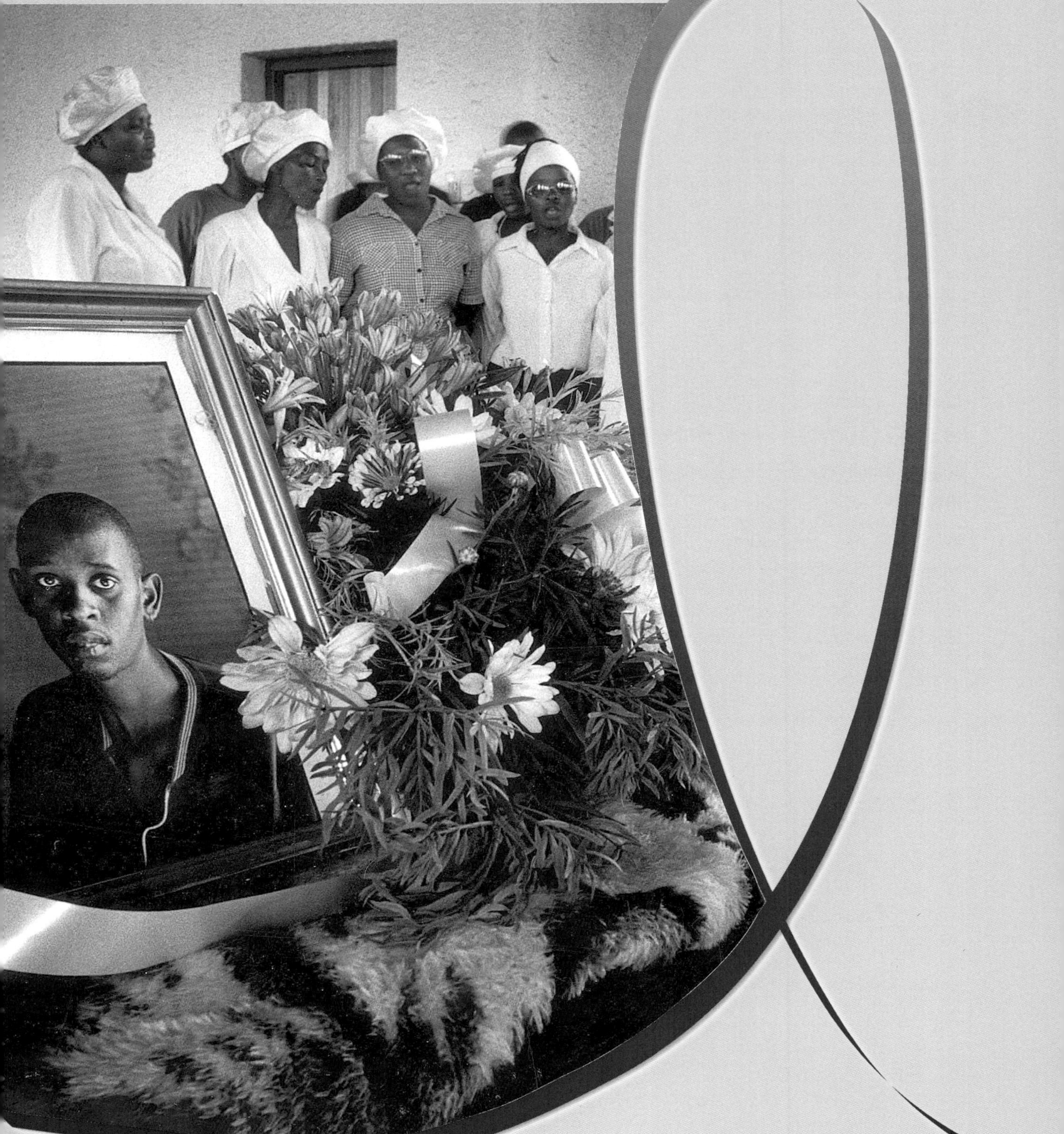

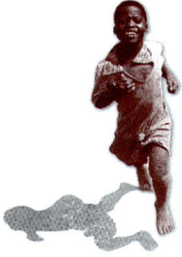

# chapter three
# community participation: advocacy & action

**Chapter 2 showed how WHO and partners are galvanizing treatment scale-up as part of a comprehensive response to the pandemic. Forming close partnerships with communities and civil society groups, particularly people living with HIV/AIDS, will be crucial to achieving the treatment target, to the success of the overall response, and to the wider goal of strengthening health systems. Such community participation will include advocacy, delivery of services and support to patients. Involving communities as full partners will require changes to the way in which public health services are delivered.**

Throughout the history of HIV/AIDS, many communities and groups have demonstrated remarkable energy in working to help all those whose lives have been affected. This chapter touches on some of the most inspirational examples of that vigour, which have made important differences to public and political perceptions of the disease and led to major and lasting benefits for the community as a whole. Today, the commitment shown by communities is an invaluable resource that can support the expansion of antiretroviral treatment. Beyond that vital objective, it will powerfully influence progress towards more general improvements in public health and access to care.

This chapter describes the emergence of community participation as a recognized dimension of public health work. It then examines some of the historical milestones of civil society involvement in the fight against HIV/AIDS. It emphasizes the power of a rights-based approach to achieving health goals. Finally, the chapter explores civil society and community participation in treatment expansion, particularly the role of community health workers.

Communities are groups of people living near each other, or with various social connections, and often with a shared sense of purpose or need. Within the wider community, specific HIV/AIDS communities exist, made up of people living with HIV/AIDS, their friends, families and advocates. These HIV/AIDS communities may or may not adopt formal organizational structures. Civil society organizations – those that do not fall within government or private industry – include associations of people living with HIV/AIDS and their advocates, faith-based organizations, and other groups such as trade unions or employer associations.

Achieving the 3 by 5 target will require building partnerships between national governments, international organizations, civil society and communities – and drawing on the specific strengths of each to get the work done on the ground. Government leadership will be indispensable, and civil society cannot replace the public sector. But part of effective government leadership will be forming partnerships with civil society groups and creating mechanisms to harness the skills available within communities. WHO and other international organizations can facilitate and support the process. By working with communities, the 3 by 5 initiative expresses the vision of Health for All affirmed at Alma-Ata (now Almaty, Kazakhstan) in 1978, which unites people's right to health with their right to participate in the decisions that affect their lives.

## COMMUNITY PARTICIPATION IN PUBLIC HEALTH

WHO's Constitution of 1948 states that "Informed opinion and active co-operation on the part of the public are of the utmost importance" in improving health, but it was in the 1960s and early 1970s that the practical benefits of community participation in, and ownership of, health projects began to attract increasing attention. Projects in areas of Guatemala, Niger and the United Republic of Tanzania demonstrated that popu-

# A choir sings farewell to Mzokonah

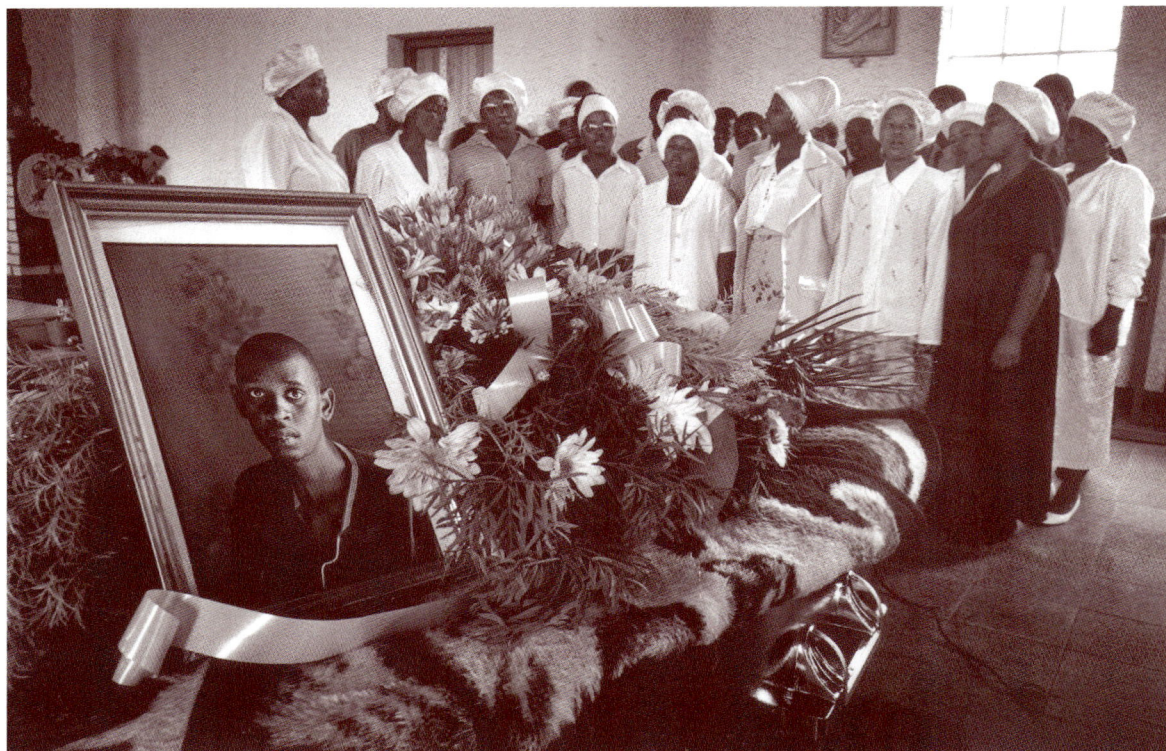

Gideon Mendel/Network

Mzokonah Malevu was ill for a long time before discovering he was HIV-positive. At first he wanted to tell only his mother, but with the guidance of a counsellor he decided to break the news to everyone in his community. At a service for the casualties of HIV/AIDS in Enseleni Township, South Africa, including orphans and carers, Mzokonah spoke in public for the first time to hundreds of people. He had a particular message for young people about how he contracted HIV/AIDS, and he stressed the need for them to protect themselves.

"I hope there will be a purpose in my death, and that my dying will help to educate my family and my community," said Mzokonah. "I want my funeral to be an HIV/AIDS education funeral, where the message can be spread far and wide." His wish was granted.

lation health gains could be made as a result of increased community involvement. In these projects, community input helped shape programme priorities and community health workers took on significant responsibilities (1). In 1978, the full participation of the community in the multidimensional work of health improvement became one of the pillars of the Health for All movement. In 1986, the Ottawa Charter, signed at the First International Conference on Health Promotion, identified strengthening community action as one of five key priorities for proactive health creation (2).

Since then, there have been both successes and setbacks. The actual capacity of communities to participate in defining and implementing health agendas has been limited by resource constraints, entrenched professional and social hierarchies, and public health models focused on individual behaviours and curative biomedical inter-ventions. Gender, race and class discrimination also play a role. Nevertheless, commu-nities have taken part in many successful public health projects, including sanitation, nutrition, vaccination and disease control programmes (3). Recent reviews of primary health care have continued to find strong support for community participation and there is evidence that such involvement has led to significant health gains (4).

## CIVIL SOCIETY RESPONDS TO THE AIDS TRAGEDY

The response to the HIV/AIDS pandemic by civil society around the world is one of the most vivid examples of community participation and self-determination. The emphasis in the Declaration of Alma-Ata on community participation "in the spirit of self-reliance and self-determination" fits with the views of early HIV/AIDS activists, expressed in the Denver Principles (5). Drafted in 1983 at a meeting of activists in Denver, USA, they assert the right of people living with HIV/AIDS to dignity in life and death and to representation and power in all decisions concerning their well-being.

In the USA, where the first HIV/AIDS cases had been reported in 1981, then in Eu-rope, Canada and Australia, organizations of gay men and women were the first to respond. The Terrence Higgins Trust was established in the United Kingdom in 1982. Helseutvalget for Homofile (Norwegian gay health association) was created in 1983. These and similar groups built on strategies and social capital developed in the gay rights and feminist movements of the preceding decades.

## Box 3.1   The Society for Women and AIDS in Africa

The Society for Women and AIDS in Africa (SWAA) is a pan-African, grass-roots nongov-ernmental organization established in 1988 in response to the impact of HIV/AIDS on women and children in Africa. It tackles the factors that lead to the unequal impact of the epidemic on women, and seeks gender equity in pre-vention and care programmes. SWAA works in 40 African countries, focusing on network-ing, research, advocacy, care and support, human rights and legal issues, orphans and vulnerable children, and prevention options for women. Some examples of its activities are described below.

In Burkina Faso, SWAA is actively involved in increasing awareness of the harmful effects of female circumcision, supports orphans and vulnerable children through the distribution of books and other school supplies, and has launched a telephone hotline. A prevention project focuses on HIV/AIDS and other sexu-ally transmitted infections among commercial sex workers. SWAA has also organized and coordinated subregional training on gender and HIV/AIDS.

An advocacy programme in Kenya focuses on men and aims to foster greater awareness of the relationships between men's behaviour and HIV/AIDS, to stimulate public debate on the issues of men and HIV/AIDS, to encour-age the adoption of safer sex practices, and to increase the perception of personal risk.

In Senegal, with the support of the National Alliance Against AIDS, SWAA provides school supplies for children affected by HIV/AIDS. It also organizes income-generating activities for women, promotion of the female condom, participation in the national programme for the reduction of mother-to-child transmission, and provision of nutritional advice and other psycho-social support.

In Ghana, the society is implementing a female condom promotion project, HIV/AIDS education, and the establishment of sup-port centres for women living with HIV/AIDS, which provide women with counselling, food and clothes.

In Nigeria, SWAA is involved in organizing counselling training and services in 28 prov-inces and in developing a counselling training manual.

Groups such as the AIDS Coalition to Unleash Power (ACT UP), formed in the USA in 1987, combined a successful advocacy strategy with the building of a formidable scientific knowledge base, which enabled members to become informed participants in medical research and the policy-making process. During the 1980s and 1990s, these groups won increased funding for antiretroviral drug research, increased AIDS services budgets at federal, state and local levels, an accelerated testing process for drugs, and expanded access to experimental drugs for people not accepted into clinical trials.

International civil society organizations, including the International Federation of Red Cross and Red Crescent Societies, began HIV/AIDS-related work in the early 1980s. In African countries with struggling health systems, numerous community-based and nongovernmental organizations were on the front lines. In many communities, women assumed key leadership roles. The AIDS Support Organisation (TASO) was founded in Uganda in 1987. TASO's work has included advocacy and community education, and also a wide variety of services to people living with HIV/AIDS and their families. Working closely with government, other nongovernmental and faith-based organizations and the private sector, TASO has been a leading contributor to Uganda's HIV/AIDS control programme. In 1988, a group of African women created the Society for Women and AIDS in Africa (SWAA), to work with and for women and their families affected by the epidemic, based on locally defined concerns and priorities. Today, SWAA has become a continent-wide network, working in 40 countries (see Box 3.1).

Other women-led groups have had a powerful impact at country and local levels. Women Fighting AIDS in Kenya, for example, was founded in 1993 by a group of women in Nairobi, many of whom were HIV-positive. In addition to advocacy for women and children affected by the pandemic, the group offers a wide range of services to women and families, including HIV education, individual counselling and support, home-based care, and training in income-generating activities. From an early stage, faith-based organizations have assumed major responsibilities for activities connected with HIV prevention, community education, care, treatment and support (see Box 3.2).

## Box 3.2  The role of faith-based organizations

Faith-based organizations have a crucial role to play in the widespread uptake of HIV/AIDS treatments, because of their influence within communities and their reach in rural and remote areas. Together with religious institutions, faith-based organizations are central to efforts to reduce stigma and discrimination. They account for around 20% of the total number of agencies working to combat HIV/AIDS. They are well positioned to offer psychosocial, moral and spiritual support to people in difficult circumstances, and they now have a growing role in treatment scale-up.

The Saint Stephen Anglican Church Widows' Group in Kisumu, Kenya, for example, helps operate a mobile voluntary counselling and testing clinic that also provides essential medicines for opportunistic infections and runs income-generating activities for women and young people. Although they have not been directly engaged in the provision of antiretroviral drugs so far, their efforts are integral components of a successful scale-up strategy.

Some faith-based organizations have designed systems for tackling inequity and gender issues in relation to access to antiretroviral drugs. They have worked to ensure that certain individuals or groups do not have privileged access to treatment, but rather that communities develop their own criteria for access.

Other organizations are involved in the direct provision of drugs. For example, the Mission for Essential Drugs and Supplies, a joint collaboration between the Christian Health Association of Kenya and the Kenya Episcopal Conference-Catholic Secretariat, is providing affordable essential medicines including antiretroviral drugs. They are importing generic drugs for the Mission and for other nongovernmental organizations at a reduced cost. The Mission's health facilities also have a home-based care component that supports monitoring of adherence to antiretroviral therapy and tuberculosis medications, and contributes to nutritional and other socioeconomic support to households and communities.

Faith-based organizations could be brought into treatment scale-up in order to combine their comparative advantages (in, for example, community mobilization, care activities, bringing about adherence and promoting confidence to seek treatment) with the training of their non-medical personnel in relevant medical skills.

## THE POWER OF A HUMAN RIGHTS APPROACH

Advocacy arguments have increasingly been grounded in a human rights framework. This draws on both fundamental moral principles and the legal obligations of states to respect, protect and fulfil human rights, including the right to health. These obligations derive from international law, regional human rights agreements and national laws *(6)*. A rights-based approach to HIV/AIDS has propelled social mobilization by civil society groups in a growing number of countries.

In Brazil, the Brazilian Interdisciplinary AIDS Association, founded in 1986, works to defend the rights of people with HIV/AIDS through research, education and policy analysis. In Bolivia, Venezuela and other Latin American countries, civil society organizations have successfully used legal action based on human rights conventions to obtain access to treatment through national health systems *(7)*.

The Treatment Action Campaign in South Africa uses community education and mobilization, mass civil protest, media campaigns, legal mechanisms, and alliances with other nongovernmental organizations and labour groups to defend the rights of people infected with and affected by HIV. Its national fight for access to HIV/AIDS therapy led to the Pan-African Treatment Action Movement, launched in August 2002.

Human rights standards and principles should also guide the planning and implementation of treatment policies and programmes. The human rights approach recognizes that rights are universal and reinforces the value of full participation of all members of society. Such an approach also requires increased accountability of decision-makers and greater equity in health care policies.

Countries have increasingly acknowledged these imperatives. At the 1994 World AIDS Summit in Paris, 42 governments declared that the enhanced involvement of people living with or affected by HIV/AIDS was critical to ethical and effective national responses to the epidemic. This principle of greater involvement is fundamental to the fairness of any policies and programmes concerning HIV/AIDS *(8)*. In 1998, the Office of the United Nations High Commissioner for Human Rights and UNAIDS jointly developed international guidelines on HIV/AIDS and human rights, a tool that applies human rights law and norms to the specific context of HIV/AIDS and identifies what states can and should do in the light of their human rights obligations *(9)*. Commitment to these principles was reinforced in the Declaration of Commitment on HIV/AIDS, adopted at the United Nations General Assembly Special Session on HIV/AIDS in 2001 *(10)*.

Nongovernmental organizations and civil society groups have led the application of human rights standards to the problem of access to medicines for the poor (see Box 3.3). Efforts such as the Access to Essential Medicines Campaign and the Drugs for Neglected Diseases Initiative of Médecins Sans Frontières have focused global attention on the medicines crisis in the developing world and helped drive public debate on the effects of trade and intellectual property rights regulations on poor people's access to treatments for a wide variety of health problems *(11–13)*.

An international coalition of activists and civil society groups worked with representatives of developing countries before and during the World Trade Organization (WTO) Ministerial Conference in Doha, Qatar, in November 2001. Civil society engagement gave impetus to the Doha Declaration, which formally clarified that the WTO Agreement on Trade-Related Aspects of Intellectual Property Rights "can and should be interpreted and implemented in a manner supportive of WTO members' right to protect public health and, in particular, to promote access to medicines for all" *(14)* (see Box 2.5). In April 2002, the United Nations High Commissioner for Human Rights welcomed the Doha Declaration and urged the international community quickly to define ways of enabling all countries to benefit from its provisions *(15)*.

## CIVIL SOCIETY AND TREATMENT EXPANSION

Civil society advocacy helped open the way for the 3 by 5 initiative. UNAIDS and WHO calculated in 2001 that it should be possible to provide 3 million people in developing countries with antiretroviral therapy by the end of 2005, but international commitment, funding and patient enrolment lagged. Energetic advocacy by activist groups in forums such as the 2002 Barcelona International AIDS Conference helped to turn the idea of expanded access to antiretroviral drugs into a definite policy commitment engaging national governments, the United Nations and other major international institutions.

Following the declaration of the global AIDS treatment emergency, representatives of people living with HIV/AIDS from Africa, Asia, the Caribbean, Europe, Latin America and North America were among the key partners consulted in the design of WHO's 3 by 5 strategy. Ongoing collaboration is vital. Catalysing innovative partnerships is one method of changing ways of thinking and working in global health. The treatment initiative is making community participation a measurable element of programme processes and outputs: an intermediate target has been set of 3000 partnerships established worldwide between formal antiretroviral therapy outlets and community-based groups by December 2004 *(16)*.

### From advocacy to service implementation

Advocacy, community education and promotion of rights will be crucial to the success of scaling up treatment. The vital role of communities in prevention and long-term care has been widely acknowledged *(17)*. In many countries aiming to expand coverage with antiretroviral therapy despite severe health workforce shortages, members of local communities will also participate directly in service provision and support *(18)*. Growing evidence from innovative treatment programmes shows that community members and their organizations are also capable of performing a broad range of essential tasks in the provision of antiretroviral treatment services.

Rapid assessments of treatment sites in a number of high-burden countries, together with a few documented programmes, suggest that the core function of communities and families lies in adherence support. In some treatment programmes, community organizations have transferred to their own settings tasks traditionally performed by facility-based formal health workers. For example, trained community members monitor side-effects and supervise pill intake in Haiti and Rwanda *(19, 20)*.

Some associations of people living with HIV/AIDS in settings with limited treatment access have, purely as a survival strategy, initiated their own services with support from organizations in richer countries. They rely on the formal health care delivery

## Box 3.3  A successful community effort in Suriname

In Suriname, as in many developing countries, HIV/AIDS medicines are not included in any public or private health insurance package and they are not subsidized by the government. Although Suriname is able to obtain relatively cheap medicines from Brazil and India, the cost of treatment (around US$ 60 per patient per month) is too high for most people living with HIV/AIDS, and many have died as a result.

The Emergency Treatment Fund for HIV/AIDS was set up in Suriname to help prevent more deaths, with the collaboration of, among others, the Pan American Health Organization. The Fund also received an initial contribution of US$ 15 000  from the Canada Fund for Africa, and in September 2002 began to purchase medication. Private donations were also solicited, by which people could "adopt" two children or one adult for US$ 600 per year. In the first six months, 50 people profited from the work of the Fund, but initial resources were insufficient to meet demand.

In collaboration with a fundraising committee, the Fund organized a mass media campaign aiming to raise US$ 70 000, which seemed to many to be an impossible goal considering the poor economic situation in the country and the stigma surrounding the subject. However, more than US$ 150 000 was raised. Since then, total donations have risen to over US$ 200 000. This is enough to sustain the Fund for 1–2 years.

system only for essential medical tasks. Many treatment-related tasks, such as the administration of laboratory monitoring, are performed by community members *(21)*. Another example of moving tasks out of formal medical facilities and into the community comes from Uganda, where TASO's Masaka branch takes responsibility for the initial selection and counselling of patients for antiretroviral treatment, then refers them to a treatment programme located in the district hospital (see Box 3.4).

In some cases, community members have worked within formal health centres. For example, in Thailand, day care centres have been set up within public health facilities, where people living with HIV/AIDS can meet and participate in various activities. Community organizations are an integral part of the care and treatment system. In Khayelitsha, South Africa, lay people have moved into the primary health care centre as counsellors, helping patients to make treatment plans in order to enhance adherence *(23)*.

Experiences in several existing antiretroviral treatment sites suggest that the relationship between health facility and community can and should be structured as a genuine partnership. A partnership model allows for regular dialogue, assigns tasks to those best suited regardless of professional status, and supports mutual feedback. Considerable investments are necessary in terms of training, staff time for supportive supervision, and additional support. A critical issue is sharing ownership of the treatment programme: health workers who are usually accustomed to maintaining control over service provision, specifically with regard to treatment, may be reluctant to share ownership of the treatment programme with communities or even accept community members' input in responding to clients' needs.

Employing people living with HIV/AIDS as paid staff members is another strategy that may allow facilities to benefit from their unique skills and knowledge and help to break down barriers between health services, communities and clients. Different disease programmes have reported that health professionals often initially resist the involvement of community members in care and treatment, but later accept this involvement when they see the positive results obtained *(24, 25)*.

Front-line facilities – health centres – are in direct contact with families and clients on a daily basis, and therefore in a position to maintain a functional partnership with communities. Evidence suggests, however, that this unique opportunity is often missed. Community organizations are frequently overlooked by health professionals, and their potential to contribute to health is often not appreciated by the health care system *(26)*.

Shared ownership – increasing the control of communities and clients over health services – is not only desirable from a human rights point of view, it is a requirement for reaching the poor with antiretroviral treatment and other health services. Many success stories exist. In Zambia, the Chikankata faith-based district hospital generated a community process that resulted in excellent joint work for HIV/AIDS prevention and care *(27)*. In one of the poorest communities in Haiti, clients and their fellow community members have become active contributors to antiretroviral treatment services *(19)*. The network of AIDS Communities in South Africa mobilized external support and built a broad partnership to set up and run a treatment clinic in KwaZulu-Natal *(28)*.

The success of the partnership model is clear at the level of small programmes, so the challenge is to scale up these models. As countries move to expand delivery of treatment, existing health service structures may be used to facilitate community partnerships. The most relevant in many settings may be those front-line structures connected with primary health care.

To establish community involvement as normal practice in existing health facilities targeted for scale-up of antiretroviral therapy, efforts are needed to change the relationships between communities and health providers. This implies fostering appropriate attitudes and skills among health professionals to work with communities and put in place incentives for this kind of work. Resource allocation must strengthen the front-line facilities that form the interface with communities. It also implies the need to build community capacity for a greater involvement, and the need to put in place specific arrangements for greater community ownership.

## COMMUNITY HEALTH WORKERS AND TREATMENT

One approach to strengthening the active engagement of communities in health development is to train and deploy people as community health workers. Antiretroviral treatment programmes in resource-limited settings have so far not often built on existing community worker programmes, but it is important that countries assess their experiences in this area and look for chances to work with community health worker cadres and recruits drawn from associations of people living with HIV/AIDS (see Box 3.5).

Community health workers have functioned successfully in small-scale nongovernmental programmes, as well as in large-scale national programmes integrated into the public health system. In many countries in sub-Saharan Africa, for example, faith-based organizations have provided quality care for 20 years. Many faith-based health care facilities have large staffs of outreach workers, home and community health workers, who function in unique networks *(29)*. Other organizations with similar networks have also played important roles in HIV/AIDS prevention and care. The 3 by 5 initiative will partly be run through these infrastructures, using the capacities and networks already in place.

Involving community health workers is a prime area for the practical approach to increasing treatment coverage. Although current knowledge is far from exhaustive, the existing evidence provides enough information to enable planners and implementers to move immediately to build programmes in a step-by-step, problem-solving manner, tackling obstacles as they arise. Operational research will be vital in providing quick feedback on lessons learnt from community health worker participation, as programmes scale up. This research must be planned and budgeted for.

Community health workers should not be viewed simply as local helpers who can temporarily take on tasks the formal health care delivery system lacks the resources to perform. They are not primarily a cheap way to deal with human resource constraints.

## Box 3.4 Partnerships for treatment in Uganda

In the Masaka district of Uganda, antiretroviral treatment has been introduced for the poor by the Uganda Cares initiative, a partnership of the Ministry of Health, the Uganda Business Coalition on HIV/AIDS and the international AIDS Healthcare Foundation Global Immunity.

The treatment programme is located in Masaka district hospital as an outpatient service. The Masaka district office of The AIDS Support Organisation (TASO) which is the national HIV/AIDS service organization founded by people living with HIV/AIDS, is also located on the hospital premises. TASO-Masaka tackles prevention, care and treatment through a combined system of employed, paid staff such as community-based counsellors, and a decentralized system of trained community volunteers who serve a number of houses in their own neighbourhood. Regular meetings between community volunteers, TASO and facility-based staff are held.

TASO fulfils various critical roles related to treatment, including:

■ Initial selection (based on agreed criteria), counselling and referral of candidates for treatment from the members enrolled in its community and home care programme. This maximizes the treatment readiness of patients before they first visit the facility for counselling and clinical review. The Kitovu mobile service (a faith-based community and home care organization) is a similar referral partner.

■ Follow-up of patients at home and at community level, thereby minimizing patient drop-out from the treatment programme.

■ Organizing transport to clinic appointments for those who are too ill to make their own arrangements.

■ Nutritional support for those requiring it.

Overall, the treatment programme reported a 97% adherence rate after one year of operation *(22)*.

# Treating children with care

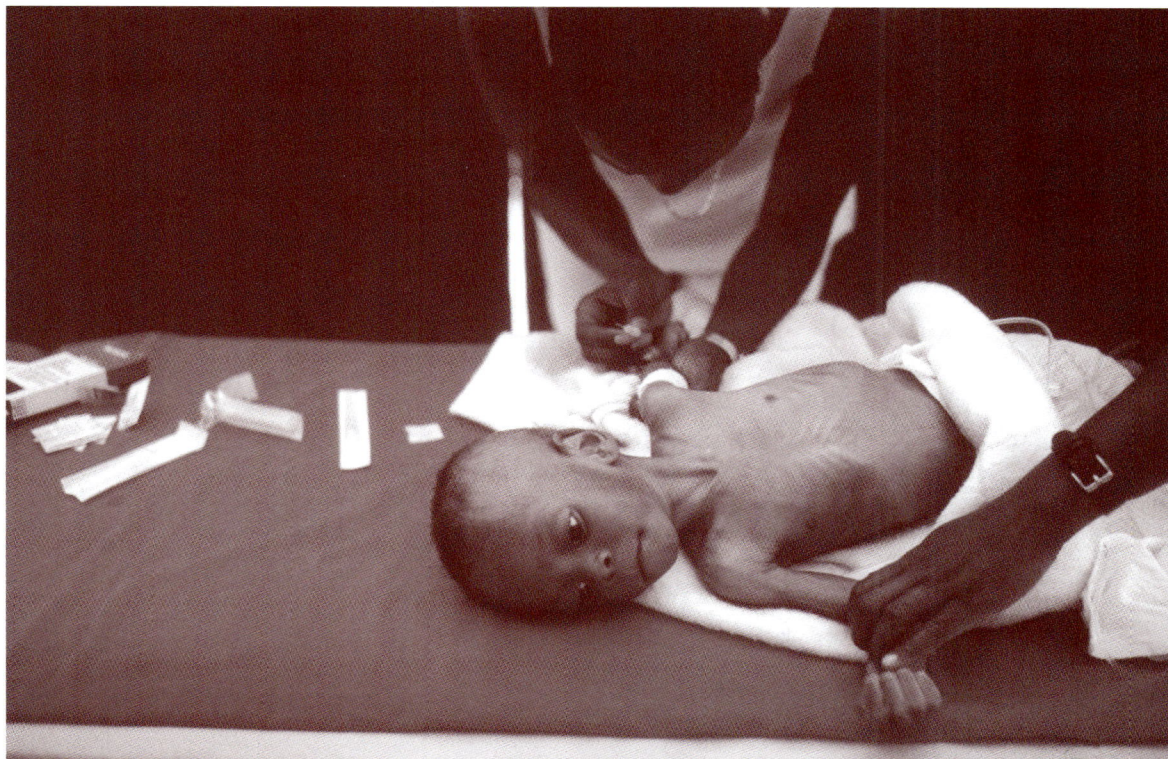

Jodi Bieber/Network

Sparrow Village in Johannesburg, South Africa, is a village community for the treatment and counselling of people living with HIV/AIDS in the terminal stages of the disease. It is home to children who play in brightly painted playgrounds. But Sparrow Village is not only a hospice, it is also a training centre and a base from which to educate the public about HIV/AIDS.

"Most of our patients were subjected to rejection and humiliation," says Dr Duncan McAulay. "But here they gain a moment of respite and a little dignity before they die."

For treatment scale-up to succeed, extensive participation of civil society organizations and communities like this is a necessity. Some community and faith-based organizations have assumed major responsibilities for activities connected with HIV/AIDS prevention, treatment and care.

Rather, community health worker programmes can and should be seen as part of a broader strategy to empower communities, enable them to achieve greater control over their health and improve the health of their members.

The following areas are vital for achieving success:

*Inclusion of curative activities:* communities are usually in direct need of curative care. If community health workers are not involved in this area, people are less interested in and supportive of their activities *(30)*. Experiences from Nepal, for example, show that when policies were established that allowed community health workers to dispense medication, community workers' motivation and their acceptance by the wider community increased *(31)*. Poor performance of community health worker programmes is also frequently associated with an insufficient supply of drugs *(32, 33)* .

*Supportive supervision, strong linkage with health professionals and referral systems:* recent experiences show that, with supervision, HIV/AIDS treatment programmes relying extensively on community health workers are able to maintain quality *(34)*. Experience in antiretroviral treatment from Haiti, Rwanda and South Africa shows that supervision is effectively provided by regular meetings, simple forms that facilitate reporting and feedback, and willingness of health professionals to engage with communities *(19, 20)*. A community health workers' programme should be integrated into a referral system that includes more advanced care centres able to respond to problems that cannot be solved at lower levels.

*Remuneration:* where financial compensation is provided to community health workers, both benefits (retention of workers) and negative effects (being viewed by communities as government employees) have been found *(28)*. Community health workers who volunteer can usually contribute only a limited time each week.

Innovative ways to compensate volunteers for their time have been introduced. For example, community volunteers involved in the onchocerciasis control programme in Kabarole district, Uganda, combined the distribution of drugs to control onchocerciasis with the retail of condoms which became an effective income-generating activity *(35)*. In several countries, volunteers receive no payment, but do receive incentives with monetary value, for example a bicycle that can be used for other purposes. Payment is needed to sustain the required level of commitment in the long run whenever community health workers are contributing an amount of time comparable to that given by professionally trained health workers. No community health workers' programme, whether relying on volunteers or paid workers, is without costs, and every such programme will need a budget to be effective and sustainable.

*Relationship with the community:* support and recognition from community organizations and leaders, and appreciation from members of the community, are identified as critical incentives for community health workers *(36)*. Fostering such relationships will mean involving associations of people living with HIV/AIDS and other community-based organizations and leaders whose support will be vital. Through their networks, community organizations may complement community health workers by tackling needs such as nutrition and income generation. Efforts to keep community health workers strongly attached to community organizations are therefore important. This can be accomplished by working through existing community-based organizations in setting up and monitoring the community health workers' programme. It will be critical to put in place arrangements that guarantee accountability. One way to achieve this is to give the community organizations, rather than the formal health care system, control over monetary or other compensation for community workers.

## COMMUNITY EMPOWERMENT AND PUBLIC HEALTH: SHAPING THE FUTURE

Community involvement is essential to all aspects of a comprehensive approach to HIV/AIDS: prevention, treatment, care, support – and research (see Chapter 5). In

## Box 3.5 Applying the expertise of people living with HIV/AIDS: Hellen's story

Hellen is the administrative clerk at an HIV/AIDS clinic in rural Uganda. As a person living with HIV who started antiretroviral treatment nine months ago, Hellen has considerable insight into the ups and downs of treatment. With this expertise, she is able to respond to many of the concerns that patients bring to the clinic.

Hellen is also an activist for the National Community of Women Living with AIDS in Uganda. In this role she organizes nutritional support for patients on treatment and contributes to treatment education at the grass-roots level. As a member of the local HIV/AIDS drama group, Hellen is also involved in community education. She is thus the kind of expert within civil society who can create effective bridges between the formal health sector, the broader community, and people living with HIV/AIDS, as well as linking prevention and treatment efforts.

Hellen says about her work in the community: *"Working at the grass-roots level is very important. People don't know much about treatment. If you look well, because of the treatment you get, people don't want to believe that you have AIDS. They think your illness was something else" (22).*

# Educating sex workers in Dhaka

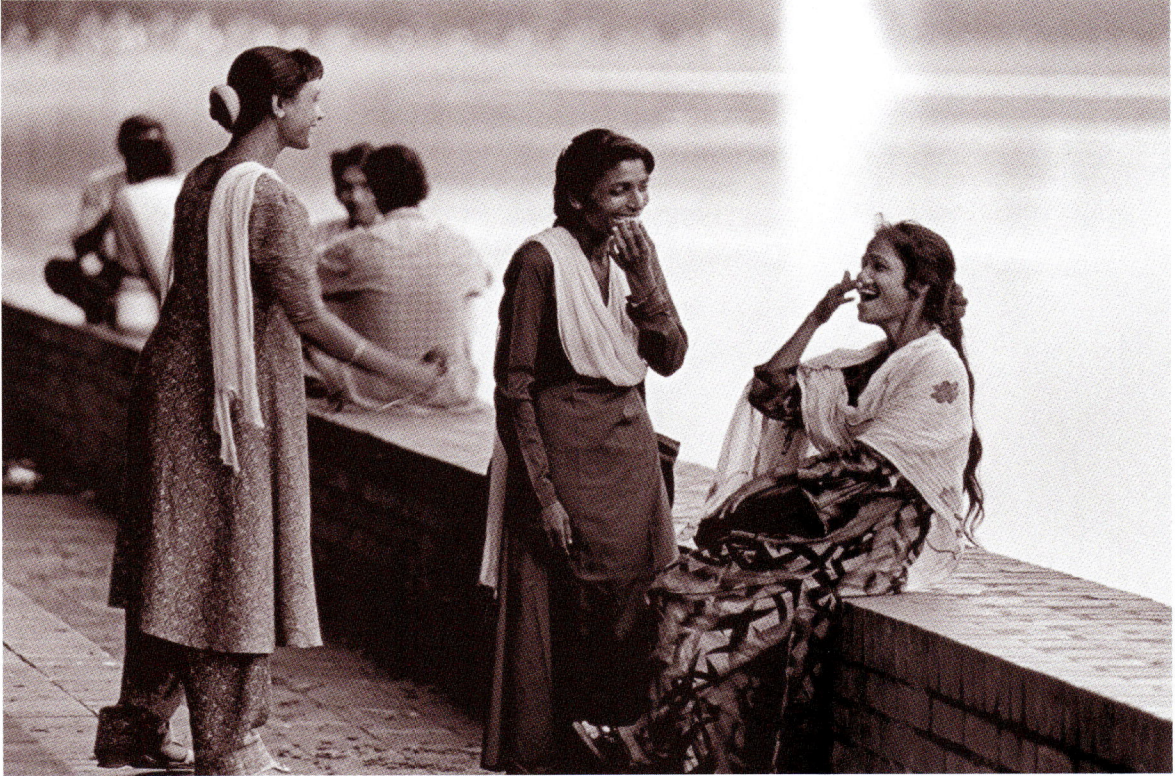

Shahidul Alam/Drik/Network

In Dhaka, Bangladesh, Hajera has established a sex workers cooperative to fight for better working conditions for her peers. She spends each evening distributing condoms to sex workers and sharing information about HIV/AIDS.

Community participation is a recognized dimension of public health work. CARE Bangladesh, a nongovernmental organization, has established a behaviour change programme that works with target groups to educate vulnerable populations, provide access to condoms and promote the use of condom distribution outlets. The distributors are paid a small stipend, are taught to read and write, and receive basic health education about HIV/AIDS.

the expansion of treatment up to and beyond the targets of the 3 by 5 initiative, civil society must raise performance demands on the public, private and nongovernmental sectors. Scale-up cannot happen without government commitment, but civil society advocacy can support this commitment.

The success of this effort in HIV/AIDS control will have important implications for the wider public health agenda. The necessity of community involvement in treatment roll-out represents an opportunity to build skills and catalyse collaboration between communities, health care providers and public health planners that can carry over into other areas of public health work, and help strengthen health systems across the board. Communities educated and mobilized around HIV/AIDS control, provision of services and support will be better able to take part in health promotion, disease control and treatment efforts that tackle other health problems. These include tuberculosis and malaria, maternal and child health, and chronic adult diseases in low-income and middle-income countries. Recognizing and building up these capacities is part of the process of strengthening health systems. Success in accelerating this process could be a lasting contribution of the 3 by 5 initiative to global health improvement.

---

This chapter has demonstrated the vital role that communities and civil society organizations play in the fight against HIV/AIDS and the success of the 3 by 5 initiative. Governments and international organizations, including WHO and its partners, will catalyse this process. The next chapter shows how the comprehensive response, with the close involvement of all these allies, aims to strengthen health systems and hence bring long-term improvements in health services for all.

## References

1. Newell KW, ed. *Health by the people*. Geneva, World Health Organization, 1975.
2. *Ottawa Charter for Health Promotion. First International Conference on Health Promotion, Ottawa, Canada, 17–21 November 1986*. Geneva, World Health Organization, 1986 (WHO/HPR/HEP/95.1; http://www.who.int/hpr/NPH/docs/ottawa_charter_hp.pdf, accessed 20 February 2004).
3. Kahssay HM, Oakley P, eds. *Community involvement in health development: a review of the concept and practice*. Geneva, World Health Organization, 1999 (Public Health in Action, No 5).
4. *A global review of primary health care: emerging messages*. Geneva, World Health Organization, 2003 (WHO/MNC/OSD/03.01, p. 17).
5. Advisory Committee of People With AIDS. *The Denver Principles*. 1983 (http://www.actupny.org/documents/Denver.html, accessed 20 February 2004).
6. *25 questions and answers on health and human rights*. Geneva, World Health Organization, 2002 (WHO Health and Human Rights Publication Series, Issue No. 1).
7. *Report on the global HIV/AIDS epidemic 2002*. Geneva, Joint United Nations Programme on HIV/AIDS and World Health Organization, 2002:64–65.
8. *From principle to practice: greater involvement of people living with or affected by HIV/AIDS*. Geneva, Joint United Nations Programme on HIV/AIDS, 1999.
9. *HIV/AIDS and human rights: international guidelines, 1998; HIV/AIDS and human rights: international guidelines – revised Guideline 6. Access to prevention, treatment, care and support, 2002*. Geneva, Office of the United Nations High Commissioner for Human Rights and Joint United Nations Programme on HIV/AIDS, 1998; 2002.
10. *Declaration of Commitment on HIV/AIDS*. New York, United Nations, 2001 (United Nations General Assembly Special Session on HIV/AIDS, 25–27 June 2001, paragraph 58).
11. Trouiller P, Olliaro P, Torreele E, Orbinski J, Laing R, Ford N. Drug development for neglected diseases: a deficient market and a public-health policy failure. *Lancet*, 2002, 359:2188–2194.
12. Kindermans JM, Matthys F. Introductory note: the Access to Essential Medicines Campaign. *Tropical Medicine and International Health*, 2001, 6:955–956.
13. *DNDi: an innovative solution (working draft)*. Geneva, Drugs for Neglected Diseases Initiative, 2003 (http://www.dndi.org/cms/public_html/images/article/268/ InnovativeSolutioncolour.pdf, accessed 20 February 2004).
14. *Declaration on the TRIPS Agreement and Public Health*. Geneva, World Trade Organization, 2001 (http://www.wto.org/english/thewto_e/minist_e/min01_e/mindecl_trips_e.htm, accessed 20 February 2004).
15. *Access to medication in the context of pandemics such as HIV/AIDS*. Geneva, Office of the United Nations High Commissioner for Human Rights, 2002 (Commission on Human Rights resolution 2002/32; http://www.unhchr.ch/huridocda/huridoca.nsf/(Symbol)/ E.CN.4.RES.2002.32.En?Opendocument, accessed 20 February 2004).
16. WHO/UNAIDS. *Treating 3 million by 2005: making it happen. The WHO strategy*. Geneva, World Health Organization, 2003:55.

17. *Community mobilization and AIDS: technical update.* Geneva, Joint United Nations Programme on HIV/AIDS, 1997.

18. *Emergency scale-up of antiretroviral therapy in resource-limited settings: technical and operational recommendations to achieve 3 by 5. Draft report from the WHO/UNAIDS Zambia Consultation, 18–21 November 2003, Lusaka, Zambia.* Geneva, World Health Organization, 2003 (http://www.who.int/3by5/publications/documents/zambia/en/, accessed 20 February 2004).

19. Farmer P, Léandre F, Mukherjee JS, Gupta R, Tarter L, Yong Kim J. Community-based treatment of advanced HIV disease: introducing DOT-HAART (directly observed therapy with highly active antiretroviral therapy). *Bulletin of the World Health Organization*, 2001, 79:1145–1151.

20. Essengue S. *Human resources and service delivery issues in antiretroviral treatment services: report of treatment site visits in Rwanda, October 2003.* Geneva, World Health Organization, 2003 (Department of Health Service Provision, unpublished report).

21. De Gagné D. Community capacity for treatment: the solidarity in treatment project. In: Goede H, Ansari W, eds. *Partnership work: the health service-community interface for HIV/AIDS prevention, care and treatment. Report of a WHO consultation.* Geneva, World Health Organization, 2003 (http://whqlibdoc.who.int/publications/2003/9241590963.pdf, accessed 20 February 2004).

22. Goede H, Matsiko C. *Human resources and service delivery issues in antiretroviral treatment services: report of treatment site visits in Uganda, October 2003.* Geneva, World Health Organization, 2003 (Department of Health Service Provision, unpublished report).

23. *Antiretroviral therapy in primary health care: experience of the Khayelitsha Programme in South Africa.* Geneva, World Health Organization, 2003 (Perspectives and Practice in Antiretroviral Treatment Series; http://www.who.int/hiv/pub/prev_care/en/South_Africa_E.pdf, accessed 16 February 2004).

24. Special Programme for Research and Training in Tropical Diseases. *Community-directed treatment of lymphatic filariasis in Africa. Report of a multicentre study in Ghana and Kenya.* Geneva, World Health Organization, 2000 (TDR/IDE/RP/CDTI/00.02).

25. Kironde S, Nasolo J. Combating tuberculosis: barriers to widespread non-governmental organisation involvement in community-based tuberculosis treatment in South Africa. *International Journal of Tuberculosis and Lung Disease*, 2002, 6:679–685.

26. Kahssay HM, Baum F, eds. *The role of civil society in district health systems: hidden resources.* Geneva, World Health Organization, 2004 (forthcoming).

27. Williams, G. *From fear to hope.* St Albans, Teaching Aids at Low Cost, 1990 (Strategies for Hope Series).

28. *Ithembalabantu "People's Hope" Clinic KwaZulu-Natal, South Africa: first year progress report, July 2003.* Amsterdam, AIDS Healthcare Foundation Global Immunity, 2003 (http://www.ahfgi.org/global_pdf/SAReport_a4.pdf, accessed 20 February 2004).

29. *The role of faith-based organizations in the fight against HIV/AIDS.* Geneva, Joint United Nations Programme on HIV/AIDS, 2004 (forthcoming).

30. Walt G, Ross D, Gilson L, Owuor-Omondi L, Knudsen T. Community health workers in national programmes: the case of the family welfare educators of Botswana. *Transactions of the Royal Society of Tropical Medicine and Hygiene*, 1989, 83:49–55.

31. Curtale F, Siwakoti B, Lagrosa C, LaRaja M, Guerra R. Improving skills and utilization of community health volunteers in Nepal. *Social Science and Medicine*, 1995, 40:1117–1125.

32. Parlato M. Favin M. *Progress and problems: an analysis of 52 A.I.D. assisted projects.* Washington, DC, American Public Health Association, 1982.

33. Stekelenburg J, Kyanamina SS, Wolffers I. Poor performance of community health workers in Kalabo district, Zambia. *Health Policy*, 2003, 65:109–118.

34. Uys LR. The practice of community caregivers in a home-based HIV/AIDS project in South Africa. *Journal of Clinical Nursing*, 2002, 11:99–108.

35. Kipp W, Burnham G, Bamuhiiga J, Weis P, Buttner DW. Ivermectin distribution using community volunteers in Kabarole district, Uganda. *Health Policy and Planning*, 1998, 13:167–173.

36. *Strengthening the performance of community health workers: interregional meeting of principal investigators, 12–16 November 1990.* Geneva, World Health Organization (SHS/DHS/91.1).

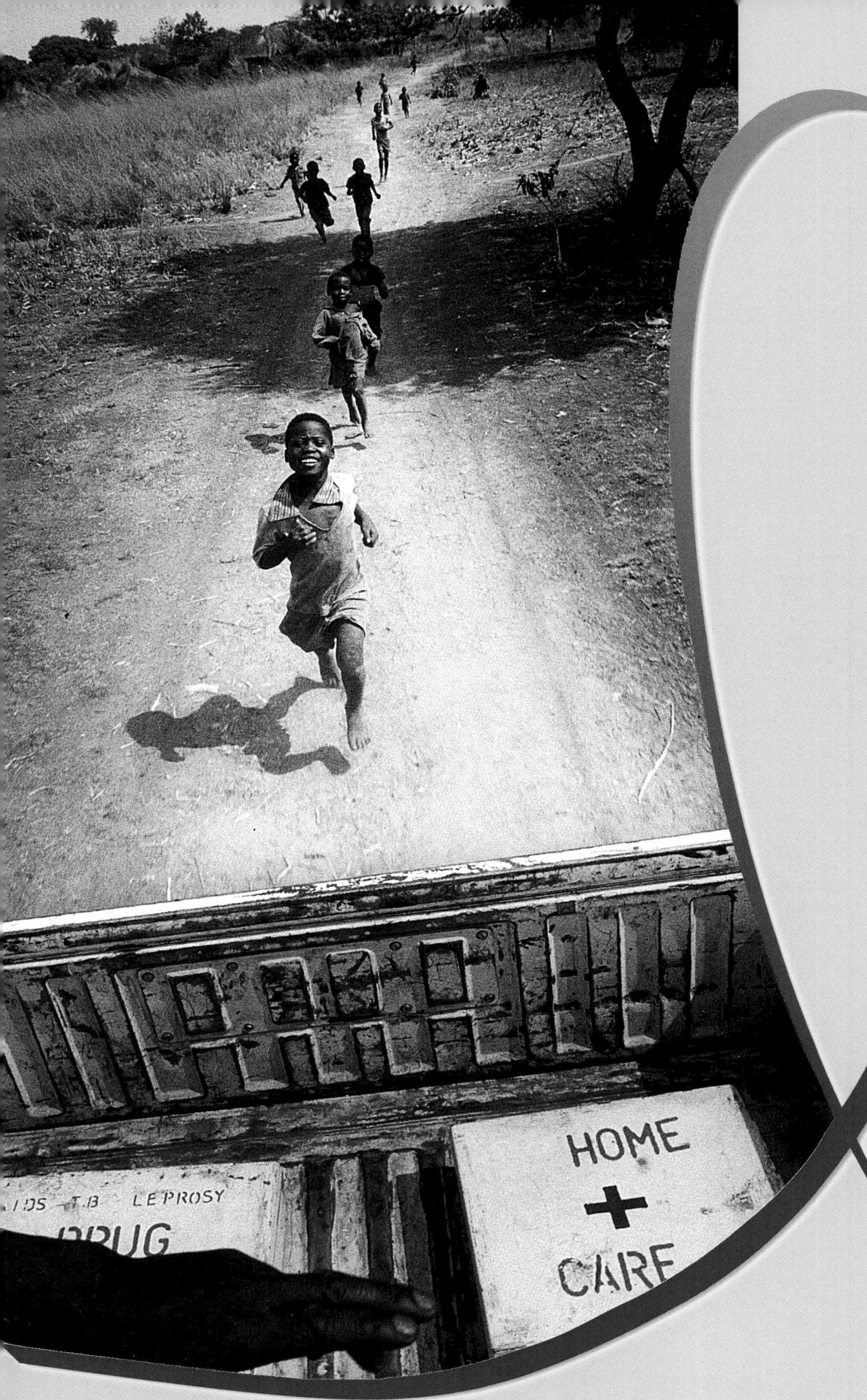
T.B LEPROSY
HOME
+
CARE

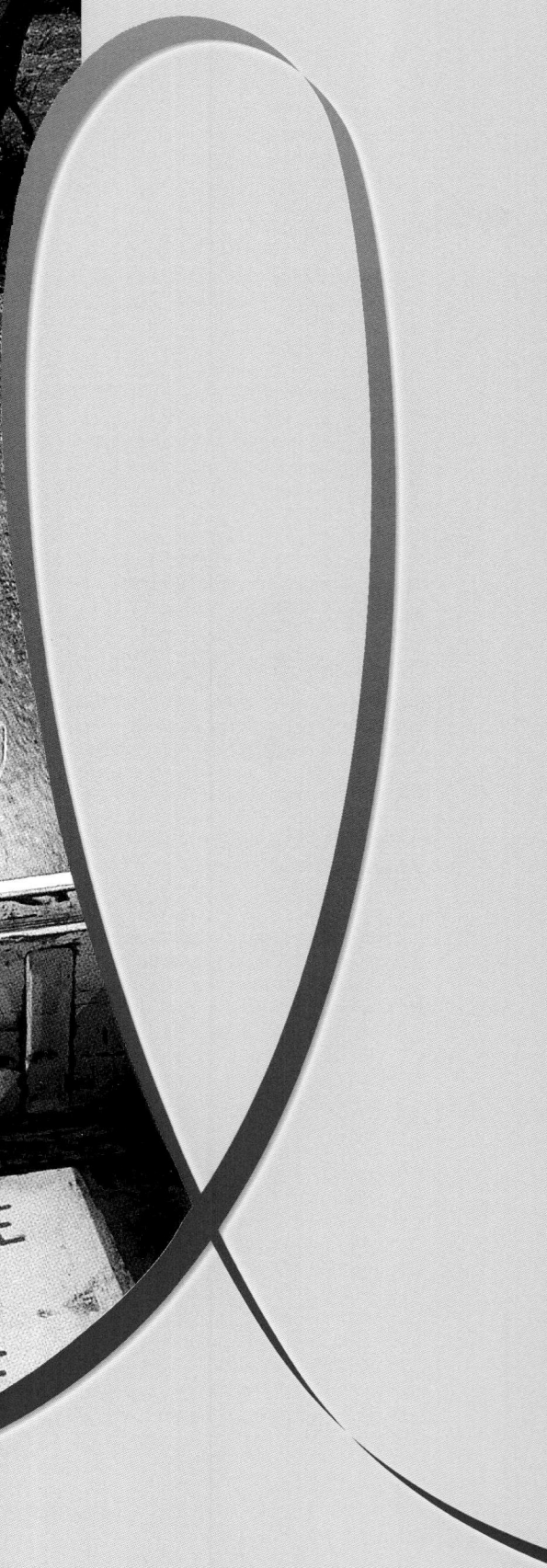

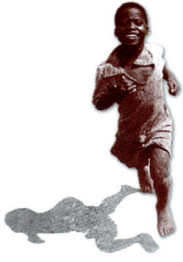

## chapter four
# health systems:
# finding new strength

**The treatment initiative presents a tremendous challenge to the health systems of countries heavily burdened by HIV/AIDS. Ideally, those systems should function effectively, efficiently and serve the entire population. In most cases, however, they are poorly run, underfunded and sometimes barely able to function at all. This chapter examines what is necessary to strengthen them in order to implement the initiative, while also improving and expanding many other health interventions related to both communicable and chronic noncommunicable diseases. It shows that a major effort is urgently needed, requiring a massive increase in resource transfers from rich to poor countries.**

Far from being a drain on resources, the 3 by 5 initiative has the potential to strengthen health systems in a number of ways. It can attract resources to the health system over and above those required for HIV/AIDS. It can spur investment in physical infrastructure, help develop procurement and distribution systems of generic products, and foster interaction with communities across a wide range of health interventions. Any possible adverse effects of the initiative on the wider health system must be anticipated so that they can be minimized.

Current levels of health expenditure in many poor countries are far below those needed to provide the bare minimum of services to their populations. In the years ahead, the financing gap will have to be filled largely by external donors. National governments and their economies are incapable of generating much more funding than they do already, while donors have still to live up to past collective undertakings.

The expansion of treatment should not divert resources and attention away from prevention and other forms of care. Indeed, the aim is for the initiative to become profoundly synergistic with those interventions [1] (see Chapter 2).

Antiretroviral therapy calls for a pattern of chronic care in which individual patients receive continuous follow-up treatment for the remainder of their lives, rather than the occasional acute interventions that characterize the response to most infectious diseases. If health systems can be strengthened to accommodate this new pattern, the management practices developed for antiretroviral therapy (appointment systems, integrated medical records, drug supply systems, and adherence support) can also be applied to the management of other common, chronic conditions such as diabetes and hypertension.

This chapter shows how both public and private providers within health systems have helped to combat HIV/AIDS in some developing countries. It then uses the conceptual framework of four principles of health systems – leadership, service delivery, resource provision and financing – to examine how health systems, and especially publicly funded systems, can be strengthened to implement the 3 by 5 initiative while continuing to improve and expand many other health interventions.

## INVESTING IN CHANGE

With only a few exceptions, HIV/AIDS epidemics have hit hardest the countries whose health systems are least able to cope. Chronic underfunding and poor management largely explain their precarious position. Efforts to reform the public health sector have tended to focus on underfunding, centralized decision-making, and inefficient delivery of services. Responses have included the introduction of user fees, decentralization and contracting with the private sector. The limited successes – and frequent unintended adverse effects – of these reform initiatives have left public health providers in great need of capacity strengthening. Two broad strategies have been proposed: increased spending to overcome deficiencies of inputs and strengthen management systems; and the use of alternative delivery systems and health service providers from outside government *(2)*.

New investments in capacity building, especially in human resources, need considerable time to mature. The alternative strategy of bypassing the public sector provider network offers the possibility of quicker benefits. This strategy has already been widely employed in a series of interventions, particularly in prevention efforts such as peer educator programmes, school education, social marketing of condoms, and mass media campaigns.

Most of the early experience with HIV/AIDS treatment in developing countries has been gained in private practice and in sites managed by nongovernmental organizations and research institutions, which are free of the bureaucracy and severe resource limitations that constrain the public system. Such providers have been prominent in demonstrating the feasibility of the treatment in resource-limited settings. However, scale-up will inevitably require a large number of treatment sites and therefore much larger participation by the public sector, which has the largest network of service delivery points. This is already apparent in many national plans, and it is inevitable that expanding treatment will entail the strengthening of public provider systems.

However, the treatment initiative will benefit from the experience of earlier disease programmes that have led to improved health system practice: collaboration between international, national and local authorities in the context of poliomyelitis eradication and SARS control; the value of monitoring systems based on outcome measures in the case of the DOTS strategy for tuberculosis control; and effective partnerships with parties outside government, also in the context of tuberculosis control. There are fewer examples of specific programmes enhancing the capacity to deliver other services, but improved disease surveillance and infection control measures for SARS *(3)* have wider application, and it has been possible to add the distribution of vitamin A supplements to polio eradication activities. There is little evidence that categorical programmes have undermined wider systems capacity. Synergistic benefits will occur if they are planned in advance and, equally, any adverse effects need to be anticipated so that their impact can be mitigated *(4)*.

It is therefore important that treatment scale-up is designed not to undermine the capacity of health systems to reach broader health goals by, for example, avoiding disproportionate diversion of existing resources into antiretroviral therapy, or refraining from the use of incentives only for staff directly engaged in HIV programmes. While the public sector will be the largest single provider of antiretroviral therapy in future, various other providers have pioneered treatment delivery and will continue to have an expanding role. The following sections indicate their potential.

## BEYOND THE PUBLIC SECTOR

Since antiretroviral drugs became available, small numbers of patients in developing countries have been able to obtain treatment from private practitioners on a fee-for-service basis, financed either directly out of pocket or by third-party payers such as insurance schemes or employers. Even if governments begin to offer free treatment, the demand for private practitioner services is likely to increase as the price of drugs continues to fall.

Faith-based organizations (see Box 3.2) have also been pioneers in offering antiretroviral therapy on a fee-for-service basis. In Kenya, for example, the founders of a pilot programme at the Nazareth Hospital, near Nairobi, have proposed a scheme to embrace 20 other faith-based hospitals in western and central Kenya *(5)*.

International nongovernmental organizations, notably Family Health International and Médecins Sans Frontières, have been associated with some of the most innovative programmes delivering antiretroviral therapy. Médecins Sans Frontières projects in Kenya and Malawi have provided free services to very poor rural populations, and in South Africa the organization has supported a community-based programme (see Box 4.1).

### The business sector contribution

Many large private firms have been providing antiretroviral therapy to their employees, either directly as part of occupational health services or indirectly by financing access

## Box 4.1  Antiretroviral therapy in the Western Cape Province, South Africa

South Africa's first public sector project offering antiretroviral therapy was established at community health centres in the Cape Town township of Khayelitsha, where clinics began treatment in May 2001. By June 2003, over 5000 patients had enrolled and over 600 children and adults had started treatment. The costs of drugs, viral load tests and the wages of half the clinical staff have been met by Médecins Sans Frontières; the remaining costs have been covered by the provincial government.

Adherence, survival and virological success in this project are comparable to if not better than those in many settings in wealthier countries. The primary care setting has contributed

greatly to a very high retention of patients. The potential to treat families in one setting, to connect with community-based support groups and nongovernmental organizations, and proximity to referring services all contribute to impressive clinical outcomes.

The province is attempting to bolster the entire primary care system in tandem with the delivery of antiretroviral therapy. To do this, management responsibility for primary care and HIV/AIDS has been located within one directorate, and aggressive staff recruitment and retention strategies try to fill posts in HIV/AIDS services and in other primary care services simultaneously.

Primary care services are benefiting from the strengthening of referral systems with hospitals, the provision of clinical support by specialists, and the increased emphasis on drug availability. Nurses with no formal training in diagnostics and curative care have rapidly become competent primary care clinicians through training and mentoring in HIV/AIDS care. Increased resources (both human and financial) have been directed at primary care as a result of the work of these projects. There has been a reinvigoration of clinical support networks, increased uptake of a range of services including voluntary counselling and testing, and more openness about HIV/AIDS *(6, 7)*.

# The health truck comes to town

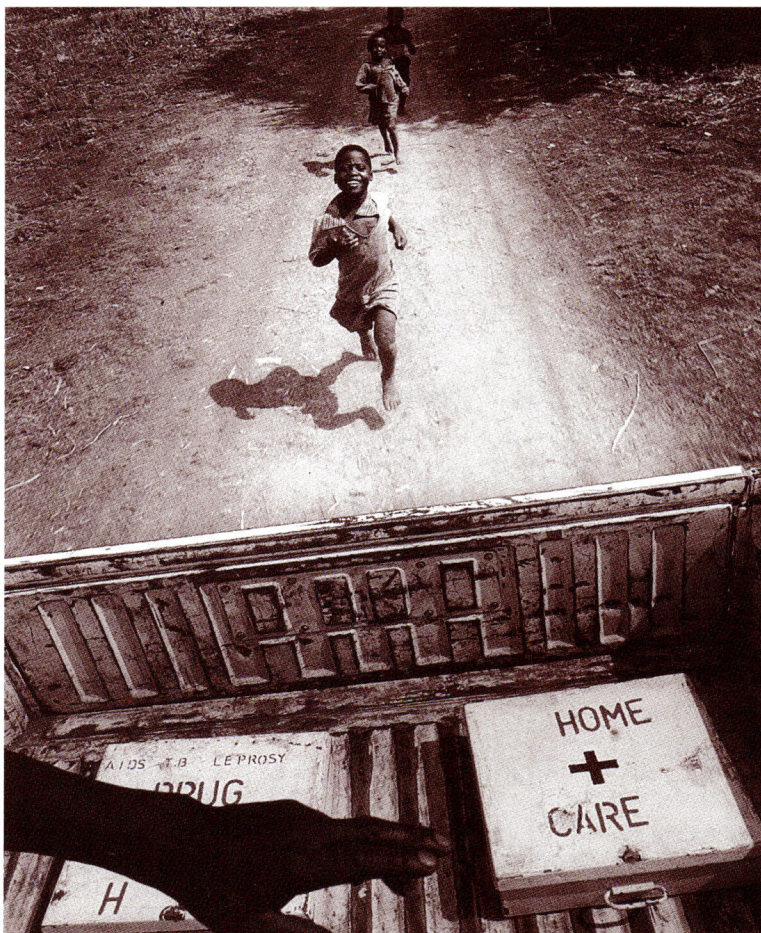

Gideon Mendel/Network

Children excitedly chase the truck delivering medicines to their village. The truck also brings health care workers from a distant hospital into this rural Zambian community where they help provide treatment.

"In Zambia it is difficult to afford aspirin. Our government spends US$ 10 per head on health per year and several hundred thousand people live with HIV/AIDS, so it is impossible to look after everyone in hospitals or hospices," says Daphetone Siame from Chikankata Hospital's AIDS Management and Training Services. "The HIV/AIDS team at our hospital decided to visit people in their own homes in order to monitor their condition and to teach their families how to care for them: it works!"

There are many benefits in caring for people at home – it can be cheaper, many patients prefer not to be in hospital, and community care can be a powerful means to break down prejudices and to educate people about HIV/AIDS.

Zambia's first home-based care programmes started in 1987, when nearly 90% of HIV/AIDS patients at the Chikankata Hospital said they would prefer to be at home. The hospital arranged for teams of health workers to visit them once a month, covering an area within an 80-km radius. In addition to delivering health care to patients, the teams counselled families and educated communities about HIV/AIDS. A key goal is to encourage acceptance of HIV/AIDS patients in the community and to stress that infection is not transmitted by ordinary household contact.

to other schemes. Very often, treatment is a logical extension of long-standing commitments to respond to HIV/AIDS in the workplace, with health education activities, condom distribution, counselling and testing, as well as long-term care and social support. In some cases, benefits extend to family members and the wider communities. However, there are two severe limitations on the contribution of the business sector. First, only a minority of businesses are implementing these enlightened policies. Second, most people who would benefit are not employed by the kind of multinational firms that can provide treatment.

The strengthening of health systems that the treatment initiative hopes to galvanize will therefore involve nongovernmental organizations and businesses, but this will not be enough. The key factor will be the leadership of governments.

## LEADERSHIP FOR CHANGE

Providing wider access to antiretroviral therapy creates a set of challenges and opportunities that will require strong government leadership and guidance, while still involving local innovation and participation. Among the essential ingredients of good leadership are the ability to mobilize institutions and individuals around common goals and give a clear sense of direction, enlisting public and political support for health actions, as well as ensuring the application of common standards. Good leadership also means facilitating communication, brokering knowledge, identifying gaps and taking steps to fill them. It means promoting partnerships where appropriate, arbitrating in conflict, actively promoting accountability, and, crucially, making sure that vulnerable groups are protected.

Four aspects of leadership are particularly relevant. The first is to define a clear *national strategic framework* for prevention, care and treatment that gives the vision and direction needed by all actors across the health system. This has to be set in the context of a broader framework for responding to threats to population health, and needs to take a long-term view. The second element is the ability to build *coalitions* and maintain stakeholders' commitment to the agreed objectives and strategies. The third is the formulation and enforcement of a *system of rules and incentives* for all providers to ensure quality care, whether in the public or the private sector. The fourth element, *oversight*, involves maintaining a strategic overview of what is happening across the health system. It also means determining whether policies are being carried out, what is on course and what is not, and responding as needed. Designing a health information system and managing a monitoring process are critical to ensuring the factual basis on which sound leadership decisions can be made.

## HEALTH INFORMATION SYSTEMS

Timely and accurate health information is the essential foundation for policy-making, and for the planning, implementation and evaluation of all health programmes. The 3 by 5 initiative needs careful and ongoing assessment of treatment requirements, programme access, coverage, quality of services and health outcomes, and operations research. Initially, health information may have to be collected as a vertical programme activity. The system will require the introduction of new technologies for patient identification and a continuous medical record, from which data can be extracted for the cohort analyses essential to the accurate measurement of treatment outcomes. Appointment systems and patient tracing are essential elements of chronic care management. The necessary investments and innovations in health information systems will assist the strengthening and reform of country health information systems towards which WHO is working, partly in the context of the Health Metrics Network *(8)*. WHO will also link the health information component to activities related to strengthening the capacity of national health research, aligning national health research production, knowledge sharing and applications, and other activities in countries.

## MONITORING 3 BY 5

A sound strategy for 3 by 5 will involve monitoring indicators such as the number of patients receiving different services, treatment adherence, quality of care and availability of drugs. It will also require monitoring indicators that assess whether the goal of strengthening the wider health system is being achieved; these indicators include overall trends in inputs, processes, outputs and outcomes.

Although much information is already being produced, some critical gaps remain: these include details of the activities of the private sector and estimates of service requirements relative to those actually delivered. Making monitoring manageable will require selectivity and creativity in the information to be collected, in the ways information flows are managed, and in the ways information is synthesized and presented.

The ability to monitor resource flows is an essential element of monitoring, evaluation and policy development. It is important to know how much is spent on health, the sources of funds, through whom they are channelled, what goods and services are purchased, and who ultimately benefits. Tracking health expenditure using the national health accounts framework is the starting point for assessing the level of domestic and international commitment to supporting health, and can be adapted to show the commitment to particular activities such as HIV/AIDS prevention and care. It is also critically important to develop ways of tracking additional external resources to make sure that they do not replace normal expenditures on health or HIV/AIDS, and that they are used efficiently and equitably. Innovative processes will be required to collect and analyse new knowledge and disseminate the findings both nationally and internationally.

## SERVICE DELIVERY

The majority of patients starting to receive antiretroviral therapy will be recruited from settings where opportunistic infections are already apparent: tuberculosis treatment services, acute medical care in outpatient departments and hospital wards, and home-based care programmes. Increasingly, patients will be identified as HIV-positive in other settings where testing is offered, such as free-standing voluntary counselling and testing centres, maternal and child health clinics where prevention of mother-to-child transmission programmes are in place, and clinics dealing with sexually transmitted infections. Patients identified at these entry points, even though asymptomatic and not eligible immediately for antiretroviral therapy, need to be inducted into a continuing review process. This will enable their opportunistic infections to be correctly diagnosed and treated. It will also ensure that they are prepared psychologically and socially for the time when they will receive treatment and that it is initiated at the right time. This continuing care might be provided in dedicated HIV clinics, in clinics specializing in tuberculosis or sexually transmitted infections, in general medical clinics, or in home care programmes. Making this continuum of services available to every community will be a tremendous challenge, and one for which all countries will need considerable assistance.

There are also geographical and institutional dimensions to the challenge of scaling up provision of antiretroviral therapy. Previously, the locations in which treatment has been provided have been predominantly urban and the facilities have been mostly hospitals. This was natural during the pilot phase, which demonstrated the feasibility of the therapy in resource-poor settings, and it remains rational to expand the service delivery network by working downwards through the hierarchy of facilities from the better-endowed to the more basic. Population coverage on the scale envisaged, however, requires a dramatic expansion in the number of service delivery points, and that inevitably means expanding into the geographical periphery of each country and district and into lower-tier facilities which lack the staff and resources of the pilot sites. This dissemination of service delivery points is also important for geographical equity of access to services. Fortunately, some pilot sites have developed services on a district-wide basis and demonstrated the feasibility of delegating tasks to mid-level health workers in primary care facilities *(9)*. The antiretroviral therapy treatment guidelines developed by WHO assume a pattern of services at district level whereby there is a central facility (hospital or major health centre) connected to a network of ambulatory care facilities by cross-referral of patients and specimens, and supportive supervision of the less skilled staff customarily found at lower-tier facilities *(10)*.

# Waiting for treatment

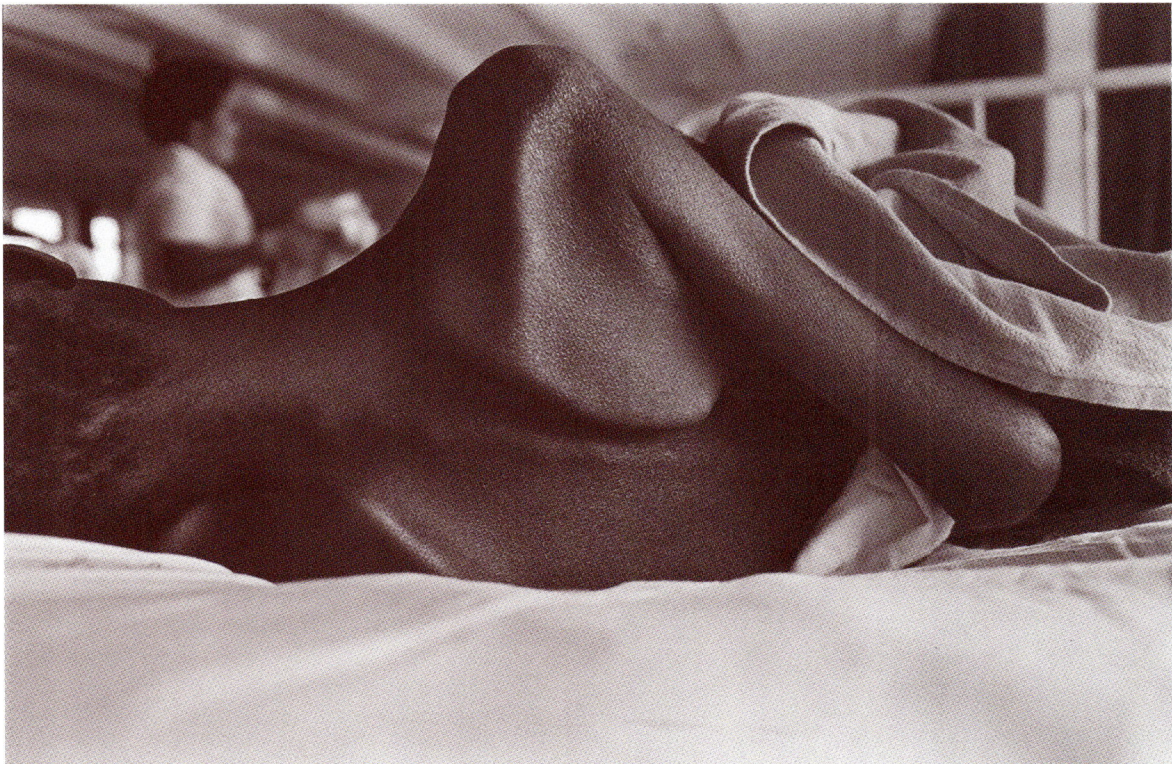

Gideon Mendel/Network

Health systems in many developing countries are as frail and vulnerable as the HIV/AIDS patients they try to help. The systems themselves are also in desperate need of treatment. As this man quietly waits for attention in hospital, chronically underfunded health services must also hope that their turn will come soon. For him, antiretroviral treatment is the answer. For health systems that are already overwhelmed, the future depends on injections of new resources.

Dissemination of service provision into primary care facilities may increase the distance to laboratories and skilled diagnosticians, but it reduces the distance (geographical and social) to the communities from which the patients come, which are themselves a crucial resource for care and treatment. Since a high level of adherence to treatment is a condition for viral load suppression, the proximity of drug re-supply and the support of community members in adherence and other tasks (as discussed in Chapter 3) are important for programme success.

## HEALTH SYSTEM RESOURCES

The capacity of health providers to deliver services is determined by the resources they can deploy. These can be divided into tangible resources such as buildings, equipment, staff and supplies, and intangible ones – the management systems that control their deployment. These are all often severely defective in high-burden countries, and will need substantial investments. It can be argued that deficiencies in human resources most severely constrain the capacity for effective service delivery.

### The human resource crisis

It is widely recognized that there now exists a health workforce crisis throughout the developing world *(11–13)*. It is characterized by a shortage and maldistribution of trained health workers caused by elevated attrition rates from, among other things, voluntary changes of occupation and emigration from poor to richer countries, a shortfall in the production of trained health workers (in part attributable to a shortage of candidates qualified by general education attainment to enter pre-service training), and a tendency to focus training efforts on the higher-level, internationally recognized cadres.

This has been a crisis in the making for several decades, and certainly existed well before the advent of HIV/AIDS, but it has been exacerbated by the epidemic *(14)*. There has been a dramatic increase in deaths within the health workforce, attributable to AIDS (see, for example, Figure 4.1). In Malawi, 44 deaths occurring in 1997–1998 among nurses represented 40% of the annual output from training; in Zambia, 185 deaths in 1999 represented 38% of the annual output from government training schools *(16)*. Absence because of ill-health has also dramatically increased. One study of laboratory workers in Malawi found that nearly half of total working time was lost to sickness and related causes. A secondary effect is increased absenteeism as health workers need time to care for sick relatives and to attend funerals.

### Systemic solutions to the workforce crisis

Human resource specialists now agree that the crisis will only yield to systemic solutions such as substantial improve-

Figure 4.1 Deaths from HIV/AIDS among health workers in Malawi, 1990–2000

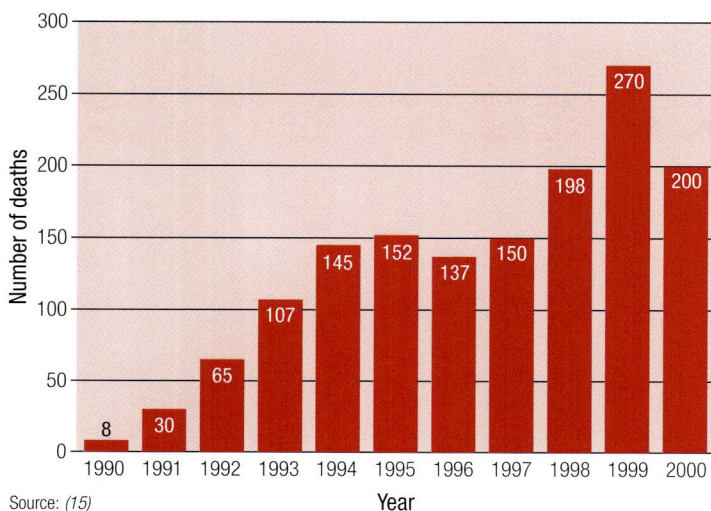

Source: *(15)*

ment in the basic package of pay and benefits, an expansion in the volume of pre-service training, decentralization of some aspects of personnel management, a programme of management training focused on supportive supervision, and adequate protection of the workforce against the risk of occupational exposure to HIV infection *(17–19)*.

Systemic solutions need to link improved rewards to improved productivity. One way to do this is to make payment conditional on the meeting of performance criteria. A good example is Médecins Sans Frontières' incentive payment scheme in Thyolo District, Malawi. The incentives are given to all health workers, not just those directly involved in activities supported by Médecins Sans Frontières; payment of the incentives is discretionary and dependent on performance criteria; and the scheme is administered by local managers, thus empowering their supervision of the workforce (see Box 4.2). This isolated example illustrates reform principles of system-wide relevance.

Given the prevailing shortages, massive expansion of human resources is needed to permit scale-up of antiretroviral therapy without excessive damage to existing programmes. This implies a large number of actions including: emergency recruitment, in some cases from abroad; relaxing fiscal constraints related to public sector hiring; introducing new cadres; increasing community input; initiating treatment-focused in-service training on a large scale; and expanding pre-service training. Although the benefits of expanded pre-service training will inevitably accrue outside the short timescale of 3 by 5, delay in tackling this crucial bottleneck will impose insuperable obstacles on efforts to maintain the momentum of expanded access.

The experience of the pilot sites delivering antiretroviral therapy provides only limited guidance for the optimum staffing of future services, since they have generally been intensive in their use of human resources. New patterns of service delivery and staffing, such as those recommended by WHO *(20)*, need to be implemented; they should entail less frequent patient contact with the provider system, rely less on skilled labour inputs, and optimize the use of inputs other than those from the formal delivery system. These new patterns imply maximum delegation of tasks within the formal health care team, and maximum involvement of community resources. On the basis of standardized treatment guidelines, competency-based training (ensuring better alignment between training and practice), adequate supervision mechanisms, and improved management systems would contribute to productivity gains. Chapter 3

## Box 4.2  Incentives to health workers in Malawi

In Malawi, Médecins Sans Frontières is working in partnership with the Thyolo District Health Office to control tuberculosis and reduce the transmission of HIV; they also provide medical care, treatment, nutritional and social support for people living with HIV/AIDS, tuberculosis or both, and respond to nutritional or medical emergencies.

As part of this collaboration, Médecins Sans Frontières has sought innovative ways of tackling human resource constraints, focusing specifically on reducing staff attrition rates within the district and improving staff management, motivation and performance.

This work includes:

- ensuring that infection control measures and materials are in place;
- using non-clinical staff to conduct activities such as health promotion and voluntary counselling and testing;
- extending its workplace policy on antiretroviral therapy to all district health staff;
- piloting a performance-related incentive to all district health staff;
- using this incentive as a mechanism to encourage and supervise staff.

Incentive payments range from US$ 6 to US$ 22 per month, adding roughly 10% to basic government salaries. They are dependent on a monthly review of performance carried out jointly by the district health management team and Médecins Sans Frontières programme managers, using a common evaluation checklist that assesses working hours, discipline, accuracy in carrying out tasks, management of resources (equipment, medicines, supplies, food) and cleanliness. Médecins Sans Frontières proposes that these innovations be carefully evaluated and considered for adoption at the national level.

described how volunteers drawn from people living with HIV/AIDS, who may already be receiving antiretroviral therapy, constitute a resource that can be deployed to good effect.

Different issues arise in the settings of middle-income countries and countries in transition, where resources are less severely constrained, the numbers of trained health workers are generally higher, and the basic capacities of health facilities are more secure. The emphasis therefore lies on ensuring, through appropriate collective financing mechanisms, universal entitlements to care that include the most vulnerable and stigmatized populations. Subsidiary concerns include reducing the cost of treatment regimes, establishing reliable diagnostic and drug distribution networks, and improving surveillance *(21)*. Box 4.3 describes a remarkable success story.

## FINANCING ISSUES

There are two interrelated levels at which the financing of HIV/AIDS interventions, including delivery of antiretroviral therapy, needs to be considered. The first, which has received the most attention, is the international division of responsibility between recipient countries and donors. The second level refers to the methods used within countries to finance provision of services.

One of the key messages of this report is that success in containing and reversing the HIV/AIDS pandemic is contingent on a massive increase in resource transfers from rich to poor countries. The 3 by 5 initiative cannot be implemented in isolation from a regeneration of health systems; this cannot be financed from the slender resources available to the poorest countries. It has been estimated that US$ 35–40 per capita per annum is needed to finance a minimum health service package including antiretroviral therapy, but actual levels of expenditure fall far short of this *(2)*. The average amount spent, per capita, on health services in low-income countries was US$ 23 in 2001, of which only US$ 6 was public spending.

## Box 4.3  Universal access to antiretroviral therapy in Brazil

Brazil is the first developing country to have implemented a universal antiretroviral distribution programme. Initiated in the early 1990s, by 2003 the programme was providing free antiretroviral medication to about 125 000 patients. The programme is credited with a dramatic reversal in the previously rising trend of AIDS mortality, averting 90 000 deaths and 358 000 AIDS-related hospital admissions.

Brazil has a population of approximately 175 million. With an adult HIV prevalence rate of 0.7% and a per capita income of US$ 4350, the challenge presented by HIV/AIDS may appear to be more manageable than in countries with higher disease burdens and lower incomes. However, this is a result of the national response: in 1990, Brazil had one of the highest reported numbers of infected individuals in the world, and the World Bank projected that 1.2 million people would become infected by 2000. The current UNAIDS estimate is that approximately 600 000 people are living with HIV/AIDS, suggesting that the Brazilian response has succeeded in halving the impact of the epidemic.

This success is attributed to a concerted and early government response, the foundations for which were laid by political and professional changes in the 1980s, strong and effective participation of civil society, multisectoral mobilization, a balance between prevention and treatment, and systematic advocacy of human rights in all strategies and actions. In particular, guidelines for prevention policies have emphasized the need to direct attention to more vulnerable populations, such as men who have sex with men, injecting drug users and commercial sex workers; to ensure access to prevention supplies, especially condoms, syringes and needles; and to introduce preventive actions in health care services. Condom use increased tenfold between 1986 and 1999, while needle and syringe exchange programmes significantly lowered HIV prevalence rates among injecting drug users.

A number of features appear to be critical to the provision of universal access to antiretroviral therapy. Most important in Brazil was the government's acceptance of responsibility in a 1996 presidential decree that guaranteed all patients free access to HIV/AIDS medications. The cost of treatment was reduced by manufacturing antiretroviral drugs domestically, and by aggressive price negotiation with international pharmaceutical companies, using the threat of compulsory licensing. A drugs logistic system supplying 450 outlets was developed, and laboratory capacity was established to monitor viral load, CD4 counts and drug resistance. Services are delivered through a network of more than 1000 public care and testing services, financed by federal, state and municipal governments *(22)*.

Even supposing that the poorest countries were able to make the greatly increased domestic fiscal effort to raise an additional 1–2% of gross national product (GNP) for health – relative to the average of 14% for all public expenditures – the per capita amounts generated would still be inadequate. With per capita incomes below US$ 300 per annum, an additional 1% of GNP raised for public health expenditure still produces less than US$ 3 per capita, leaving a substantial gap between resources required and those available. The shortfall can be made good only by transfers from the rich world. One estimate of the amount required is US$ 22 billion annually by 2007 *(1)*, against which current transfers, though supplemented by innovative mechanisms (see Box 4.4), remain inadequate.

This response would be attended by four important considerations:

- First is the need for ongoing work to maintain and enhance the recent substantial increases in donor assistance for HIV/AIDS. This will require the involvement of the donor community in broad planning and monitoring at the international level.
- Second, poor countries themselves need reassurance that that the aid flows linked to HIV/AIDS will not experience the volatility that has been known in some other areas in the past.
- Third, some donor funds need to be available to repair deficiencies in basic system capacity and, above all, in the vital areas of staff salaries and pre-service training. If an expansion of aid is to be constructively used to build basic system capacities, it will have to be in more flexible forms that allow a jointly agreed programme of work to be undertaken. There has been some limited experience with the sector-wide approach, with notable success in Uganda and the United Republic of

## Box 4.4  New international sources of finance

Billions of dollars of additional resource transfers from rich to poor countries are needed annually to support the 3 by 5 initiative and its associated investments in prevention, care and health systems strengthening. Some of this money will flow through long-established bilateral and multilateral channels, but increasing sums are expected to be channelled through newly established mechanisms. Prominent among these are the Global Fund to Fight AIDS, Tuberculosis and Malaria, the World Bank's Multi-Country HIV/AIDS Program, the President's Emergency Plan for AIDS Relief, and the contributions of private foundations such as the Bill and Melinda Gates Foundation and the William J. Clinton Foundation.

So far the Global Fund has received pledges totalling US$ 4.8 billion and has committed expenditure of US$ 2.1 billion as a result of applications received in the first three rounds (of which 60% has been allocated for combating HIV/AIDS). It had disbursed US$ 178 million by the end of November 2003, its first year of expenditure. The Global Fund anticipates that commitments in relation to the first three rounds of applications will reach US$ 2.5

billion by the end of 2004 and over US$ 3.5 billion by the end of 2005, while disbursements (which necessarily lag behind commitments) will reach US$ 1 billion by the end of 2004 and US$ 2 billion by the end of 2005.

The President's Emergency Plan for AIDS Relief, announced in the 2003 State of the Union address, committed the USA to spending US$ 15 billion to fight the HIV/AIDS pandemic over the following five years. Of this total, nearly US$ 10 billion represents new commitments, to be disbursed through a number of federal government agencies, of which the largest are USAID and the Department of Health and Human Services, which oversees the Centers for Disease Control and Prevention and the National Institutes of Health. Through bilateral and multilateral channels, the US government plans to spend US$ 2 billion on HIV/AIDS in the year to June 2004, and expenditure will clearly rise in the future. Some funding from the President's Emergency Plan will be disbursed through the Global Fund, to which US$ 1.6 billion has been pledged, with the possibility of more to come if the pledge is matched by other donors' contributions.

The World Bank committed approximately US$ 2 billion to HIV/AIDS programmes over the period 1988–2003. Most of this expenditure has been in the form of concessional loans. UNAIDS estimated the grant component of these loans to have reached US$ 75 million annually by 2002.

Private foundations have begun to make significant contributions, some via the Global Fund and some acting in broad partnership within recipient countries. The Bill and Melinda Gates Foundation, in partnership with the pharmaceutical Merck Company Foundation and the Government of Botswana, established the US$ 100 million African Comprehensive HIV/AIDS Partnership, which has supported a broad range of prevention and care interventions and has helped fund the largest public sector antiretroviral therapy programme in Africa. The William J. Clinton Foundation has developed programmes in several African and Caribbean countries, leveraging the contributions of other partners and successfully brokering access to cheaper generic medicines.

Tanzania *(23)*, and across all development areas with poverty reduction strategy implementation using the proceeds of debt relief, with positive results in Ghana, Mozambique and Uganda *(24)*.

■ Fourth, it must be recognized that there is a potential problem with a massive increase in external aid threatening to produce adverse effects on macroeconomic stability and development by inducing domestic inflation and appreciation of the exchange rate.

The potential adverse effects may be transitory and more than offset by the effective use of aid to improve national productivity.

There is an obvious link between the international and domestic financing of health programmes. Smaller contributions from external sources mean that poor countries have to provide more funding from their own resources, either through collective mechanisms such as taxation or insurance, or individually out of pocket. South Africa receives very little external aid for its health sector, but it has recently seen some important changes in its domestic financing arrangements for antiretroviral therapy. In November 2003, the government committed itself to spending more than US$ 1.73 billion over three years to combat HIV/AIDS, more than tripling the amount spent during the preceding three years. Of this, US$ 270 million will be set aside for antiretroviral drugs. These funds will be insufficient, however, to cover all people who need medication, and multiple funding sources will be required to provide ongoing treatment.

In low-income developing countries, which generally do not have extensive insurance mechanisms, most personal health services are financed by a mix of taxation and user fees in the public sector. With the exceptions of Botswana and Brazil (both middle-income countries which have decided to meet the cost from public sources), developing country governments have not been greatly involved in financing antiretroviral therapy, probably because of its high unit cost. Private providers have been financing antiretroviral therapy through user fees for some time; international nongovernmental organizations and research-funded sites have received substantial external funds and have been able to provide either free or heavily subsidized treatment. Private-sector employers have provided free access to antiretroviral therapy, either directly through occupational health services or indirectly through private insurance intermediaries. A mixture of public and private financing is desirable, but only if it ensures equal access.

## Box 4.5  Health financing reform in Kenya

Until recently, patients in Kenya paid fees at the point of treatment for government-provided health services, which worsened the plight of poor people. A situation in which private providers served all sections of the community on a fee-for-service basis led to out-of-pocket payments reaching 75% of total health expenditures. Recently, however, social health insurance reforms have been proposed, aiming at adequate, accessible and affordable health services, including antiretroviral treatment. The draft law was scheduled to be submitted to parliament in early 2004.

The new insurance system will be funded by prepaid contributions from active and retired workers, enterprises and the self-employed, with government subsidies to enable participation by the poor. These contributions constitute the revenue of a new National Social Health Insurance Fund. When insured members seek treatment, they will no longer have to pay fees at the time and point of treatment. Health facilities will be paid by the Fund for the health services they provide to insured patients. Both outpatient and inpatient health services will be part of the insurance benefit package.

A series of financial projections for the period 2004–2008 have been undertaken to determine whether treatment costs for HIV/AIDS might overly burden the proposed health insurance system. It is projected that the number of patients treated will rise from 108 000 in 2004 to 186 000 in 2008. For the poorest Kenyans, this treatment would be paid for via government subsidies to the National Social Health Insurance Fund, while the better off would pay half of the cost. The cost of antiretroviral drugs will occupy an increasing share of the Fund's revenues: from 5.4% in 2004 to 13.4% in 2008. It has been determined that up to 2007, inclusion of treatment in the benefit package is financially feasible. But from 2008 onwards the government subsidies would have to be revised upwards in order to secure financial equilibrium in the Fund.

Thus, scaling up the provision of antiretroviral therapy with greater public provider involvement presents a considerable challenge to governments.

Some governments are not confident that the costs will be adequately met by donors, they do not expect to be able to afford free provision from domestic resources (even with the dramatically reduced drug prices now in prospect), and do not see a basis for discrimination between antiretroviral therapy and other life-saving treatments for which user fees are charged. It is the stated intention of some governments to apply to antiretroviral therapy the standard regime of partial cost recovery (that is, user fees meet some but not all costs of service provision, the balance being borne by taxation) in public facilities. Almost all governments that operate user fees have some system of fee waivers which, in theory at least, allows very poor people to be exempt from payment.

In other quarters, there is an expectation that antiretroviral therapy will be provided free or at only nominal cost to all who need it, financed by external aid or other solidarity mechanisms. Inability to pay should not be a barrier to access. There is now evidence that out-of-pocket payment has undermined adherence to treatment and increased the risk of drug resistance. There are precedents for free treatment, for example for tuberculosis, even in countries which otherwise charge user fees in public facilities.

In most countries a mixed regime in financing antiretroviral therapy will probably continue, the argument being that people who are able to pay should do so and free treatment should be reserved for when payment could undermine access and adherence to treatment. This is a critical matter, because out-of-pocket payments for health already result in a substantial number of households facing financial catastrophe and poverty in the countries most affected by HIV/AIDS. The attention given to 3 by 5 may drive health financing reforms designed to improve access to all health services for the poor, an endeavour actively supported by WHO. An example of such reform is the proposal to develop a social health insurance scheme in Kenya (see Box 4.5).

## MEETING THE CHALLENGE: HOPE FOR THE FUTURE

The 3 by 5 initiative presents a tremendous challenge to the health systems of countries with a high burden of HIV/AIDS, given the magnitude and urgency of the changes that will be initiated against a background of chronic incapacity and under-performance. An inspiring vision exists, based on the work of the treatment pioneers, of how health service and community resources can be combined in comprehensive prevention, treatment and care programmes, even in resource-poor settings. It must be hoped that this inspiration will reignite the determination of governments and people all over the world to invest sufficiently in health systems so that they can reverse the course of the HIV/AIDS epidemic. By doing so, strengthened health systems will gain the capacity to confront successfully the ancient enemy of infectious disease and the growing burden of chronic diseases.

The next chapter looks beyond 2005 and considers how advances in many areas of research, together with new approaches to gathering and sharing information, can assist international efforts in the prevention, treatment and control of HIV/AIDS and also contribute to building stronger health systems.

## References

1. WHO/UNAIDS. *Treating 3 million by 2005: making it happen. The WHO strategy.* Geneva, World Health Organization, 2003.
2. *Macroeconomics and health: investing in health for economic development. Report of the Commission on Macroeconomics and Health.* Geneva, World Health Organization, 2001.
3. *Severe acute respiratory syndrome (SARS).* Geneva, World Health Organization, 2003 (http://www.who.int/csr/sars/en, accessed 16 February 2004).
4. Mogedal S, Stenson B. *Disease eradication: friend or foe to the health system?* Geneva, World Health Organization, 2000 (WHO/V&B/00.28; http://www.who.int/vaccines-documents/DocsPDF00/www552.pdf, accessed 16 February 2004).
5. Brown RG. Kenyan faith-based initiative AIDS project, Nazareth Hospital, Limuru, Kenya. 2003 (unpublished manuscript).
6. Orrell C, Bangsberg DR, Badri M, Wood R. Adherence is not a barrier to successful antiretroviral therapy in South Africa. *AIDS*, 2003, 17:1369–1375.
7. Bekker LG, Orrell C, Reader L, Matoti K, Cohen K, Martell R et al. Antiretroviral therapy in a community clinic – early lessons from a pilot project. *South African Medical Journal*, 2003, 93:458–462.
8. *Health Metrics Network: an update after 50 days.* Geneva, World Health Organization, 2003 (http://www.who.int/mip/2003/other_documents/en/health_metrics-boerma.pdf, accessed 16 February 2004).
9. *Projet: Malawi.* Luxembourg, Médecins Sans Frontières, 2003 (http://www.msf.lu/projets/malawi [in French], accessed 16 February 2004).
10. *Antiretroviral treatment (ART) guidelines and technical and operational recommendations for ART.* Geneva, World Health Organization (http://www.who.int/3by5/publications/briefs/arv_guidelines/en, accessed 16 February 2004).
11. *The world health report 2003 – Shaping the future.* Geneva, World Health Organization, 2003.
12. *The health sector human resource crisis in Africa.* Washington, DC, United States Agency for International Development, 2003.
13. Liese B, Blanchet N, Dussault G. *The human resource crisis in health services in sub-Saharan Africa.* Washington, DC, World Bank, 2003.
14. Tawfik L, Kinoti SN. *The impact of HIV/AIDS on the health sector in sub-Saharan Africa: the issue of human resources.* Washington, DC, Academy for Educational Development, 2001.
15. Government of Malawi/UNDP. *The impact of HIV/AIDS on human resources in the Malawi public sector.* New York, United Nations Development Programme, 2002.
16. Aitken J-M, Kemp J. *HIV/AIDS, equity and health sector personnel in southern Africa.* Harare, Regional Network for Equity in Health in Southern Africa, 2003 (Equinet Discussion Paper No. 12).
17. Ferrinho P, Dal Poz M, eds. *Towards a global health workforce strategy.* Antwerp, ITG Press, 2003.
18. Bhattarai MD. Proper HIV/AIDS care not possible without basic safety in health set-up. *Bulletin of the World Health Organization*, 2002, 80:333.
19. *Improving health workforce performance.* Geneva, World Health Organization, 2003 (WHO/World Bank High Level Forum on the Health Millennium Development Goals, Issue Paper No.4).
20. *Scaling up antiretroviral therapy in resource-limited settings: guidelines for a public health approach.* Geneva, World Health Organization, 2003 (Department of HIV/AIDS, 2003 revision).

21. *Scaling up health systems to respond to the challenge of HIV/AIDS in Latin America and the Caribbean.* Washington, DC, Pan American Health Organization, 2003.
22. Teixeira PR, Vitoria MA, Barcarolo J. The Brazilian experience in providing universal access to antiretroviral therapy. In: Moatti JP, Coriat B, Souteyrand Y, Barnett T, Dumoulin J, Flori YA, eds. *Economics of AIDS and access to HIV/AIDS care in developing countries. Issues and challenges.* Paris, Agence Nationale de Recherches sur le Sida, 2003.
23. *Harmonization and MDGs: a perspective from Tanzania and Uganda.* Geneva, World Health Organization, 2003 (WHO/World Bank High Level Forum on the Health Millennium Development Goals, Case study).
24. *Poverty reduction strategy papers – progress in implementation.* Washington, DC, International Monetary Fund, 2000 (http://www.imf.org/external/np/prsp/2000/prsp.htm, accessed 16 February 2004).

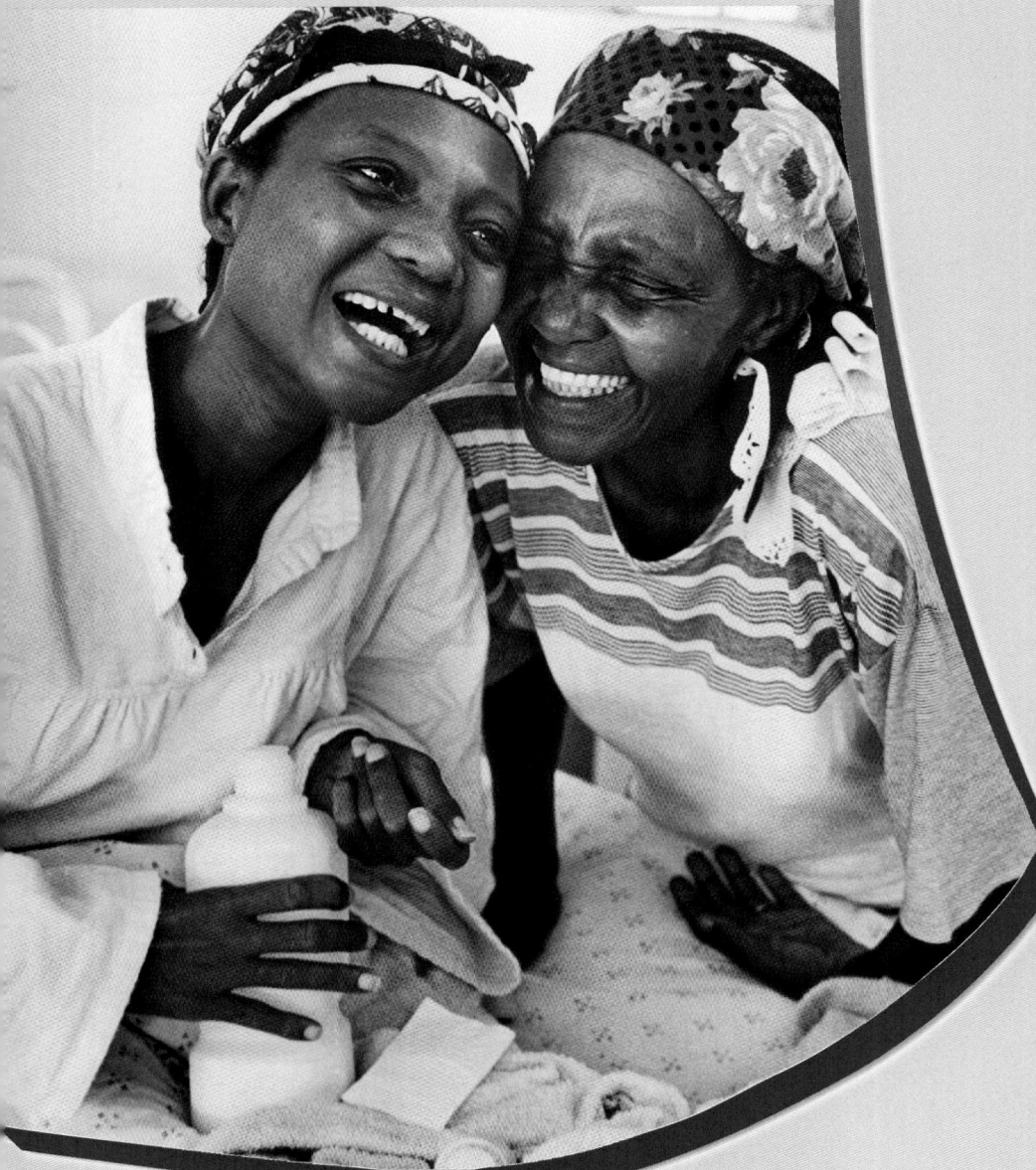

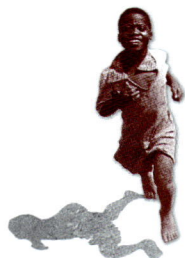

chapter five
# sharing
# research & knowledge

**Harnessing the power of research to achieve treatment targets and to build health systems that respond to the broad array of complex health issues requires an innovative approach to gathering and sharing information. Existing, classic methods of research and dissemination of new knowledge – while still necessary – will not be sufficient to achieve these goals. In the short term, new methods of assessing the performance of treatment programmes are essential. So, too, is the rapid sharing of information in order for countries to benefit from the most recent and most relevant experience elsewhere and adapt it to local circumstances.**

The HIV/AIDS treatment initiative is generating many urgent new research questions for which answers must be found quickly and communicated without delay. The fast progress that is simultaneously occurring in information and knowledge technologies will help. Innovative routes are already beginning to overtake and bypass standard research publishing processes and other conventional forms of knowledge sharing.

Traditional notions of research and publication are insufficient to bridge the wide gap between current knowledge and its successful application. A new approach is required which recognizes that useful knowledge can expand beyond formal research designs and can be quickly shared and applied through social networks and other channels, rather than simply through traditional publication methods. These applications of knowledge management in the public health sector are relatively new, but early efforts show promise [1].

A modern approach to knowledge management strengthens existing information and research networks through the Internet and other means of communication, and builds vibrant new networks that allow the rapid sharing of knowledge and practical experience at the front line – among clinicians, researchers, health workers and others. Thus, the people most closely involved in achieving wider access to antiretroviral therapy can learn from each other's successes – and also from their failures – especially if this takes place in an atmosphere of transparency.

Both successes and failures have characterized much of the history of HIV/AIDS research in all its forms. Since scientists first identified the human immunodeficiency virus (HIV) as the cause of AIDS in 1983, many remarkable research achievements, spanning the understanding, treatment and prevention of the disease, have benefited many millions of people. Twenty years ago no effective treatment was known; today a range of antiretroviral drugs exists – treatments that dramatically improve patients' quality and length of life, though they are still reaching only a tiny fraction of those who need them. Meanwhile, despite high hopes 20 years ago for an HIV vaccine, the world is still waiting. Notwithstanding significant advances, it will be several years at least before a safe and effective vaccine becomes widely available.

The development, licensing and delivery of such a vaccine remains the greatest hope for the eventual control of HIV/AIDS, and realizing this hope depends on scientific research. In examining the continuing quest for a vaccine, this chapter reviews research into other important areas of HIV/AIDS prevention, treatment and care. Even while awaiting effective vaccines, the moral obligation is unambiguous: to scale up activities to treat and care for people living with HIV/AIDS – whoever they are and wherever they live – and to contain the spread of the disease. Such ethically sound actions require new tools that can be produced only by research of the highest quality, research which must extend far beyond the laboratory to include multidisciplinary operational and health policy research.

HIV/AIDS researchers face four broad categories of challenge, all crucial to present and future success:

- Prevention research – slowing down the growth and geographical expansion of the epidemic: a challenge for epidemiology and sociobehavioural aspects of prevention.
- Vaccine research – designing a safe and effective preventive vaccine: the best hope for the long-term prevention and control of HIV/AIDS.
- Treatment research – generating new antiretroviral drugs and designing new therapeutic strategies that would be active on "wild" and resistant strains of viruses, be easy to take and better tolerated than currently available drugs: a challenge for basic and clinical research.
- Delivery system research (operational research) – making care and antiretroviral treatment available to all those who need it worldwide: a multidisciplinary undertaking. This is the greatest research challenge because it must deliver results on the ground, often more complicated than the relatively straightforward task of scientific discovery. Furthermore, this aspect of research has, until now, been largely neglected by both researchers and funding organizations. Here, too, a knowledge management framework may prove useful.

## PREVENTION RESEARCH

### Linking prevention and access to treatment

As efforts to provide treatment are scaled up, concerns have been voiced regarding its potential impact on preventive behaviours. The availability of treatment, some fear, may lower people's perception of risk and hence lead to lower vigilance; in contrast, others argue that the strengthening of health-related interventions will encourage testing and counselling, and that the knowledge of HIV status may increase protective behaviour. Studies of people living with HIV in developing countries indicate that treatment is, indeed, associated with increased sexual activity but, at the same time, it is associated with more consistent condom use. In developed countries, an increase in risky behaviour was documented among certain population groups after the introduction of effective antiretroviral therapy, without clear evidence of why this happens *(2, 3)*. The epidemiological data are only suggestive, and trends need to be documented across settings, over time, and among key subpopulations, in particular in people living with HIV/AIDS and other highly exposed groups.

Treatment may directly contribute to prevention of new infections to the extent that lowering of viral load decreases the probability of sexual transmission. Decreased infectiousness is likely to be counterbalanced by increases in the life expectancy of patients. Research must contribute to the adaptation of interventions in order to ensure the sustainability of prevention over the long term *(4, 5)*.

More generally, better evidence is needed on how preventive behaviours can be promoted across age groups, sexes, social strata and different categories of serological status, especially in the context of scaling up access to treatment. The mechanisms linking risk perceptions to behavioural change are shaped by contextual variables and are situation-specific and partner-specific *(6)*. Better evidence is also needed on the extent to which the findings from developed countries are valid for developing countries. There are also indications that gender influences the selection of strategies to reduce risk *(7)*. It is important to investigate whether such differences in perceived risks and protection represent a general gendered pattern.

# Treatment and care for children with HIV

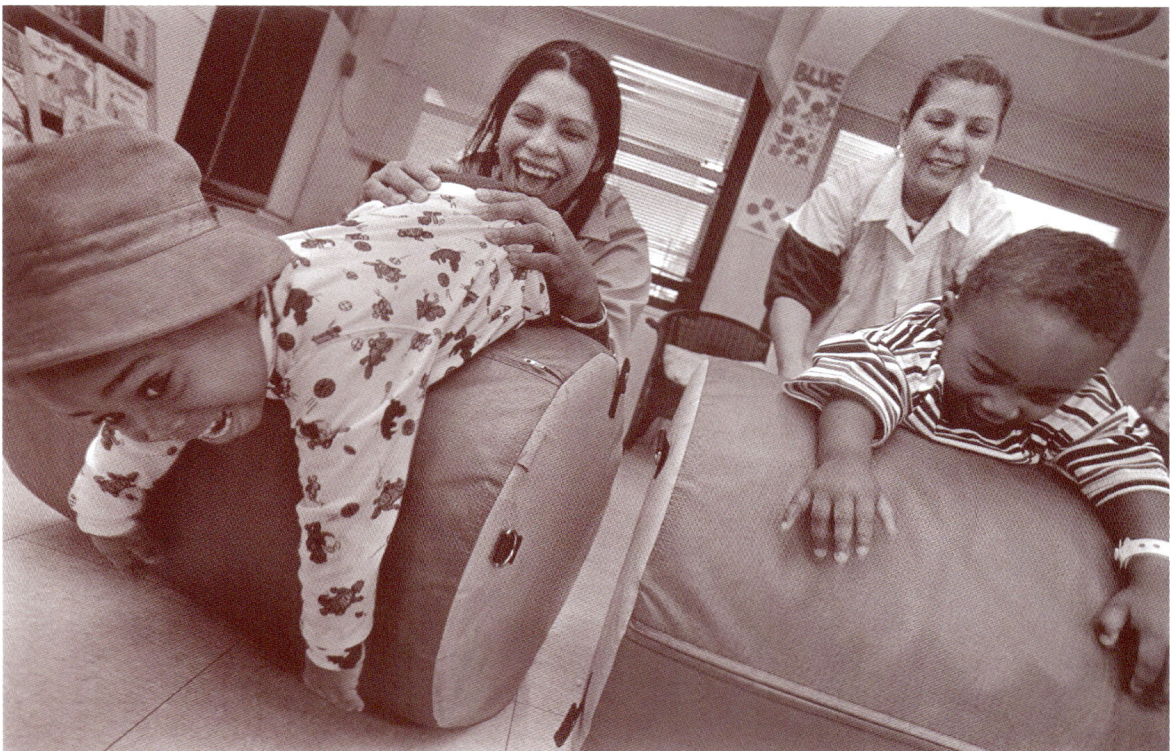

*Eugene Richards/Network*

Young HIV-positive children at the Incarnation Children's Center, New York, USA, play with their carers. The Center is funded to conduct clinical trials of new treatment options, including antiretroviral therapy.

Many children with HIV have lost a parent to the disease. They are likely to have behavioural and emotional difficulties, which can complicate their treatment as they grow older.

Microlevel studies indicate that medical information and public health recommendations are not automatically accepted by the general public and that people interpret professional advice in the light of local notions and past experience with health care *(8)*. Investigations of beliefs and practices that are contrary to public health recommendations can suggest ways to communicate better with the public. The availability of effective treatments should contribute to furthering confidence in medicine and public health.

## Preventing transmission from mother to child

Among the issues that urgently require further research are better methods of ensuring the prevention of HIV transmission from mother to child, particularly in developing countries and in the postnatal period. Every year, an estimated 700 000 children become infected with HIV. The overwhelming majority acquire the virus through mother-to-child transmission, which can occur either during pregnancy and delivery or postnatally during breastfeeding. In the absence of any intervention, rates of this form of transmission can vary from 15% to 30% without breastfeeding, and reach as high as 45% with prolonged breastfeeding *(9)*. Transmission during the peripartum period accounts for one-third to two-thirds of overall numbers infected, depending on whether breastfeeding transmission occurs or not, and this period has therefore become a focus of prevention efforts.

Transmission of HIV from mother to child can be prevented almost entirely by antiretroviral drug prophylaxis (usually now given in combinations), elective caesarean section before onset of labour and rupture of membranes, and refraining from breastfeeding *(10, 11)*. In resource-poor countries, however, elective caesarean section is not a safe option, and refraining from breastfeeding is often not feasible or acceptable. In Africa, no more than 5% of HIV-infected women and neonates who could benefit from interventions are receiving them.

Antiretrovirals, either alone or in combinations of two or three drugs, have been shown to be highly effective in reducing mother-to-child transmission of HIV. Evidence of the efficacy of antiretroviral prophylaxis from Africa, Europe, Thailand and the USA has been demonstrated for short-course drug regimens. The substantial efficacy of triple combinations has been shown in observational studies in industrialized countries *(10, 11)*, where rates of transmission are now below 2% in the absence of breastfeeding. There is an urgent need for evidence from breastfeeding mothers in sub-Saharan Africa, one of the most affected populations. Short-term safety and tolerance of the prophylactic regimens have been demonstrated in all the controlled clinical trials on mother-to-child transmission *(12)*. Further studies of these issues are required, especially on the long-term implications of potential antiretroviral resistance for HIV-infected mothers and their children.

Preventive interventions with antiretrovirals have not yet been successfully implemented on the scale required *(13)*. Even where antiretroviral treatment is applied peripartum, infants remain at substantial risk of acquiring infection in the breastfeeding period. These facts also require investigation; they demonstrate once again the need to strengthen health systems, while integrating HIV/AIDS interventions with reproductive and maternal and child health services.

## Protecting women with microbicides

Protecting women against HIV infection is another important area for researchers. Microbicides are anti-infective products such as gels, creams, impregnated sponges and similar devices that women apply before sexual intercourse to prevent HIV transmission and other sexual infections. Unlike the condom, their use is controlled by the woman and they will not necessarily be contraceptive. Attempts are also being made to incorporate microbicides into silicone intravaginal rings that are left in the vagina for several weeks to ensure contraception, with sustained release of the agent providing continuous protection against infection.

Microbicides could make a very substantial difference by widening people's choice of protective interventions. To achieve high levels of use will require a continuing education process aimed at women as well as health policy officials and providers. Epidemiological modelling based on data from over 70 low-income countries suggests that even a partially effective microbicide is likely to have a significant impact on the epidemic: a product that is only 60% effective in protecting against HIV could avert 2.5 million new infections over a three-year period, even if it is used in only 50% of sex acts not protected by condoms, and assuming it is used by only 20% of people easily reached by existing health services *(14)*. However, the microbicide concept has only recently received sufficient support to allow progress to be made. Pharmaceutical companies have not so far regarded microbicides as providing economic incentives for substantial investment, though the Bill and Melinda Gates Foundation is now giving serious consideration to this matter.

## VACCINE RESEARCH

Although advances have been made in both prevention and treatment, the best hope for prevention and control of HIV/AIDS lies in the development, licensing and delivery of a safe and effective preventive vaccine.

The existence of globally diverse strains of HIV remains one of the greatest obstacles to HIV vaccine development. Attempts to design immunogens capable of eliciting effective neutralizing antibodies against those strains have been unsuccessful. In the absence of such immunogens, the main focus has been on developing vaccines to elicit cell-mediated immunity against HIV. This type of vaccine could suppress viral load, slow the progression of disease, and potentially blunt transmission *(15)*.

The design of improved next-generation candidate HIV vaccines faces many scientific challenges. The mechanisms for protective immunity are unknown, as are the necessary antigens. Despite the failure of one of the most hopeful candidates in recent efficacy trials, however, it is now clear that circulating HIV strains can in fact be neutralized. Another challenge is the extensive genetic diversity of HIV, suggesting that successful vaccines may need to contain cocktails of antigens from across different clades of the virus. Recent clinical data on some vaccines currently in clinical trials have been encouraging, but whether the responses elicited by the vaccines correlate with clinical protection awaits human efficacy trials.

The development of an HIV vaccine faces hurdles of manufacturing, clinical trials, regulation and delivery. These aspects will need to be tackled to ensure that safe and effective HIV vaccines are licensed and delivered as quickly as possible. The development of vaccines is hampered by the limited capacity for efficacy trials, particularly in the developing world. There is also limited regulatory capacity to facilitate the testing and eventual licensure of successfully developed HIV vaccines.

The next five years will probably see the first results from efficacy trials testing the concept of vaccines that aim to suppress viral load, slow disease and potentially blunt transmission of HIV. Several new candidates are expected to be evaluated in clinical trials for safety and immunogenicity. It is likely, however, that to achieve significant improvements in HIV vaccine design and improve the prospects for success, solutions to the major scientific questions will need to be found. As a result, the major stakeholders in HIV vaccine development have recently come together to propose a "global enterprise" to accelerate HIV vaccine development *(16)*. Achievement of this vision will probably require significantly greater resources. The International AIDS Vaccine Initiative recently found that worldwide expenditure for research on HIV vaccines was, in 2001, between US$ 500 million and US$ 600 million, which represented only 10% of the expenditure for research in other areas of HIV/AIDS. Creative strategies to enhance coordination and collaboration among the many stakeholders are also required.

## TREATMENT RESEARCH

A cornerstone of efforts to reach universal access targets is sustained dedication to basic research and to the understanding of AIDS pathogenesis, in order for new drugs, novel therapeutic strategies and vaccines to be designed and developed.

The availability of potent combinations of antiretroviral drugs in the developed world has resulted in a steep decline in HIV-associated morbidity and mortality. Death rates from AIDS fell by 80% over the four years following the launch of highly active antiretroviral therapies in Europe and North America. Following their more widespread introduction in the second half of the 1990s, it also became clear that issues relating to adherence, toxicities, immunological and virological failure of treatment, and occurrence of resistance all needed to be tackled.

### Sustaining long-term adherence

Effective treatment with antiretroviral drugs requires long-term adherence. From an operational research point of view, monitoring the uptake of treatment involves: defining optimal measures of adherence which can be used in resource-poor countries; assessing the validity of self-reports, compared with other methods such as pharmacy records or electronic monitoring systems; and identifying ways to encourage more accurate reporting by patients.

Evidence shows that the variables with the strongest effect on adherence are treatment-related. These include the complexity of the regimen, side-effects, the "battle fatigue" that results from long-term use, and patients' attempts to remedy these problems by modifying the dosage or administration of drugs. Misperceptions and lack of trust regarding the medication's effectiveness further compound these problems. Women face unique obstacles related to child care, lack of partner support, and the attitudes of peers and family members. Among the social variables that are found to affect adherence, stigma and fear of disclosure have the strongest effects *(17)*. In addition, costs matter: copayment is detrimental to long-term adherence *(18)*.

Questions about long-term use remain, despite new ideas regarding barriers to adherence. The increased availability and lower costs of drugs, and the advent of fixed-dose combinations, have raised hopes of reducing access problems by lowering cost.

Initiation and continued use are influenced by different factors, however, so attention has to be focused on use over the long term. Recent studies show that patients in Haiti and a number of African countries take about 90% or more of their drugs *(19, 20)*. This gives cause for optimism. At the same time, however, lifelong use of drugs raises the question of sustainability, for which operational research may provide some insights *(21)*.

A number of interventions (most of them tested in developed countries) have been conducted with antiretrovirals. Individualized education and advice have proved to be successful, especially when associated with participation in support groups. Scaling up treatment will mean sharing responsibilities with health workers who lack formal medical training – allowing health workers to monitor and follow up patients – and this will have profound implications. The extent to which the lessons from successful programmes can be rapidly implemented in diverse settings indicates a rich agenda for operational research, and the key role of innovative knowledge-sharing mechanisms.

## Coping with toxicities

The importance of treatment-associated adverse effects in current HIV therapy is illustrated by several studies demonstrating that 40% or more of patients initiating highly active antiretroviral therapies will experience one or more forms of drug toxicity, and consequently may need to modify their regimen within the first year of treatment *(22)*. Examples include hepatic toxicity, rash, diarrhoea, anaemia and peripheral neuropathy. Other adverse effects may become noticeable clinically only after more prolonged exposure to therapy (one to two years) *(23, 24)*.

Innovative ways of assessing the potential toxicity of new drugs are needed at all preclinical and clinical phases of drug development. To ensure that millions of people get the best, sustained treatment, it is imperative that issues of resistance and longer-term safety and tolerability of treatment receive sufficient attention as treatment expansion unfolds. However, drug toxicities will always be preferable to inevitable death in the absence of drug treatment, particularly if concerns over toxicities prevent availablity of treatment in resource-poor settings.

## Preventing drug resistance

The issue of resistance by HIV to antiretroviral drugs is a major concern. Evidence from clinics, apart from clinical treatment trials, suggests that the frequency of incomplete virological suppression in people treated with combination therapies may exceed 50% *(25)*. Incomplete suppression results in acquired viral resistance to antiretrovirals. Resistance often occurs to more than one or two of the three drugs that are being taken by the patient, because of cross-reactivity between drugs within a given antiretroviral family. While the emergence of a drug-resistant virus may be associated with a slower immunological decline in some people, virological failure of treatment places people at risk of developing resistance to antiretroviral drugs. They are also at risk of losing treatment options after treatment has been modified several times, and of ultimate immunological failure and morbidity.

Methods are needed that ensure the effectiveness of antiretroviral therapies in preventing virological treatment failure, and novel, more potent drugs will have to be designed that are active on both "wild" and resistant strains of viruses. Since current therapy is capable of suppressing viral replication but not capable of viral eradication from the host, no current therapeutic regimen will be completely successful. Thus, reservoirs of infection are established early and apparently persist in all HIV-infected people irrespective of therapy *(26)*. A systematic and rigorous approach to treatment offers the best opportunity to study and promote adherence and thereby reduce drug resistance and treatment failure (see Chapter 2).

## Developing new drugs and strategies

Dozens of new drugs are being researched, including those belonging to the three currently available families of antiretrovirals: nucleosidic and non-nucleosidic reverse transcriptase inhibitors and protease inhibitors. Research and development of new compounds in these three families aims at providing drugs that are more potent, easier to take and better tolerated, as well as new formulations combining several of the drugs in one pill.

The first of a new class of "entry inhibitor" drugs that prevent the virus getting into cells in the first place was launched in 2003. These drugs will probably be the most important new antiretrovirals. They target human cell components, rather than viral components, and therefore the virus should find it more difficult to develop resistance to them. The next class of drugs expected is that of inhibitors of the integration of viral DNA into the host's genome.

The issues of toxicities and insufficient virological and immunological potency are not being solved by current treatment strategies. Therefore, new strategies need to be targeted at immune-based approaches to the treatment of HIV-1 infection, such as therapeutic vaccination, passive immunization or eradication of the "reservoirs" of infection. These approaches represent a vital area of basic and clinical research for the coming years.

## Tackling tuberculosis and HIV/AIDS together

Tuberculosis (TB) impacts heavily on HIV morbidity and mortality, as HIV is the most potent risk factor for reactivation of latent tuberculosis infection to active disease. A person dually infected with HIV and *Mycobacterium tuberculosis* has an annual risk of developing TB ranging from 5% to 15%, compared with the lifetime risk of 10% for someone with an intact immune system.

One component of the strategy to decrease TB-related morbidity in people living with HIV/AIDS is to prevent the progression of latent TB infection to active disease, by offering isoniazide preventive therapy as part of the clinical package of HIV care. This treatment has been shown to reduce the risk of TB in tuberculin test positive HIV-infected individuals by 67% *(27)*. Because of reinfection, however, the effect is relatively brief in communities where TB is endemic. The BCG vaccine for TB does not protect against primary infection and, on average, has a protective effect against active disease of only 50%. A crucial means of improving HIV-related morbidity will be the development of an improved TB vaccine. The many steps needed to identify TB infection, and the need to take treatment for at least six months with periodic evaluations for adverse reactions, mean that the proportion of individuals who complete treatment, even under the best conditions, is small.

In order for isoniazide preventive therapy to be an effective public health measure, further research is needed to understand how to diminish the loss of treatment candidates at each step of the process, and how to find effective, shorter-term treatment with few side-effects. New medication delivery methods (for example, medication skin patches and other depo-preparations) are also required, as are new methods other than tuberculin skin tests to determine cases of infection.

## OPERATIONAL RESEARCH

Pilot treatment programmes have been successfully conducted in several countries including Côte d'Ivoire, Senegal, Thailand and Uganda, clearly demonstrating that treatment in those settings is feasible, and that adherence to treatment, tolerance of therapy and incidence of resistance are no different from those found in developed countries *(20, 28, 29)*. Expanding care and antiretroviral therapy to all those who need them worldwide raises a number of challenges for sociobehavioural, clinical and operational research. The term "operational research" refers here to an array of subjects and disciplines supporting the design and improvement of the systems that allow effective prevention, treatment, care and, ultimately, vaccines to reach all those who need them. It denotes the sciences underlying the rational organization of care, and might also be called "delivery system research". In its own way, its enquiries tackle problems as difficult and as intellectually challenging as those in the other three areas of research summarized above; the methods are not those of biomedical science, but rather of social science, economics, statistics, engineering, psychology and anthropology, among others.

Operational research, so defined, can help to involve, guide and coordinate the roles of care providers from government, the private sector, nongovernmental organizations, communities, faith-based organizations and the workplace, and to deliver antiretroviral therapy. Equally importantly, such research is needed to measure and monitor in a standardized way the impact of antiretroviral therapy in terms of parameters such as additional years of healthy life, fewer deaths, economic progress across society,

## Box 5.1  Learning by doing – the operational research agenda

In treatment programmes it is critical to obtain data about what works, what does not work and why, and to have this information available as quickly as possible. This is implicit in the 3 by 5 strategy, where one of the two strategic elements in Pillar Five, "The rapid identification and reapplication of new knowledge and successes" (see Chapter 2), is to learn continuously by doing – with ongoing evaluation and analysis of programme performance and a focused operational research agenda.

The treatment initiative's operational research agenda has six areas of activity.

■ *Coordinating and helping to develop an appropriate operational research agenda.* Consensus will be developed with programme managers about the immediate needs of antiretroviral therapy programmes, and the agenda will be reviewed regularly as data and evidence are generated and new issues emerge.

■ *Seeking data on the impact of scaling up antiretroviral therapy.* While treatment is expected to accelerate prevention, clear evidence is required that this does happen. Any negative interactions, such as stigma and discrimination, must also be identified rapidly so that they can be halted.

■ *Identifying ways to define the effects of scaling up therapy on health systems performance.* The resource inputs and capacity building called for in line with the targets are expected to strengthen health systems. It is important to provide clear evidence that this does indeed happen, and to seek ways to facilitate it. It is equally important to see where the opposite is happening and to identify ways to minimize any negative impacts.

■ *Identifying ways to cost and analyse antiretroviral therapy programmes.* The debate about whether treatment or prevention is more cost effective has been made redundant by the universal recognition of the merits of a comprehensive approach. Nevertheless, solid cost data and cost-effectiveness analysis must be made available to help develop sustainable systems and their long-term financing.

■ *Improving programme design and finding better tools.* The results of all operational research and other strategic information-gathering on risky behaviour and the evolution of drug resistance need to be analysed rapidly. The capacity of research groups in developing countries will be supported to enable most data analysis to be done nationally.

■ *Incorporating new knowledge into policy and practice.* Data and new knowledge need to be fed back rapidly both to the centres where the research was carried out (an ethical obligation) and, more widely, to any programmes facing a similar situation. This core activity of WHO underpins the entire operational research approach.

development of drug resistance, and adherence to treatment (see Box 5.1).

Key issues to be tackled through operational research include:

- optimizing therapeutic regimens for scaling up therapy, for example by performing clinical trials and following up cohorts of treated patients;
- monitoring tolerance of therapy in trials and open patient cohorts;
- establishing optimal ways of monitoring therapy in the context of resource-limited settings; specifically, improving means of enumerating CD4 cell counts, measuring plasma HIV viral load and assessing viral resistance;
- building surveillance programmes to monitor resistance to antiretroviral drugs: when resistance develops to today's drugs, new treatments will be needed;
- improving diagnosis and treatment of opportunistic infections;
- seeking data on the impact of scaling up antiretroviral therapy on prevention and risky behaviour, mitigation, and stigma and discrimination, and using the data to improve programmes designed to reduce risky behaviours;
- identifying the consequences of antiretroviral treatment scale-up on health systems performance;
- creating peer-to-peer learning systems at the clinic, district and country levels so that new findings discovered in the field, combined with existing knowledge, can be quickly disseminated and applied;
- developing innovative, scalable models of how human resources in resource-poor settings can best be mobilized and trained to tackle HIV/AIDS prevention, care and treatment.

## Economic issues

Economic research is essential to ensure that therapeutic strategies using antiretrovirals are successful in developing countries. Earlier cost–effectiveness analyses erroneously concluded that such treatment is not cost effective compared with other interventions, especially prevention. These studies did not adequately consider major issues such as the strong link between treatment and prevention (which are not substitutes but are complementary activities); the economic law of diminishing returns that makes prevention very effective at low levels of coverage but each additional input less effective as coverage approaches 100%; and the underestimation of the impact of HIV/AIDS on economic activity and development. Furthermore, they are now rendered obsolete by the huge fall in the cost of antiretrovirals that has since taken place.

Researchers have already linked the dynamic relationship between potential famine and the spread of HIV among rural agricultural workers; the relationship between HIV and malnutrition in general; and the effect of food insecurity on the autonomy of individuals, particularly women. Understanding the complex intersectoral relationships gives a better picture of HIV's true impact, and illuminates possible points of intervention *(30, 31)*.

To discover and improve methods of scaling up access to treatment, economic analysis must be coupled with clinical data provided by longitudinal follow-up of patients in resource-poor settings. The cost-effectiveness ratio of different clinical and economic strategies will provide information that will help answer questions, such as: at what level can treatment ideally be initiated? What are the most effective strategies for switching regimens? How can biological monitoring be optimized? Economic research will also contribute to the identification and evaluation of different strategies of funding access to treatment. At the macroeconomic level, it will be important to establish how the cost burden is distributed between domestic and international sources and, among domestic contributions, the share and incidence of out-of-pocket payments. At the microeconomic level, the effect of different financing arrangements on treatment adherence, the development of drug resistance, and final treatment outcomes will be significant topics of study.

## Health policy analysis

It will be important to identify the factors that affect efforts to increase access to treatment, particularly in the context of health services. Some of the key factors are: leadership and management skills; sufficient and sustained funds for antiretroviral medications; technical competence in drugs and commodities procurement; training; monitoring of outcomes; and, in the public sector, a functioning district health system capable of delivering services. Research should include: identifying which factors increase or hinder integration of HIV/AIDS control programmes with public health policy and collaboration with other programmes; developing policies that support such collaboration and integration; and analysing the roles and comparative advantages of all the stakeholders involved in implementation of HIV/AIDS and other interventions.

# Unsafe blood practices transmit infection

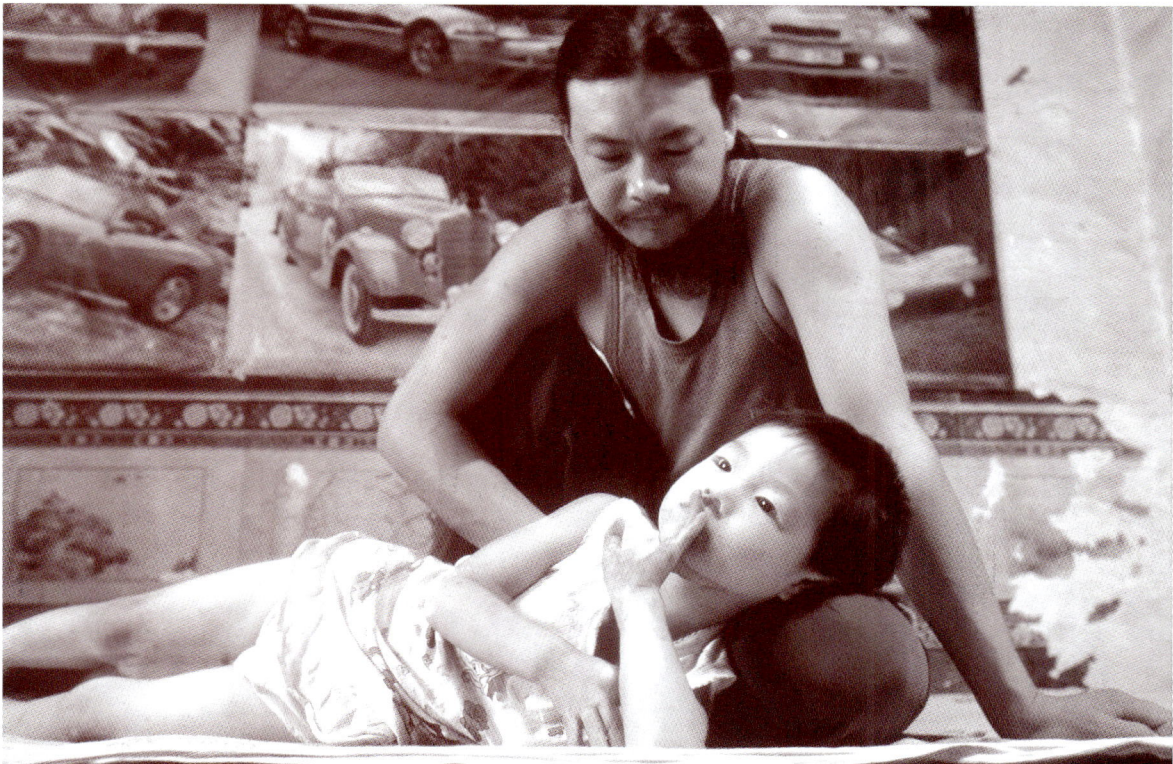

Fritz Hoffman/Network

Wang Kai Jai's mother contracted HIV/AIDS after selling her blood to a hospital. In turn, Wang Kai Jai, now four years old, from Licheng, Hebei Province, China, became infected.

Many people living with HIV/AIDS have acquired the virus through infected blood or blood products or by using unsafe blood donation facilities. In some areas of China, people eager to escape poverty sold their blood through middlemen who often reused needles.

Scaling up access to treatment must be used as an opportunity to promote global health reforms at the country level with benefits that go beyond HIV care. There is the potential to create effective incentives to improve health infrastructure in resource-limited settings. Research is needed to identify all the potentially negative and positive externalities of scaling up access and their effects on health systems.

## Equity issues

Social inequality in the settings where care is to be implemented, the constraints on resources available for treatment, and the need to define eligibility criteria for the provision of antiretroviral drugs, all call for special attention to the equity dimension of the intervention. Special measures need to be taken in order to avoid the possibility of unwittingly reinforcing existing inequalities, setting up a two-tier system in allocating resources, or weakening other disease control efforts by giving priority to HIV/AIDS. In addition, care must be taken to protect the rights of patients when measures such as partner notification and disclosure are deemed to be necessary, and attention must be directed to the local conditions that may hamper confidentiality, especially when treatment is implemented on a large scale.

Many of the barriers that prevent disadvantaged members of society from accessing health care and obtaining treatment are a result of the deficiencies of health services, and there is a growing awareness that the treatment scale-up initiative represents an opportunity to tackle some of these shortcomings. Hence, it will be necessary regularly to review socioeconomic information about treated patients in order to make sure that poorer people have equal access to medication. More work is needed on the appropriate indicators of equity and how information can be collected about them.

Special consideration should be given to gender as it affects the provision of care. A better understanding is required of the particular circumstances that lead to discrimination against HIV-positive women, and of those conditions that enable women to respond and take control of their own affairs. It would be useful to keep track of programmes that have sought to integrate gender considerations into health services, which have an important role to play.

Another obstacle to care comes from the stigma that is attached to seropositive status, and concerted efforts to assess this information can help define locally effective strategies. There is little doubt that stigma and avoidance of testing and treatment are mutually reinforcing, and that it is precisely the individuals who are marginalized because of their status who are not reached by prevention and care efforts. The evidence base for what works in order to reduce stigma and why is, however, thin and has to be strengthened by well-designed studies, both to substantiate the effect of multiple interventions and to define the packages that are effective in different contexts *(32, 33)*.

## INTERNATIONAL COLLABORATION

Progress has been accelerating in international collaboration and coordination in HIV/AIDS research, which is critical to achieving the Millennium Development Goal of halting and reversing the pandemic by 2015.

Joint innovative actions, through global research networks and partnerships between the public sector, academic institutions, communities, the private commercial sector and civil society organizations, bring benefits greater than the sum of current high-quality but separate research projects. The benefits include quicker generation of research findings, consensus on international standards for the conduct of research, and research capacity strengthening.

Collaboration permits parallel, concurrent efforts to obtain more timely answers to critical questions. Partnership across sectors through creative public–private alliances can contribute to faster progress in research by linking together diverse approaches and different stages of the research process (see Box 5.2).

International collaboration can lead to consensus on standards for the conduct of research which respect the human rights of study participants, support the research priorities of host countries, and promote community involvement in the design and conduct of research. Collaboration can also ensure that prevention and care interventions that are demonstrated to be safe and effective are rapidly made available to all study participants and to other members of the high-risk populations from which they were drawn.

International collaboration to strengthen research capacity enables the creation of a critical mass of researchers who can focus on national priorities, participate in policy-making bodies, and contribute to international research efforts. International and regional training partnerships must be complemented by active efforts to stem the brain drain from developing to developed countries, as Brazil, China and India are doing. This is achieved through investment in research and development to construct strategic knowledge-based industries that can employ nationals educated at home and abroad and attract expatriates to return.

Building national and international research infrastructures, laboratory capacity and improved surveillance systems; collecting, processing and disseminating data; and training basic and clinical researchers, social scientists, health care providers and technicians are all essential to efforts to accelerate knowledge creation. Such acceleration is required to respond to the scale of the HIV/AIDS pandemic. The substantial remaining challenge, and one to which the 3 by 5 initiative is directed, is to ensure that this knowledge immediately improves the lives of people most in need *(34)*.

## Box 5.2  Building partnerships in the fight against disease

The long-term struggles against poliomyelitis and tuberculosis (TB) have shown how international and multisectoral partnerships can work effectively to combat major diseases.

When the World Health Assembly established the goal of polio eradication in 1988, the need for a new kind of partnership was evident. The pioneering work to eliminate polio from the WHO Region of the Americas was initially carried out by a small group of partners, consisting of WHO, Rotary International, the United Nations Children's Fund (UNICEF) and the US Centers for Disease Control and Prevention. This group then grew to include the government of every country in the world, 30 major donor partners (contributing more than US$ 1 million) and dozens of implementing partners, including national and international

humanitarian organizations and nongovernmental organizations.

To ensure effectiveness, a number of basic principles have guided work over the 15 years during which this group has worked together in pursuit of its common goal of a polio-free world:
- multisectoral representation;
- long-term commitment;
- top-level institutional representation;
- full use of comparative advantages;
- common operating principles and forums (for example, the work of the partnership was guided by a series of common, strategic plans covering several years, resource requirement documents and workplans at the international, regional and national levels).

As part of the campaign to combat TB, the Stop TB Partnership has become greatly respected globally. It includes WHO and the World Bank, and its strategic objectives have been formulated in close consultation with high-burden countries themselves. These objectives are directed towards the problems and policy priorities of the principal stakeholders, for example in relation to the United Nations Millennium Development Goals.

The Partnership has an increasing number of active participants. It has made significant progress against TB, highlighted work on new diagnostics, drugs and vaccines, and rapidly operationalized the Green Light Committee and Global Drug Facility to tackle lack of access to TB drugs.

## Sharing knowledge

Extending treatment opportunities needs a faster research process than is available through traditional notions of research. The nature of the HIV/AIDS epidemic is changing quickly in many countries – too quickly to be effectively countered through standard research processes, whose timeline is typically measured in years. In addition, many of the decisions on which research projects are to be funded and pursued are made by policy-makers at some distance from the problem. As a result, resources and efforts are invested in work that may have little or no relevance to actual implementation in the field.

The public health community must rethink its definition of knowledge and the structure by which it is generated, shared and applied. The aims of knowledge management are to collect all relevant information and intellectual capital into a common system, and provide equal access to that information, ensuring that it can be synthesized with local needs. Such a system enables members of the public health community to

# A mother's story

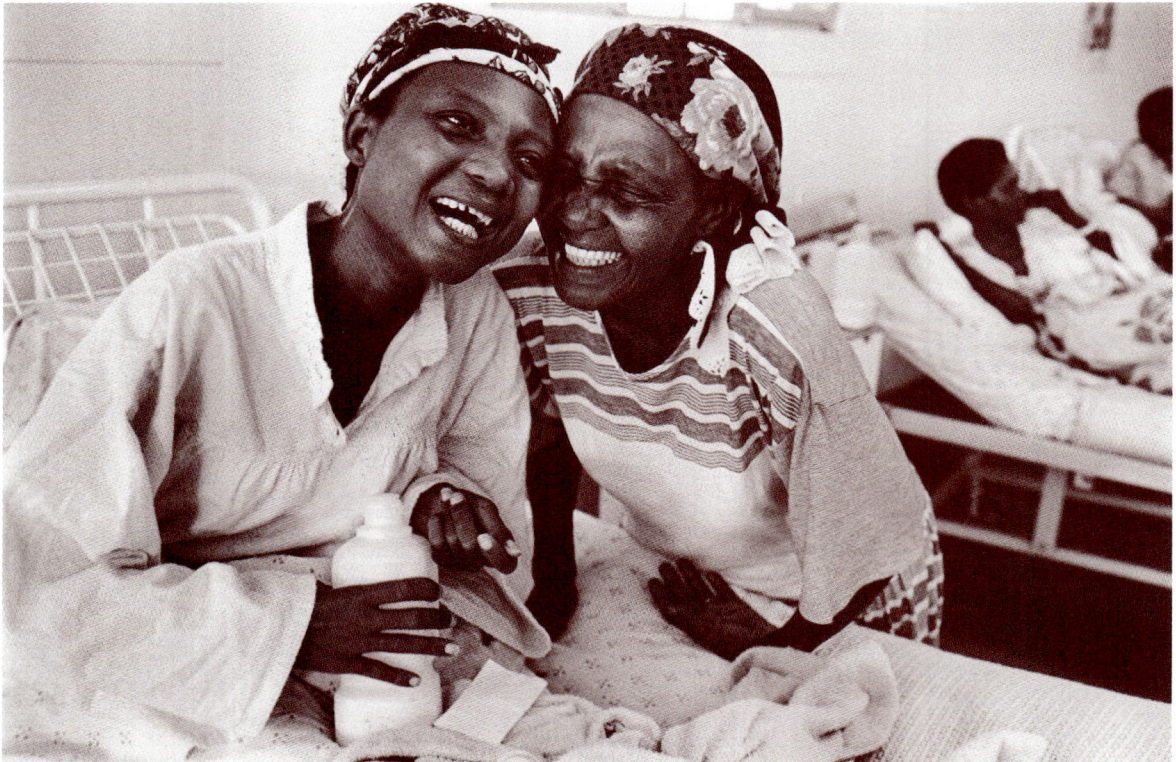

Gideon Mendel/Network

Nesta Mkhwanazi comforts her daughter, Samkelisiwe, who has been receiving antiretroviral treatment in the tuberculosis ward of Ngwelezane Hospital, KwaZulu-Natal, South Africa (see Samkelisiwe's story in Chapter 1).

"My daughter's recurring tuberculosis cannot be cured," says Nesta. "She has also been tested and diagnosed with HIV/AIDS. This has made life very difficult for us, as I have only a monthly pension of 500 rand [approximately US$ 75] with which to support and care for my two daughters and four grandchildren. At 51 I find it hard to be a mother again to all these children. However, I am proud that my daughter has decided to disclose her HIV/AIDS status to our community and to help educate others about this disease."

communicate directly with their peers on matters of mutual interest, such as effective practice in their own localities.

The 3 by 5 goal prompts public health practitioners to share and exploit experiential knowledge in a much more direct way, for example through "communities of practice" – informal networks linking individuals and groups who share common professional interests and who benefit from frequent exchanges of knowledge through the Internet or other telecommunication methods. Progress in information and communication technologies and other learning systems such as communities of practice gives cause for optimism. Improved communication can spur a knowledge revolution that will particularly benefit poor countries and communities, through greater use of the Internet, e-mail and telephone, and better satellite and wireless technology. By whatever means, the promotion and improvement of learning systems at all levels should greatly assist the achievement of public health goals as well as helping to strengthen health systems in general.

# References

1. Bailey C. Using knowledge management to make health systems work. *Bulletin of the World Health Organization*, 2003, 81:777.

2. Msellati P, Juillet-Amari A, Prudhomme J, Akribi HA, Coulibaly-Traore D, Souville M et al. Socio-economic and health characteristics of HIV-infected patients seeking care in relation to access to the Drug Access Initiative and to antiretroviral treatment in Côte d'Ivoire. *AIDS*, 2003, 17(Suppl. 3):S63–S68.

3. Katz MH, Schwarcz SK, Kellogg TA, Klausner JD, Dilley JW, Gibson S et al. Impact of highly active antiretroviral treatment on HIV seroincidence among men who have sex with men: San Francisco. *American Journal of Public Health*, 2002, 92:388–394.

4. Blower S, Schwartz EJ, Mills J. Forecasting the future of HIV epidemics: the impact of antiretroviral therapies and imperfect vaccines. *AIDS Reviews*, 2003, 5:113–125.

5. Moatti JP, Souteyrand Y. HIV/AIDS social and behavioural research: past advances and thoughts about the future. *Social Science and Medicine*, 2000, 50:1519–1532.

6. Poppen PJ, Reisen CA. Perception of risk and sexual self-protective behavior: a methodological critique. *AIDS Education and Prevention*, 1997, 9:373–390.

7. Bajos N. Social factors and the process of risk construction in HIV sexual transmission. *AIDS Care*, 1997, 9:227–237.

8. Schoepf B. International AIDS research in anthropology: taking a critical perspective on the crisis. *Annual Review of Anthropology*, 2001, 30:335–361.

9. De Cock K, Fowler MG, Mercier E, de Vincenzi I, Saba J, Hoff E et al. Prevention of mother-to-child HIV transmission in resource-poor countries: translating research into policy and practice. *JAMA*, 2000, 283:1175–1182.

10. Cooper ER, Charurat M, Mofenson L, Hanson IC, Pitt J, Diaz C et al. Combination antiretroviral strategies for the treatment of pregnant HIV-1-infected women and prevention of perinatal HIV-1 transmission. *AIDS*, 2002, 29:484–494.

11. Dorenbaum A, Cunningham CK, Gelber RD, Culnane M, Mofenson L, Britto P et al. Two-dose intrapartum/newborn nevirapine and standard ARV therapy to reduce perinatal HIV transmission: a randomized trial. *JAMA*, 2002, 288:189–198.

12. Mofenson LM, Munderi P. Safety of antiretroviral prophylaxis of perinatal transmission for HIV–infected pregnant women and their infants. *AIDS*, 2002, 30:200–215.

13. Dabis F, Ekpini ER. HIV-1/AIDS and maternal and child health in Africa. *Lancet*, 2002, 359:2097–2104.

14. *The public health benefits of microbicides: model projections*. New York, Rockefeller Foundation, 2002.

15. Shiver JW, Fu TM, Chen L, Casimiro DR, Davies ME, Evans RK et al. Replication-incompetent adenoviral vaccine vector elicits effective anti-immunodeficiency-virus immunity. *Nature*, 2002, 415:331–335.

16. Klausner RD, Fauci AS, Corey L, Nabel GJ, Gayle H, Berkley S et al. Medicine. The need for a global HIV vaccine enterprise. *Science*, 2003, 300:2036–2039.

17. *Adherence to HIV treatment*. Geneva, World Health Organization, 2003 (Department of HIV/AIDS unpublished internal technical brief).

18. Lanièce I, Ciss M, Desclaux A, Diop K, Mbodj F, Ndiaye B et al. Adherence to HAART and its principal determinants in a cohort of Senegalese adults. *AIDS*, 2003, 17(Suppl. 3): S103–S108.

19. Farmer P, Leandre F, Mukherjee JS, Claude M, Nevil P, Smith-Fawzi MC et al. Community-based approaches to HIV treatment in resource-poor settings. *Lancet*, 2001, 358:404–409.

20. Katzenstein D, Laga M, Moatti JP. The evaluation of the HIV/AIDS Drug Access Initiatives in Côte d'Ivoire, Senegal and Uganda: how access to antiretroviral treatment can become feasible in Africa. *AIDS*, 2003, 17(Suppl. 3):S1–S4.

21. Spire B, Duran S, Souville M, Leport C, Raffi F, Moatti JP et al. Adherence to highly active antiretroviral therapies (HAART) in HIV-infected patients: from a predictive to a dynamic approach. *Social Science and Medicine*, 2002, 54:1481–1496.

22. Fellay J, Boubaker K, Ledergerber B, Bernasconi E, Furrer H, Battegay M et al. Prevalence of adverse events associated with potent antiretroviral treatment: Swiss HIV Cohort Study. *Lancet*, 2001, 358:1322–1327. Erratum 358:2088.

23. Fliers E, Sauerwein HP, Romijn JA, Reiss P, van der Valk M, Kalsbeek A et al. HIV-associated adipose redistribution syndrome as a selective autonomic neuropathy. *Lancet*, 2003, 362:1758–1760.

24. Reiss P. How bad is HAART for the heart? *AIDS*, 2003, 17:2529–2531.

25. Valdez H, Lederman MM, Woolley I, Walker CJ, Vernon LT, Hise A et al. Human immunodeficiency virus 1 protease inhibitors in clinical practice: predictors of virological outcome. *Archives of Internal Medicine*, 1999, 159:1771–1776.

26. Siliciano JD, Kajdas J, Finzi D, Quinn TC, Chadwick K, Margolick JB et al. Long-term follow-up studies confirm the stability of the latent reservoir for HIV-1 in resting CD4+ T cells. *Nature Medicine*, 2003, 9:727–728.

27. Siliciano JD, Kajdas J, Finzi D, Quinn TC, Chadwick K, Margolick JB et al. A trial of three regimens to prevent tuberculosis in Ugandan adults infected with the human immunodeficiency virus. *New England Journal of Medicine*, 1997, 337:801–808.

28. *L'accès aux traitements du VIH/SIDA en Côte d'Ivoire [Access to treatment for HIV/AIDS in Côte d'Ivoire]*. Paris, Agence Nationale de Recherches sur le Sida, 2001.

29. *L'initiative sénégalaise d'accès aux traitements antiretroviraux. Analyses économiques, sociales, comportementales et médicales [The Senegalese initiative to provide access to antiretroviral treatment: economic, social, behavioural and medical analyses]*. Paris, Agence Nationale de Recherches sur le Sida, 2002.

30. Loevinsohn M, Gillespie S. *An 'HIV/AIDS lens' to guide agricultural and food policy in Africa*. Washington, DC, International Food Policy Research Institute, 2003.

31. Moatti JP, Coriat B, Souteyrand Y, Barnett T, Dumoulin J, Flori YA, eds. *Economics of AIDS and access to HIV/AIDS care in developing countries. Issues and challenges*. Paris, Agence Nationale de Recherches sur le Sida, 2003.

32. *Disentangling HIV and AIDS stigma in Ethiopia, Tanzania, and Zambia*. Washington, DC, International Center for Research on Women, 2003.

33. Parker R, Aggleton P. HIV and AIDS-related stigma and discrimination: a conceptual framework and implications for action. *Social Science and Medicine*, 2003, 57:13–24.

34. *Declaration of Commitment on HIV/AIDS*. New York, United Nations, 2001 (United Nations General Assembly Special Session on HIV/AIDS, 25–27 June 2001).

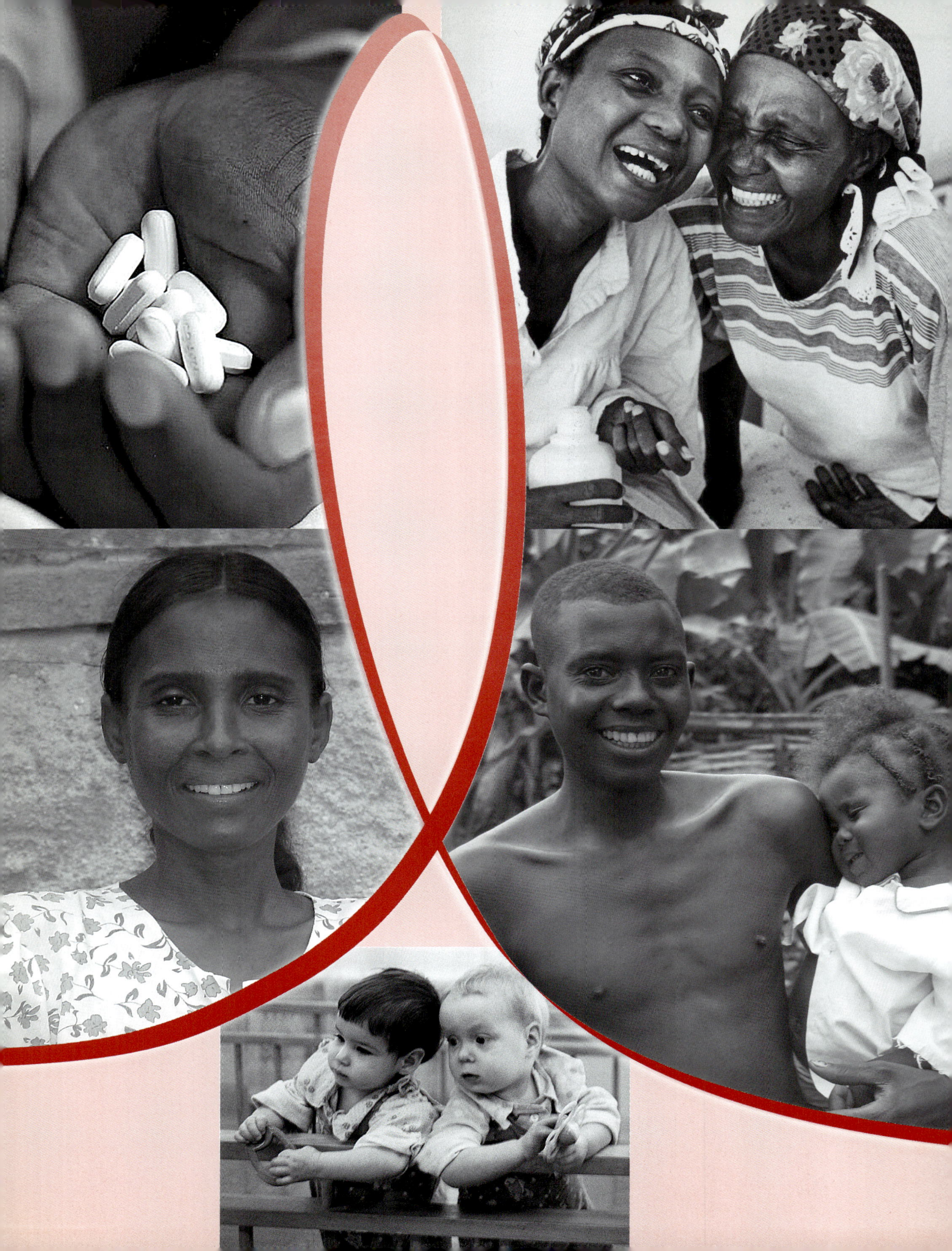

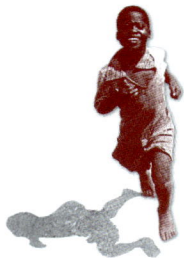

# conclusion

This report began with the story of Joseph Jeune, a 26-year-old peasant farmer in Haiti. It is a story of how hope can triumph over despair, and it also is an example of how people can fight back successfully against HIV/AIDS.

This is a crucial moment in the history of HIV/AIDS, and an unprecedented opportunity to alter its course. The most important message of this report is that, today, the international community has the chance to change the history of health for generations to come and to open the door to better health for all.

*The World Health Report 2004* has chronicled the global spread of HIV/AIDS over the last quarter of a century. It has also traced the efforts of advocacy groups, civil society organizations, community health care workers, researchers and many others to control it and to combat its many side-effects, including stigma and discrimination. Despite those often heroic efforts, more than 20 million people have died from HIV/AIDS and an estimated 34–46 million others are now infected with the causative virus, for which there is as yet no vaccine and no cure.

But there is treatment. Joseph Jeune owes his life to it, as do many others. The pictures of Joseph before and after treatment illustrate what can be done. Antiretroviral therapy saved him from an early grave and enabled him to return to work in his fields and care for his family.

Effectively tackling HIV/AIDS is the world's most urgent public health challenge. In advocating a comprehensive strategy which links prevention, treatment, care and support, this report makes a special case for treatment, which has been the most neglected element in most developing countries.

Treatment is the key to change. It is now possible to save the lives of millions of people who need that treatment but do not yet have access to it. Almost 6 million people now need antiretroviral drugs but only about 400 000 received them in 2003. This knowledge underpins the commitment of WHO and its partners to help provide 3 million people in developing countries with antiretroviral therapy by the end of 2005 – and not to stop there.

The treatment expansion initiative far outreaches the capacities of any single organization. It is one of the most ambitious public health projects in history, and is fraught with difficulties. But within the multiple partnerships of the international community, the knowledge that this *can* be done is leading to the recognition that it *must* be done.

The moral imperative needs no reinforcement, yet there are other excellent reasons to support the treatment initiative. As this report has shown, the long-term economic and social costs of HIV/AIDS in many countries have been seriously underestimated, and some countries in sub-Saharan Africa may be brought to the brink of economic collapse. Treatment expansion is vital to protect their stability and security and to strengthen the foundations of their future development. Furthermore, and of inestimable importance, treatment can be the accelerator that drives efforts to strengthen health systems in all developing countries.

Building up health systems is essential, not just in the fight against HIV/AIDS but also in generally improving access to better health care for those most in need. This report has demonstrated how international organizations, national governments, the private sector and communities can combine their strengths to achieve this objective.

Advocacy by WHO and its partners for increased international investment in health is beginning to bear fruit. Countries should get the maximum public health benefit from new funds that are now becoming available. Although largely intended for HIV/AIDS, these resources can simultaneously strengthen some of the world's most fragile health systems.

Beyond 2005 lies the challenge of extending treatment to many more millions of people, and of maintaining it for the rest of their lives, while simultaneously building and sustaining the health infrastructures to make that huge task possible. The success of this action cannot be guaranteed. But inaction will not be forgiven. It will be judged by those who suffer and die needlessly today, and by the historians of tomorrow. They will have a right to ask why, if we let the chance of changing history slip through our fingers, we did not act in time.

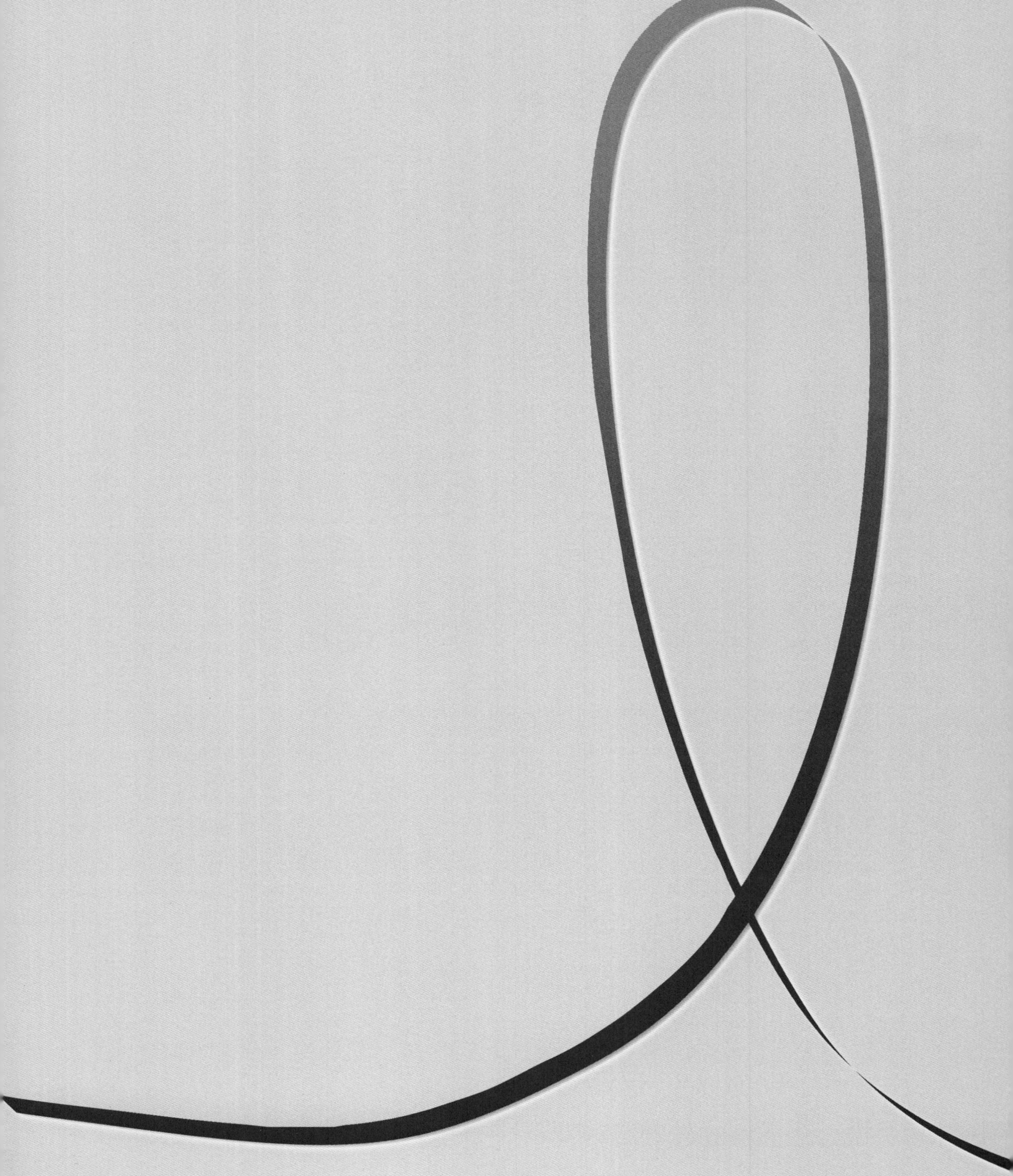

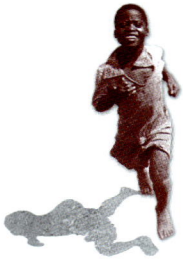

## statistical annex
# explanatory notes

The tables in this technical annex present information on core indicators of population health in WHO Member States and regions for the year 2002, selected national health accounts aggregates for 1997–2001, and baseline estimates for health-related Millennium Development Goal indicators in WHO Member States. These notes provide an overview of concepts, methods and data sources, together with references to more detailed documentation. It is hoped that careful scrutiny and use of the results will lead to progressively better measurement of core indicators of population health and health system financing. The main results in the population health tables are reported with uncertainty intervals in order to communicate to the user the plausible range of estimates for each country on each measure.

Because the production time of *The World Health Report 2004* has been much shorter than usual, it was not possible to carry out consultations on new figures with Member States. Annex Tables 1–6 thus present figures for the same years as the Annex Tables published in *The World Health Report 2003*. Initial WHO estimates and technical explanations were sent to Member States for comment. Comments or data provided in response were discussed with them and incorporated where possible. The estimates reported here should, however, still be interpreted as the best estimates of WHO rather than the official viewpoint of Member States. Only new information received from Member States following consultations in 2003, which was received too late for inclusion in *The World Heath Report 2003*, has been used to update Annex

Tables 1–6. Additionally, revisions to Annex Tables 2 and 3 have taken into account new data for some causes of death as described below.

The work leading to the production of these annex tables was undertaken mostly by the WHO Evidence and Information for Policy cluster in collaboration with counterparts from the WHO regional offices and WHO representatives in Member States. All six WHO regional offices provided updated health expenditure information obtained from Member States in their regions. The WHO Regional Offices for the Americas and Europe also provided cause-of-death data from their Member States.

## ANNEX TABLE 1

To assess overall levels of health achievement, it is crucial to develop the best possible assessment of the life table for each country. Life tables have been developed for all 192 Member States for 2002, starting with a systematic review of all available evidence from surveys, censuses, sample registration systems, population laboratories and vital registration on levels of and trends in child mortality and adult mortality *(1)*. This review benefited greatly from a collaborative assessment of child mortality levels for 2001 by WHO and UNICEF and from analyses of general mortality by the United States Census Bureau *(2)* and the United Nations Population Division *(3)*. WHO uses a standard method to estimate and project life tables for all Member States using comparable data. This may lead to minor differences compared with official life tables prepared by Member States.

All estimates of population size and structure for 2002 are based on the 2002 demographic assessments prepared by the United Nations Population Division *(3)*. These estimates refer to the de facto population, and not the de jure population in each Member State. The annual growth rate, the dependency ratio, the percentage of population aged 60 years and more, and the total fertility rate are also derived from the United Nations Population Division database. To aid in demographic, cause-of-death and burden of disease analyses, the 192 Member States have been divided into five mortality strata on the basis of their levels of child and adult male mortality. The matrix defined by the six WHO regions and the five mortality strata leads to 14 epidemiological subregions, since not every mortality stratum is represented in every region. These subregions are defined on pages 156–157 and used in Annex Tables 2 and 3 for presentation of results.

Because of increasing heterogeneity of patterns of adult and child mortality, WHO has developed a model life table system of two-parameter logit life tables using a global standard, and with additional age-specific parameters to correct for systematic biases in the application of a two-parameter system *(4)*. This system of model life tables has been used extensively in the development of life tables for those Member States without adequate vital registration and in projecting life tables to 2002 when the most recent data available are from earlier years.

Demographic techniques (Preston–Coale method, Brass Growth–Balance method, Generalized Growth–Balance method and Bennett–Horiuchi method) have been applied, as appropriate, to assess the level of completeness of recorded mortality data for Member States with vital registration systems. For Member States without national vital registration systems, all available survey, census and vital registration data were assessed, adjusted and averaged to estimate the probable trend in child mortality over the past few decades. This trend was projected to estimate child mortality levels in 2002. In addition, adult sibling survival data from available population surveys were analysed to obtain additional information on adult mortality. Life expectancy, under-five mortality in terms of probability of dying by five years of age and adult mortality in terms of probability of dying between 15 and 60 years of age derive directly from the life tables.

To capture the uncertainty resulting from sampling, indirect estimation technique or projection to 2002, a total of 1000 life tables have been developed for each Member State. Uncertainty bounds are reported in Annex Table 1 by giving key life table values at the 2.5th percentile and the 97.5th percentile. This uncertainty analysis was facilitated by the development of new methods and software tools *(5)*. In countries with a substantial HIV/AIDS epidemic, recent estimates of the level and uncertainty range of the magnitude of the epidemic have been incorporated into the life table uncertainty analysis.

## ANNEX TABLES 2 AND 3

Causes of death for the 14 epidemiological subregions and the world have been estimated based on data from 112 national vital registration systems that capture about
18.6 million deaths annually, representing one-third of all deaths occurring in the
world. In addition, information from sample registration systems, population laboratories and epidemiological analyses of specific conditions has been used to improve
estimates of the cause-of-death patterns *(6–16)*. These data are used to estimate
death rates by age and sex for underlying causes of death as defined by the International Statistical Classification of Diseases and Related Health Problems (ICD) classification rules.

Cause-of-death data have been carefully analysed to take into account incomplete
coverage of vital registration in countries and the likely differences in cause-of-death
patterns that would be expected in the uncovered and often poorer subpopulations.
Techniques to undertake this analysis have been developed based on the Global Burden of Disease study *(17)* and further refined using a much more extensive database
and more robust modelling techniques *(18)*.

Special attention has been paid to problems of misattribution or miscoding of causes
of death in cardiovascular diseases, cancer, injuries and general ill-defined categories.
A correction algorithm for reclassifying ill-defined cardiovascular codes has been developed *(19)*. Cancer mortality by site has been evaluated using both vital registration
data and population-based cancer incidence registries. The latter have been analysed
using a complete age, period cohort model of cancer survival in each region *(15)*.

The regional and global estimates of mortality and burden of disease by cause for
2002 published in Annex Tables 2 and 3 have been updated from those published in
*The World Health Report 2003*, not only to take into account revisions to life tables for
a few countries but also to include revised estimates of mortality for some causes,
based on improved data and recent evidence.

Estimates of HIV/AIDS mortality have been revised to take into account new and
different sources of data, such as national household surveys, as well as improved
information on emerging epidemics in the Americas, Asia and eastern Europe *(8)*.
Latest estimates available for countries (as at February 2004) have been incorporated into the revision of Annex Tables 2 and 3. Tuberculosis prevalence and mortality
for 2002 have been revised based on latest tuberculosis notification data, treatment
rates, and case-fatality rate data, as published in WHO's *Global tuberculosis control
report 2004*.

Estimates of measles mortality have been revised to take into account new information on the effects of supplemental immunization campaigns in reducing measles
mortality. The number and quality of supplemental immunization campaigns have
substantially increased since 2000 in Africa. Estimates of deaths from pertussis and
poliomyelitis for 2002 have also been revised to take into account new information
on notifications and immunization coverage. Neonatal tetanus and maternal tetanus
incidence and mortality have been revised, to take into account the implementation of
tetanus toxoid supplemental immunization activities. These activities target all women
of childbearing age in the highest-risk districts, and have been implemented in 29
countries since 1999.

Annex Table 3 provides estimates of the burden of disease for the 14 epidemiological subregions using disability-adjusted life years (DALYs). One DALY can be thought
of as one lost year of "healthy" life and the burden of disease as a measurement
of the gap between the current health of a population and an ideal situation where
everyone in the population lives into old age in full health *(20, 21)*. DALYs for a disease

or health condition are calculated as the sum of the years of life lost (YLL) owing to premature mortality in the population and the years lost through disability (YLD) for incident cases of the health condition. DALYs for 2002 have been estimated based on cause-of-death information for each subregion and regional or country-level assessments of the incidence and prevalence of diseases and injuries. The latter are based on a systematic assessment and analysis of data on major diseases and injuries available to WHO technical programmes and through collaboration with scientists worldwide *(16)*. WHO programme participation in the development of these estimates and consultation with Member States ensure that estimates reflect all information and knowledge available to WHO. Estimates of incidence and point prevalence for selected major causes by subregion are also available on the WHO web site at www.who.int/evidence/bod.

## ANNEX TABLE 4

Annex Table 4 reports the average level of population health for WHO Member States in terms of healthy life expectancy (HALE). HALE is based on life expectancy at birth (Annex Table 1) but includes an adjustment for *time spent in poor health*. It is most easily understood as the equivalent number of years in full health that a newborn can expect to live based on current rates of ill-health and mortality *(22, 23)*. The methods used by WHO to calculate HALE have been developed to maximize comparability across populations. WHO analyses of over 50 existing national health surveys for the calculation of healthy life expectancy identified severe limitations in the comparability of self-reported health status data from different populations, even when identical survey instruments and methods were used *(24)*. These comparability problems are a result of unmeasured differences in expectations and norms for health, so that the meaning that different populations attach to the labels used for response categories in self-reported questions (such as mild, moderate or severe) can vary greatly *(25)*. To resolve these problems, WHO undertook a Multi-Country Survey Study (MCSS) in 2000–2001 in collaboration with Member States, using a standardized health status survey instrument together with new statistical methods for adjusting biases in self-reported health *(25, 26)*.

The MCSS carried out 71 representative household surveys in 61 Member States in 2000 and 2001, using a new health status instrument based on the *International classification of functioning, disability and health (27)*, which seeks information from a representative sample of respondents on their current states of health according to seven core domains. To overcome the problem of comparability of self-report health data, the WHO survey instrument used performance tests and vignettes to calibrate self-reported health in each of the core domains *(26)*. The calibrated responses are used to estimate the prevalence of different states of health by age and sex.

The measurement of *time spent in poor health* is based on combining condition-specific estimates from the Global Burden of Disease study with estimates of the prevalence of different health states by age and sex derived from the MCSS, and weighted using health state valuations *(28)*. Data from the Global Burden of Disease study were used to estimate severity-adjusted prevalences for health conditions by age and sex for all 192 WHO Member States for 2002. Data from 62 surveys in the MCSS were used to make independent estimates of severity-adjusted prevalences by age and sex. Finally, posterior prevalences for all Member States for 2002 were calculated based on the Global Burden of Disease study and survey prevalences.

Household surveys including a valuation module were conducted in fourteen countries: China, Colombia, Egypt, Georgia, India, Indonesia, Islamic Republic of Iran,

Lebanon, Mexico, Nigeria, Singapore, Slovakia, Syrian Arab Republic and Turkey. Data on nearly 500 000 health state valuations from over 46 000 respondents were used to develop average global health state valuations for the calculation of HALE *(29)*.

The methods used by WHO to calculate healthy life expectancy were peer-reviewed during 2001 and 2002 by the Scientific Peer Review Group (SPRG) constituted by the Director-General, in response to a request by the WHO Executive Board (EB107.R8). The SPRG's final report to the Director-General *(30)* considered that the methodology for the measurement of HALE was well advanced, and made a number of technical recommendations which have been followed for the calculations reported in Annex Table 4. In particular, steps have been taken to include residents in health institutions and dependent comorbidity *(16)*.

Annex Table 4 reports for all Member States for 2002 the following: average HALE at birth, HALE at age 60, expected lost healthy years (LHE) at birth, percentage of total life expectancy (LE) lost, and 95% uncertainty intervals. LHE is calculated as LE minus HALE and is the expected equivalent number of years of full health lost through living in health states other than full health. LHE expressed as a percentage of total LE represents the proportion of total life expectancy that is lost through living in health states of less than full health.

## ANNEX TABLE 5

National health accounts (NHA) are a synthesis of the financing and spending flows recorded in the operation of a health system, with the potential to monitor all transactions from funding sources to the distribution of benefits across geographical, demographic, socioeconomic and epidemiological dimensions. NHA are related to the macroeconomic and macrosocial accounts whose methodology they borrow.

Annex Table 5 provides the best estimates that were available to WHO up to July 2003 for each of its 192 Member States. Although more and more countries collect health expenditure data, only a limited number have produced full national health accounts. Nationally and internationally available information that has been identified and obtained has been compiled for each country. Standard accounting estimation and extrapolation techniques have been applied to provide adequate time series. A policy-relevant breakdown of the data (for example, public/private expenditure) is also provided. Each year draft templates are sent to ministers of health for their comments and their assistance in obtaining additional information as appropriate. The constructive responses from ministries have provided valuable information for the NHA estimates reported here.

An important methodological contribution to producing national health accounts is now available in the *Guide to producing national health accounts with special applications for low-income and middle-income countries (31)*. This guide is based on the Organisation for Economic Co-operation and Development (OECD) *System of health accounts (32)*. Both reports are built on the principles of the United Nations *System of national accounts* (commonly referred to as SNA93) *(33)*.

The principal international references used to produce the tables are the International Monetary Fund (IMF) *Government finance statistics yearbook, 2002 (34)*, *International financial statistics yearbook, 2003 (35)* and *International financial statistics* (September 2003) *(36)*; the Asian Development Bank *Key indicators 2002 (37)*; *OECD Health Data 2003 (38)* and *International development statistics (39)*; and the United Nations *National accounts statistics: main aggregates and detailed tables, 2000 (40)*. The organizations charged with producing these reports facilitated the supply of advance copies for WHO and gave additional related information, and their contributions are acknowledged here with gratitude.

National sources include: national health accounts reports, public expenditure reports, statistical yearbooks and other periodicals, budgetary documents, national accounts reports, statistical data on official web sites, nongovernmental organization reports, academic studies, and reports and data provided by central statistical offices, ministries of health, ministries of finance and economic development, planning offices, and professional and trade associations.

Annex Table 5 provides both updated and revised figures for 1997–2001. Figures have been updated when new information that changes the original estimates has become available. This category includes benchmarking revisions, whereby an occasional wholesale revision is made by a country owing to a change in methodology, when a more extensive NHA effort is undertaken, or when shifting the denominator from SNA68 to SNA93. Colombia is a case in point.

Total expenditure on health has been defined as the sum of general government expenditure on health (GGHE or public expenditure on health), and private expenditure on health (PvtHE). All estimates are calculated in millions of national currency units (million NCU). The estimates are presented as ratios to gross domestic product (GDP), to total health expenditure (THE), to total general government expenditure (GGE), or to private expenditure on health (PvtHE).

GDP is the value of all goods and services provided in a country by residents and non-residents without regard to their allocation among domestic and foreign claims. This (with small adjustments) corresponds to the total sum of expenditure (consumption and investment) of the private and government agents of the economy during the reference year. The United Nations *National accounts statistics: main aggregates and detailed tables, 2000 (40)*, Table 1.1, was the main source of GDP estimates. For the 30 Member countries of the OECD, the macroeconomic accounts have been imported from the *National accounts of OECD countries: detailed tables 1990/2001*, 2003 edition, Volume II *(41)*, Table 1. Collaborative arrangements between WHO and the United Nations Statistics Division and the Economic Commission for Europe of the United Nations have permitted the receipt of advance information on 2001. For Iraq, Lebanon and the United Arab Emirates, United Nations Economic and Social Commission for Western Asia data were used.

When United Nations data were unavailable, GDP data reported by the IMF (*International financial statistics*, September 2003) as well as unpublished data from the IMF Research Department have been used. They included Cape Verde, Comoros, Djibouti, Eritrea, the Gambia, Ghana, Guinea, Mauritania, and Sao Tome and Principe. In the few cases where none of the preceding institutions reported updated GDP information, WHO has used data from other institutions or national series. National series were used for Andorra, Federated States of Micronesia, Nicaragua, Niue, Palau, Samoa, Solomon Islands and Tonga. Figures for Kiribati were obtained from the Asian Development Bank. The estimates for the Democratic People's Republic of Korea and Timor-Leste originate from policy reports, as no standard statistical sources had any information on these countries. Likewise, the estimates for Afghanistan, Liberia and Somalia orginate from the web site of the United Nations Statistical Department (UNSTAT). Estimates for Equatorial Guinea originate from the Banque des Etats de l'Afrique Centrale (BEAC).

The data for China exclude estimates for Hong Kong Special Administrative Region and Macao Special Administrative Region. The health expenditure data for Jordan exclude the contributions from United Nations Relief and Works Agency for Palestine Refugees in the Near East (UNRWA), which provided basic health services support to

Palestinian refugees residing on Jordanian territories, but include UNRWA expenditures to UNRWA clinics. The 1997 and 1998 health expenditure data for Serbia and Montenegro included the provinces of Kosovo and Metohia, but for 1999 and 2000 the data excluded them, since these territories have been placed under the administration of the United Nations. The estimate for 2001 was also extrapolated without Kosovo and Metohia.

General government expenditure (GGE) includes consolidated direct outlays and indirect outlays (for example, subsidies to producers, transfers to households), including capital of all levels of government (central/federal, provincial/regional/state/district, and municipal/local authorities), social security institutions, autonomous bodies, and other extrabudgetary funds. *National accounts of OECD countries: detailed tables 1990/2001*, 2003 edition, Volume II, Table 12, row 51, supplies the information for 27 member countries. The IMF *Government finance statistics yearbook* supplies an aggregate figure for 133 central/federal governments with complements for 23 regional and 45 local/municipal governments (as well as some social security payments for health data received from the IMF). It reports central government disbursement figures in its *International financial statistics*, row 82. Several other public finance audits, executed budgets, budget plans, statistical yearbooks, web sites, World Bank and Regional Development Bank reports, and academic studies have been consulted to verify total government expenditure. Extrapolations were made on incomplete time series using, inter alia, the differential between current disbursement plus savings in the United Nations *National accounts* up to 1995 and the IMF central government disbursement level. Several national authorities have also confirmed the GGE series during the consultative process.

GGHE comprises the outlays earmarked for the enhancement of the health status of population segments and/or the distribution of medical care goods and services among population segments by:

■ central/federal, state/provincial/regional, and local/municipal authorities;
■ extrabudgetary agencies, principally social security schemes, which operate in several countries;
■ external resources (mainly grants and credits with high grant components to governments).


The figures for social security and extrabudgetary expenditure on health include purchases of health goods and services by schemes that are compulsory and under governmental control. A major hurdle has been the need to verify that no double counting occurs and that no cash benefits for sickness and/or loss of employment are included in the estimates, as these are classified as income maintenance expenditure.

All expenditures are to be accounted for, including final consumption, subsidies to producers, transfers to households (chiefly reimbursements for medical and pharmaceutical bills), investment and investment grants (also referred to as capital transfers). The classification of the functions of government, promoted by the United Nations, IMF, OECD and other institutions, sets the boundaries. In many instances, the data contained in the publications are limited to those supplied by ministries of health. Expenditures on health, however, should include expenditures where the primary intent is for health regardless of the implementing entity. An effort has been made to obtain data on health expenditures by other ministries, the armed forces, prisons, schools, universities and others, to ensure that all resources accounting for health expenditures are included. Information on external resources was received courtesy of the Development Action Committee of the OECD (DAC/OECD). A quarter of Member States explicitly monitor the external resources entering their health system, information that has been used to validate or amend the order of magnitude derived from the DAC entries.

*OECD health data 2003* supplies GGHE entries for its member countries, with some gaps for the year 2001. In addition, the data for the year 2001 for Austria, Belgium, Iceland, Japan, Luxembourg, Republic of Korea and Turkey have been largely developed by WHO as they were not yet available through the OECD. Those have been projected by WHO. NHA studies were available for 54 non-OECD countries for one or more years. The detailed information in these reports permitted a more reliable basis for estimation than in other years. The IMF *Government finance statistics* reports central government expenditure on health for 122 countries, regional government outlays for health for 23 countries, and local government outlays on health for 45 countries. The entries are not continuous time series for all countries, but the document serves as an indicator that a reporting system exists in the 122 countries. A thorough search was conducted for the relevant national publications in those countries. In some cases it was observed that expenditures reported under the government finance classification were limited to those of the ministry of health rather than all expenditures on health regardless of ministry. In such cases, other series were used to supplement that source. Government finance data, together with external resources data, statistical yearbooks, public finance reports, and analyses reporting on the implementation of health policies, have led to GGHE estimates for most WHO Member States. Information on Brunei Darussalam, for example, was accessed from national sources, but also from an International Medical Foundation of Japan data compendium *(42)*. This source provided a means for double checking health budget data for seven countries.

Several processes have been used to judge the validity of the data. For example, the aggregate expenditure obtained has been compared against inpatient care expenditure, pharmaceutical expenditure data and other records (including programme administration and other costs entering the *System of health accounts* classifications) to cross-validate the information, in order to ensure: that the outlays for which details have been assembled constitute the bulk of the government expenditure on health; that intra-government transfers are consolidated; and that the estimates obtained are judged plausible in terms of systems' descriptions. The aggregate governmental health expenditure data have also been compared with total GGE, providing an additional source of verification. Sometimes the GGHE and, therefore, the figures for total health expenditure, may be an underestimate if it is not possible to estimate for local government, nongovernmental organizations and insurance. For example THE for India may not include some agents leading to a possible underestimate of between 0.3% and 0.6% of GDP. Information for Afghanistan and Iraq was received from the Regional Office for the Eastern Mediterranean, and for Cambodia from the country office.

Private expenditure on health has been defined as the sum of expenditures by the following entities:

■ Prepaid plans and risk-pooling arrangements: the outlays of private and private social (with no government control over payment rates and participating providers but with broad guidelines from government) insurance schemes, commercial and non-profit (mutual) insurance schemes, health maintenance organizations, and other agents managing prepaid medical and paramedical benefits (including the operating costs of these schemes).

- Firms' expenditure on health: outlays by public and private enterprises for medical care and health-enhancing benefits other than payment to social security.
- Non-profit institutions serving mainly households: resources used to purchase health goods and services by entities whose status does not permit them to be a source of income, profit or other financial gain for the units that establish, control or finance them. This includes funding from internal and external sources.
- Household out-of-pocket spending: the direct outlays of households, including gratuities and in-kind payments made to health practitioners and suppliers of pharmaceuticals, therapeutic appliances, and other goods and services, whose primary intent is to contribute to the restoration or the enhancement of the health status of individuals or population groups. This includes household payments to public services, non-profit institutions or nongovernmental organizations and non-reimbursable cost sharing, deductibles, copayments and fee-for-service. It excludes payments made by enterprises which deliver medical and paramedical benefits, mandated by law or not, to their employees and payments for overseas treatment.

Most of the information on private health expenditures comes from NHA reports, statistical yearbooks and other periodicals, statistical data on official web sites, reports of nongovernmental organizations, household expenditure surveys, academic studies, and relevant reports of and data provided by central statistical offices, ministries of health, professional and trade associations. For the 30 OECD member countries they are obtained from the *OECD health data 2003*. Standard extrapolation and estimation techniques were used to obtain the figures for missing years.

## ANNEX TABLE 6

Annex Table 6 presents total expenditure on health and general government expenditure on health in per capita terms. The methodology and sources to derive THE and GGHE have been discussed in the notes to Annex Table 5. Ratios are represented in per capita terms by dividing the expenditure figures by population figures. These per capita figures are expressed first in US dollars at an average exchange rate, which is the observed annual average number of units at which a currency is traded in the banking system. It is then also presented in international dollar estimates, derived by dividing local currency units by an estimate of their purchasing power parity (PPP) compared to US dollars, i.e. a rate or measure that minimizes the consequences of differences in price levels existing between countries.

*OECD health data 2003* is the major source for population estimates for the 30 OECD member countries, just as it is for other health expenditure and macroeconomic variables. All estimates of population size and structure, other than for OECD countries, are based on demographic assessments prepared by the United Nations Population Division *(3)*. This report uses the estimates referred to as the de facto population, and not the de jure population, in each Member State. An exception was made for Serbia and Montenegro for 2001, as expenditure figures excluded the provinces of Kosovo and Metohia, which became territories under the administration of the United Nations. Estimates for Serbia and Montenegro, excluding the populations of Kosovo and Metohia, were obtained from the *Statistical yearbook of Yugoslavia 2002*, thus ensuring consistency of the basis for the numerator and denominator.

Three-quarters of the exchange rates (average for the year) have been obtained from the IMF's *International financial statistics, September 2003*, row rf. Where information was lacking, available data from the United Nations, the World Bank and ad hoc donor reports (in the case of Afghanistan for example) were used. The euro:US dollar rate has been applied for Andorra, Monaco and San Marino. The New Zealand dollar:US dollar rate has been applied for Niue. The Australian dollar:US dollar rate has been applied for Nauru and Palau. Ecuador dollarized its economy in 2000, but the entire dataset has been recalculated in dollar terms for the five-year period reported.

For OECD member countries, the OECD PPP has been used to calculate international dollars. For countries that are part of the UNECE but are not members of OECD, the UNECE PPPs were calculated on the same basis as the OECD PPP. The remaining calculations for international dollars have been estimated by WHO using methods similar to those used by the World Bank.

## ANNEX TABLE 7

In September 2000, representatives of 189 countries met at the Millennium Summit in New York and committed themselves to working towards a world in which sustaining development and eliminating poverty would have the highest priority. The Millennium Development Goals (MDGs) summarize these commitments and have been commonly accepted as a framework for measuring development progress. They are an integral part of the *Road map towards the implementation of the United Nations Millennium Declaration*, which was endorsed by the United Nations General Assembly *(43)*. The MDGs give high prominence to health: three of the eight goals and 17 indicators of progress are health-related. They assist in the development of national policy frameworks, such as poverty reduction strategies and national health policies focusing on the poor, and help track the performance of health programmes and systems. Although the MDGs do not cover the whole range of public health domains, a broad interpretation of the goals provides an opportunity to tackle important cross-cutting issues and key constraints to health and development. Some common constraints include human resources for health, health care financing and government capacity, especially in the area of stewardship.

WHO is working closely with other United Nations agencies in reporting on the health-related MDGs. WHO shares lead agency responsibility with UNICEF for reporting on child mortality, maternal health, childhood nutritional status, malaria prevention measures and access to clean water, and with UNAIDS on HIV prevention. At global level, interagency mechanisms have been established to ensure technical coherence in the collection, analysis and validation of MDG-related data, and to define reporting responsibilities. At country level, WHO, through its country representatives, is the lead authority for the health content of the MDGs within United Nations country teams.

Annex Table 7 provides baseline information for WHO Member States for selected MDG health indicators. The notes below summarize definitions, measurement methods, sources of information and give further references for the MDG health indicators.

### Percentage of underweight children among children under five years of age

The internationally recommended way to assess malnutrition at population level is to take body measurements (e.g. weight and height) and to relate them to an individual's age or height. In children the three most commonly used anthropometric indices are weight-for-height, height-for-age and weight-for-age. Anthropometric values are compared across individuals or populations in relation to a set of reference values and the choice of the reference population has a significant impact on the proportion of children identified as being undernourished and overnourished. Since the late 1970s WHO has been recommending the National Center for Health Statistics (NCHS) growth reference, the so-called NCHS/WHO international reference population, for the comparison of child growth data.

The data sources presented in Annex Table 7 are population-based surveys which fulfil the following main criteria:

- a defined population-based sampling frame;
- a probabilistic sampling procedure involving at least 400 children;
- use of standard anthropometric measurement techniques;
- presentation of prevalence of underweight in z-scores cut-off points (i.e. standard deviation scores) in relation to the NCHS/WHO international reference or availability of the raw data, allowing a standardized analysis.

The figures shown in the table are estimated for each Member State from the most recent population-based survey available that fulfil these criteria *(44–46)*.

## Under-five mortality rate

Under-five mortality rate is the probability (expressed as rate per 1000 live births) of a child born in a specific year dying before reaching five years of age, if subject to current age-specific mortality rates. Under-five mortality represents over 90% of child deaths under the age of 18 worldwide.

Age-specific mortality rates calculated from birth and death data are derived from vital registration, census, and/or household surveys. When using household surveys, under-five mortality estimates are obtained in a direct Multiple Indicators Cluster Survey (MICS) (using birth history as in demographic and health surveys) or in an indirect way (such as in MICS Brass method). When mortality is high, the indirect method tends to overestimate infant mortality and underestimate child mortality.

Sources used for the calculation of child mortality rates for WHO Member States include the demographic and health surveys, MICS, national vital registration systems and national censuses *(16)*. Under-five mortality rates for 2000 published here have been revised for consistency with the 2002 figures given in Annex Table 1, using the same cycle of information, and may differ from previously published estimates of under-five mortality for the year 2000.

## Infant mortality rate

Infant mortality rate is the probability (expressed as rate per 1000 live births) of a child born in a specific year dying before reaching one year of age, if subject to current age-specific mortality rates.

When using household surveys, infant mortality estimates are obtained in a direct (using birth history as in demographic and health surveys) or indirect way (such as in MICS Brass method ). When using indirect estimates, the infant mortality estimates must be consistent with the under-five mortality estimates. Sources used for the calculation of infant mortality rates for WHO Member States include national vital registration systems, demographic and health surveys, MICS, and national censuses *(16)*.

## Percentage of one-year-old children immunized against measles

Estimates of immunization coverage are generally based on two sources of empirical data: reports of vaccinations performed by service providers (routinely recorded data) and surveys containing items on children's vaccination history (coverage surveys). For estimates based on routinely recorded data, the immunization coverage is derived by dividing the total number of vaccinations given by the number of children in the target population. For most vaccines the target population is the national annual number of births or number of surviving infants (this may vary depending on countries' policies and the specific vaccine).

For estimates based on immunization coverage surveys the denominator corresponds to children aged 12–23 months who had received at least one measles vaccination by the time of the survey or had done so before the age of 12 months.

Measles immunization coverage for 2001 is based on the WHO and UNICEF review of coverage data based on administrative records, surveys, national reports and consultation with local and regional experts *(47–49)*.

## Maternal mortality ratio

*The International statistical classification of diseases and related health problems, tenth revision* (ICD-10) defines a maternal death as: the death of a woman while pregnant or within 42 days of termination of pregnancy, irrespective of the duration and site of the pregnancy, from any cause related to or aggravated by the pregnancy or its management, but not from accidental or incidental causes. Measuring maternal mortality both reliably and in a cost-effective way is not possible except where comprehensive registration of deaths and causes of death exists. Elsewhere, survey methods or models have to be used to estimate levels of maternal mortality. WHO recommends a variety of measurement methods depending on a country's vital registration system and its capacity to provide direct observation of maternal deaths.

For Member States with good vital registration (90% coverage, medical certification of cause of death), the vital registration system is the main source for direct counting of maternal deaths in a given period. Misclassification and miscoding of maternal deaths are frequent, especially where the pregnancy status of the woman is not included in the death certificate. Adjustment methods are therefore required to produce a more accurate estimate of maternal mortality (reported maternal deaths are adjusted by a nationally reported adjustment factor if available, or by 1.5 if not).

For Member States with incomplete vital registration, but with maternal mortality estimates derived from population-based surveys, demographic and health survey and the MICS use a sibling survival method, asking respondents questions about the survival of their adult sisters in relation to the period around pregnancy and childbirth.

For Member States with no reliable national data on maternal mortality, statistical modelling is the only possibility. WHO, UNICEF and UNFPA have developed model-based estimates. A statistical model is used to estimate the proportion of deaths of women of reproductive age from maternal causes. Estimates of the number of maternal deaths are then obtained by applying this proportion to the best available figure of the total number of deaths among women in reproductive age, which is currently the WHO HIV-adjusted envelope of female deaths.

Alternative methods used include reviews of all deaths of women of reproductive age (Reproductive Age Mortality Study (RAMOS)), longitudinal studies of pregnant women, repeated large-scale household surveys and inclusion of maternal mortality-related questions in national censuses. All these methods, however, still rely on accurate reporting of deaths of pregnant women and of the cause of death, which are difficult to obtain.

Full details of methods and data sources used by WHO, UNICEF and UNFPA are given in a recent joint publication, *Maternal mortality in 2000: estimates developed by WHO, UNICEF and UNFPA (14)*.

## Percentage of live births attended by skilled health personnel

The term skilled attendant refers exclusively to people with midwifery skills (for example doctors, midwives and nurses) who have been trained to proficiency in the skills necessary to manage normal deliveries and diagnose or manage obstetric complications. They must be able to manage normal labour and delivery, recognize the onset of complications, perform essential interventions, start treatment, and supervise the referral of mother and baby for interventions that are beyond their competence or not possible in the setting in question. Traditional birth attendants, trained or not, are excluded from the category of skilled attendant at delivery.

For most countries, the main sources of information on skilled attendance at delivery are household surveys *(14)*. While efforts are made to standardize definitions of skilled birth attendants, there are concerns about the comparability of some of the results across countries and within countries at different times. Although WHO has defined the specific competencies that the skilled attendant should have, there have been no systematic efforts to ensure that the groups classified under the heading of skilled attendant actually have them. In some settings, groups of providers in the skilled attendant category include those unlikely to have the skills and experience required to manage childbirth complications safely.

Issues related to the way data on skilled attendance at delivery are collected include:

- the extent to which respondents can accurately report the skills of the birth attendant;
- potential bias introduced by the fact that most household surveys report on live births in the past five years, thus missing many adverse health outcomes which are disproportionately concentrated among women experiencing adverse outcomes such as stillbirths or miscarriages;
- the potential overrepresentation of women with short birth intervals who are almost certain to exhibit other risk factors for adverse pregnancy outcome, including high parity, low levels of education and absence of contact with other health services such as family planning. Surveys should only include the most recent birth for the survey period.

## HIV prevalence among adults aged 15 to 49 years

This indicator measures the proportion of the total population aged 15 to 49 years infected with HIV. It includes people who have progressed to AIDS, but does not include people who have died from the disease. Estimates of HIV prevalence have been developed by UNAIDS and WHO for most Member States and revised periodically to account for new data and improved methods *(7, 8, 50)*. For the most recent round of estimates, two different types of model have been used, depending on the nature of the epidemic in a particular country. For generalized epidemics, in which infection is spread primarily through heterosexual contact, a simple epidemiological model was used to estimate epidemic curves based on sentinel surveillance data on HIV seroprevalence. For countries with epidemics concentrated in high-risk groups, prevalence estimates were derived from the estimated population size and prevalence surveillance data in each high-risk category.

The HIV prevalence figures shown for 2000 have been revised from previously published figures to take into account new data and are consistent with the latest UNAIDS and WHO estimates of prevalences for 2003.

For a few countries where prevalence estimates for HIV seropositive cases (including

AIDS) are not directly available, they have been derived by scaling regional prevalence estimates by the ratio of country-specific HIV mortality to regional HIV mortality. Because different countries may be at different phases of the epidemic, the relationship between prevalence and mortality may vary across countries.

## Malaria mortality rate

Malaria-specific mortality cannot be monitored routinely in most malaria endemic African countries since there are few systems in place for reliable measurement of malaria deaths. Symptoms and signs of malaria (such as fever or convulsions) are non-specific and overlap with other diseases, so verbal autopsy methods have low sensitivity and specificity for malaria. Since malaria may increase the susceptibility of young children to other infections, many child deaths may be malaria-related rather than directly attributable to malaria. Moreover, a majority of deaths do not occur in hospitals and are not routinely recorded in the health information system, and these are unlikely to be picked up in the – usually incomplete – vital registration.

Malaria mortality estimates for all regions except the African Region were derived from the cause-of-death data sources described above in the notes to Annex Table 2. For Africa, country-specific estimates of malaria mortality were based on analyses by Snow et al. *(13)* and updated using the most recent geographical distributions produced by malaria risks in Africa (MARA) mapping, together with available information on total child mortality rates, and the contributions of other specific causes. Work is currently under way in collaboration with expert groups to refine and revise these country-specific estimates of malaria mortality.

## Tuberculosis prevalence (excluding HIV-infected people)

In 1997 WHO began to develop country estimates of tuberculosis incidence, prevalence and mortality. The data sources and methods have been described in detail elsewhere *(6)*. Briefly, estimates of incidence are derived from case notifications adjusted by estimated case detection rates, prevalence data on active disease combined with estimates of average case durations, or estimates of infection risk multiplied by a scalar factor relating incidence of smear-positive pulmonary tuberculosis to annual risks of infection.

Since the original estimates for 1997 were completed, revised and updated estimates have been prepared. The majority of countries reporting to WHO have provided notification data with interpretable trends, and with no other evidence for a significant change in the case detection rate. For most countries, therefore, except those with evidence of changes in case detection rates, it has been assumed that trends in notification rates represent trends in incidence rates. Annual reports on tuberculosis control have included further details on surveillance methods, case notifications and incidence estimates by country *(51)*.

Tuberculosis cases include all people in whom tuberculosis has been bacteriologically confirmed or diagnosed by a clinician: *definite cases* (positive culture for the mycobacterium tuberculosis), *smear-positive pulmonary cases, smear-negative pulmonary cases with clinical evidence, extrapulmonary tuberculosis*, and *relapse cases* (previously declared cured case with new episode).

Tuberculosis prevalence rates reported here are for all forms of tuberculosis excluding cases in HIV-positive people. Under the rules of the International Classification of Diseases, HIV is classified as the underlying cause of morbidity or death in HIV-positive people with tuberculosis. Although total tuberculosis prevalence rates, including cases of tuberculosis in HIV-positive people, have been reported elsewhere for this MDG indicator, Annex Table 7 reports the prevalence of tuberculosis not associated with HIV infection, for consistency with the tuberculosis mortality indicator. The total prevalence of tuberculosis in 2000 is estimated at approximately 8 million; an additional 700 000 HIV-positive people have the disease.

Estimated prevalence of all forms of tuberculosis (excluding HIV-positive people) for 2000 was calculated by multiplying estimated incidence by estimated duration. Country-specific estimates of duration were weighted for the proportion of cases treated and the proportion smear-positive. These prevalences may differ from previously published figures for 2000, as they have been updated to take into account new data from Member States. For Member States where vital registration data have been used to estimate tuberculosis mortality, incidence and prevalence estimates have been revised to be consistent with estimated deaths, estimated case-fatality rates for treated and untreated cases, and the proportion of incident cases treated.

## Tuberculosis mortality rate

The *death rate* from tuberculosis is estimated from incidence by multiplying by the estimated case-fatality rate, weighted for the proportion of cases treated and the proportion of smear-positive cases *(6, 51)*. Tuberculosis deaths in HIV-infected individuals are not included but are attributed to HIV/AIDS. For Member States with reasonably good-quality or complete death registration data, death rates are derived from direct observation and counting of registered tuberculosis deaths. These death rates may differ from previously published figures for 2000, as they have been updated to take into account new data from Member States.

## Proportions of smear-positive tuberculosis cases detected and successfully treated under DOTS

The recommended approach to tuberculosis control is via DOTS, an inexpensive strategy that could prevent millions of cases and deaths in years to come. DOTS is a five-pronged strategy for tuberculosis control consisting of: (i) sustained government commitment; (ii) detection of cases through sputum smear microscopy among symptomatic people; (iii) regular and uninterrupted supply of high-quality drugs; (iv) 6–8 months of regularly supervised treatment (including direct observation of drug-taking for at least the first two months); (v) reporting systems to monitor treatment progress and programme performance.

The success of DOTS depends on expanding case detection while ensuring high treatment success rates. These two indicators reflect the two main national targets of the strategy to be achieved for each implementing country: 85% treatment success rate and 70% case detection rate. Many of the 155 national DOTS programmes in existence by the end of 2001 have shown that they can achieve high treatment success rates, close to or exceeding the target of 85%. The global average treatment success rate for DOTS programmes was 82% for the cohort of patients registered in 2000, though cure rates tend to be lower, and death rates higher, where drug resistance is frequent or HIV prevalence is high.

These indicators are constructed from country notification of cases detected and successfully treated *(51)*. The *DOTS detection rate* is the percentage of estimated new infectious tuberculosis cases detected under the DOTS case detection and treatment strategy. Case notifications represent only a fraction of the true number of cases arising in a country because of incomplete coverage by health services, inaccurate diagnosis, or deficient recording and reporting.

The *DOTS treatment success rate* is the percentage of new, registered smear-positive (infectious) cases that were cured (identified as a bacteriological conversion from positive to negative) or in which a full course of DOTS treatment was completed. "Successfully treated" is therefore the sum of "cured" cases and the cases that "completed the full treatment course". WHO routinely compiles data on the six standard, mutually exclusive outcomes of treatment. Figures are reported as percentages of all registered cases, so that the six possible outcomes plus the fraction of cases not evaluated sum to 100%. Although treatment success is expressed as a percentage, it is usually referred to as the "treatment success rate".

## Percentage of population using solid fuels

Solid fuels include biomass fuels such as wood, agricultural residues, animal dung, charcoal and coal. In many countries in which a large proportion of the population cooks with solid fuels, household energy data are widely, although not universally, available. This is the case for around 60 countries. For countries where there are no data, WHO has developed a statistical model to predict household solid fuel use from development-related parameters. As countries develop, people gradually shift from solid to cleaner fuels.

A wide range of development indicators were tested in the modelling process, including average annual growth rates, per capita electricity and petroleum consumption, Gini coefficient, per capita fuel wood production, and traditional fuel use at the national level. As information on traditional fuel use at the national level performs similarly to gross national product (GNP) per capita, but GNP per capita is more reliable, more routinely updated, and widely available, the model uses per capita GNP rather than traditional fuel use. The final model includes percentage rural population, location within the WHO Eastern Mediterranean Region (thought to be important as it indicates oil production), GNP per capita (log transformed), and per capita petroleum use *(52)*. This is consistent with the theory that household solid fuel use declines with increases in economic growth and urbanization.

## Percentage of population with sustainable access to an improved water source

The monitoring of the population with access to adequate water supply has proved problematic, because the data are often limited when estimated by service providers. Therefore WHO and UNICEF have now turned to consumer-based information to estimate water and sanitation coverage *(53)*. For data collection, two main sources are used: household surveys and assessment questionnaires (to complement survey data or to provide estimates where survey data are not available). This allows for a far more detailed picture of the water supply technologies being used. It also captures information related to use and breakdown of self-built water facilities, of which service providers may be unaware.

Population-based surveys do not provide specific information on the adequacy of water supply facilities. It is assumed that certain types of technology are safer than others and that some of them cannot be considered as "coverage". The term "safe" was replaced with "improved". The population with access to improved water supply is considered to be covered. It is assumed that if the user has access to an "improved source" then such a source would be likely to provide 20 litres per capita per day at a distance no longer than 1000 metres. The following technologies represent improved water supply: household connection, public standpipe, borehole, protected dug well, protected spring, rainwater collection.

## Percentage of urban population with access to improved sanitation

The monitoring of access to adequate sanitation facilities has proved to be complicated for the same reasons that apply to water source. WHO and UNICEF have now turned to consumer-based information to estimate sanitation coverage by using household surveys and assessment questionnaires (to complement survey data or to provide estimates where survey data are not available) as the two main sources *(53)*. This allows for a far more detailed picture of the sanitation technologies being used. It also captures information related to usage and breakdown of self-built facilities, of which service providers may be unaware.

As for access to improved water, population-based surveys do not provide specific information on the adequacy of sanitation facilities. By assuming that certain types of technology are better than others and that some of them cannot be considered as "coverage", the term "adequate" was replaced with "improved" to accommodate these limitations. The following technologies represent improved sanitation: connection to a public sewer, connection to septic system, pour-flush latrine, simple pit latrine, ventilated improved pit latrine.

## References

1. Lopez AD, Ahmad O, Guillot M, Ferguson BD, Salomon JA, Murray CJL et al. *World mortality in 2000: life tables for 191 countries*. Geneva, World Health Organization, 2002.
2. *International database*. Washington, DC, United States Census Bureau (http://www. census.gov/ipc/www/idbnew.html, accessed 23 February 2004).
3. *World population prospects – the 2002 revision*. New York, United Nations Population Division, 2003.
4. Murray CJL, Ferguson BD, Lopez AD, Guillot M, Salomon JA, Ahmad O. Modified logit life table system: principles, empirical validation and application. *Population Studies*, 2003, 57:1–18.
5. Salomon JA, Mathers CD, Murray CJL, Ferguson B. *Methods for life expectancy and healthy life expectancy uncertainty analysis*. Geneva, World Health Organization, 2002 (GPE Discussion Paper No. 10; http://www.who.int/evidence, accessed 23 February 2004).
6. Dye C, Scheele S, Dolin P, Pathania V, Raviglione M. Global burden of tuberculosis: estimated incidence, prevalence and mortality by country. *JAMA*, 2002, 282:677–686.
7. UNAIDS Reference Group on Estimates Modelling and Projections. Improved methods and assumptions for estimation and projection of HIV/AIDS epidemics. *AIDS*, 2002, 16:1–16.
8. UNAIDS/WHO. *AIDS epidemic update 2003*. Geneva, Joint United Nations Programme on HIV/AIDS and World Health Organization, 2003.
9. Boschi-Pinto C, Tomaskovic L, Gouws E, Shibuya K. *Diarrhoea mortality in under-fives in the developing world*. Geneva, World Health Organization (in press).
10. Stein C, Birmingham M, Kurian M, Duclos P, Strebel P. The global burden of measles in the year 2000 – a model that uses country-specific indicators. *Journal of Infectious Diseases*, 2003, 187(Suppl. 1):S8–S14.
11. Crowcroft NS, Stein C, Duclos P, Birmingham M. How to best estimate the global burden of pertussis? *Lancet Infectious Diseases*, 2003, 3:413–418.
12. Williams BG, Gouws E, Boschi-Pinto C, Bryce J, Dye C. Estimates of world-wide distribution of child deaths from acute respiratory infections. *Lancet*, 2002, 2:25–32.
13. Snow RW, Craig M, Deichmann U, Marsh K. Estimating mortality, morbidity and disability due to malaria among Africa's non-pregnant population. *Bulletin of the World Health*

*Organization*, 1999, 77:624–640.

14. Abouzahr C, Wardlaw T. *Maternal mortality in 2000: estimates developed by WHO, UNICEF and UNFPA*. Geneva, World Health Organization, 2003. (http://wwwstage/reproductive-health/publications/maternal_mortality_2000/index.html, accessed 25 February 2004).

15. Mathers CD, Shibuya K, Boschi-Pinto C, Lopez AD, Murray CJ. Global and regional estimates of cancer mortality and incidence by site: I. Application of regional cancer survival model to estimate cancer mortality distribution by site. *BMC Cancer*, 2002, 2:36.

16. Mathers CD, Bernard C, Iburg K, Inoue M, Ma Fat D, Shibuya K et al. *The global burden of disease in 2002: data sources, methods and results*. Geneva, World Health Organization, 2003 (GPE Discussion Paper No. 54; http://www.who.int/evidence, accessed 23 February 2004).

17. Murray CJL, Lopez AD, eds. *The global burden of disease: a comprehensive assessment of mortality and disability from diseases, injuries and risk factors in 1990 and projected to 2020*. Cambridge, MA, Harvard School of Public Health on behalf of the World Health Organization and the World Bank, 1996 (Global Burden of Disease and Injury Series, Vol. 1).

18. Salomon JA, Murray CJL. The epidemiologic transition revisited: compositional models for causes of death by age and sex. *Population and Development Review*, 2002, 28:205–228.

19. Lozano R, Murray CJL, Lopez AD, Satoh T. *Miscoding and misclassification of ischaemic heart disease mortality*. Geneva, World Health Organization, 2001 (GPE Discussion Paper No. 12).

20. Murray CJL, Salomon JA, Mathers CD. A critical examination of summary measures of population health. *Bulletin of the World Health Organization*, 2000, 78:981–994.

21. Murray CJL, Mathers CD, Salomon JA, Lopez AD. Health gaps: an overview and critical appraisal. In: Murray CJL, Salomon JA, Mathers CD, Lopez AD, eds. *Summary measures of population health: concepts, ethics, measurement and applications*. Geneva, World Health Organization, 2002 (http://www.who.int/pub/smph/en/index.html, accessed 23 February 2004).

22. Mathers CD, Sadana R, Salomon JA, Murray CJL, Lopez AD. Healthy life expectancy in 191 countries, 1999. *Lancet*, 2001, 357:1685–1691.

23. Mathers CD, Murray CJL, Salomon JA, Sadana R, Tandon A, Lopez AD et al. Healthy life expectancy: comparison of OECD countries in 2001. *Australian and New Zealand Journal of Public Health*, 2003, 27:5–11.

24. Sadana R, Mathers CD, Lopez AD, Murray CJL, Moesgaard-Iburg K. Comparative analysis of more than 50 household surveys of health status. In: Murray CJL, Salomon JA, Mathers CD, Lopez AD, eds. *Summary measures of population health: concepts, ethics, measurement and applications*. Geneva, World Health Organization, 2002 (http://www.who.int/pub/smph/en/index.html, accessed 23 February 2004)

25. King G, Murray CJL, Salomon JA, Tandon A. Enhancing the validity and cross-cultural comparability of measurement in survey research. *American Political Science Review*, 2003, 93:567–583.

26. Üstün TB, Chatterji S, Villanueva M, Bendib L, Çelik C, Sadana R et al. WHO multi-country survey study on health and responsiveness, 2000–2001. In: Murray CJL, Evans D, eds. *Health systems performance assessment: debates, methods and empiricism*. Geneva, World Health Organization, 2003 (http://www.who.int/health-systems-performance, accessed 23 February 2004).

27. *International classification of functioning, disability and health* (ICF). Geneva, World Health Organization, 2001.

28. Mathers CD, Murray CJL, Salomon JA. Methods for measuring healthy life expectancy. In: Murray CJL, Evans D, eds. *Health systems performance assessment: debates, methods and empiricism*. Geneva, World Health Organization, 2003 (http://www.who.int/health-systems-performance, accessed 23 February 2004).

29. Salomon JA, Murray CJL, Üstün TB, Chatterji S. Health state valuations in summary measures of population health. In: Murray CJL, Evans D, eds. *Health systems performance assessment: debates, methods and empiricism*. Geneva, World Health Organization, 2003 (http://www.who.int/health-systems-performance, accessed 23 February 2004).

30. Anand S, Ammar W, Evans T, Hasegawa T, Kissimova-Skarbek K, Langer A et al. Report on the Scientific Peer Review Group on Health Systems Performance Assessment. In: Murray CJL, Evans D, eds. *Health systems performance assessment: debates, methods and empiricism*. Geneva, World Health Organization, 2003 (http://www.who.int/health-systems-performance, accessed 23 February 2004).

31. WHO/World Bank/USAID. *Guide to producing national health accounts with special applications for low-income and middle-income countries*. Geneva, World Health Organization, 2003 (http://whqlibdoc.who.int/publications/2003/9241546077.pdf, accessed 23 February 2004).

32. *A system of health accounts*. Paris, Organisation for Economic Co-operation and Development, 2000 (http://www.oecd.org/dataoecd/41/4/1841456.pdf, accessed 23 February 2004).

33. OECD/IMF/World Bank/United Nations/Eurostat. *System of national accounts 1993*. New York, United Nations, 1994.

34. *Government finance statistics yearbook, 2002*. Washington, DC, International Monetary Fund, 2002.

35. *International financial statistics yearbook, 2003*. Washington, DC, International Monetary Fund, 2003.

36. *International financial statistics, September 2003*. Washington, DC, International Monetary Fund.

37. *Key indicators 2002*. Manila, Asian Development Bank, 2002.

38. *OECD health data 2003*. Paris, Organisation for Economic Co-operation and Development, 2003.

39. *International development statistics* [CD-ROM]. Paris, Organisation for Economic Co-operation and Development, Development Assistance Committee, 2003.

40. *National accounts statistics: main aggregates and detailed tables*, 2000. New York, United Nations, 2002.

41. *National accounts of OECD countries: detailed tables 1990/2001*, 2003 edition, Volume II. Paris, Organisation for Economic Co-operation and Development, 2003.

42. *Southeast Asian Medical Information Center health statistics 2002*. Tokyo, The International Medical Foundation of Japan, 2003.

43. *Road map towards the implementation of the United Nations Millennium Declaration*. New York, United Nations, 2002 (United Nations General Assembly document A56/326).

44. *Physical status: the use and interpretation of anthropometry. Report of a WHO Expert Committee*. Geneva, World Health Organization, 1995 (WHO Technical Report Series, No. 854).

45. WHO Department of Nutrition for Health and Development. *WHO Global Database on Child Growth and Malnutrition* (www.who.int/nutgrowthdb, accessed 23 February 2004).

46. de Onis M, Blössner M. The World Health Organization Global Database on Child Growth and Malnutrition: methodology and applications. *International Journal of Epidemiology*, 2003, 32:518–526.

47. UNICEF. *UNICEF statistics: routine immunization* (http://www.childinfo.org/eddb/immuni/index.htm, accessed 23 February 2004).

48. WHO/UNICEF. *WHO and UNICEF estimates of national immunization coverage* (http://www.who.int/vaccines-surveillance/WHOUNICEF_Coverage_Review/, accessed 23 February 2004).

49. WHO. *Vaccines, immunizations and biologicals* (http://www.who.int/vaccines-surveillance/DataInfo.htm, accessed 23 February 2004).

50. *HIV/AIDS epidemiological surveillance update for the WHO African Region 2002*. Harare, World Health Organization Regional Office for Africa, 2003.

51. *WHO report 2003: global tuberculosis control. Surveillance, planning and financing*. Geneva, World Health Organization, 2003 (WHO/CDS/TB/2003.316).

52. *The world health report 2002 – Reducing risks, promoting healthy life*. Geneva, World Health Organization, 2002.

53. WHO/UNICEF. *Global water supply and sanitation assessment 2000 report*. New York, United Nations children's Fund; Geneva, World Health Organization, 2000.

## Annex Table 1 Basic indicators for all WHO Member States

Figures computed by WHO to assure comparability;[a] they are not necessarily the official statistics of Member States, which may use alternative rigorous methods.

| | | POPULATION ESTIMATES | | | | | | | | | LIFE EXPECTANCY AT BIRTH (YEARS) |
|---|---|---|---|---|---|---|---|---|---|---|---|
| | | Total population (000) | Annual growth rate (%) | Dependency ratio (per 100) | | Percentage of population aged 60+ years | | Total fertility rate | | | Both sexes |
| | Member State | 2002 | 1992–2002 | 1992 | 2002 | 1992 | 2002 | 1992 | 2002 | | 2002 |
| 1 | Afghanistan | 22 930 | 3.8 | 88 | 86 | 4.7 | 4.7 | 7.0 | 6.8 | | 42.6 |
| 2 | Albania | 3 141 | -0.4 | 60 | 53 | 7.9 | 9.5 | 2.9 | 2.3 | | 70.4 |
| 3 | Algeria | 31 266 | 1.8 | 82 | 60 | 5.7 | 6.1 | 4.2 | 2.8 | | 69.4 |
| 4 | Andorra | 69 | 1.8 | 48 | 46 | 20.0 | 21.6 | 1.4 | 1.3 | | 80.3 |
| 5 | Angola | 13 184 | 2.9 | 97 | 101 | 4.6 | 4.4 | 7.2 | 7.2 | | 39.9 |
| 6 | Antigua and Barbuda | 73 | 1.2 | 63 | 56 | 9.2 | 10.5 | 1.8 | 1.6 | | 71.4 |
| 7 | Argentina | 37 981 | 1.3 | 64 | 59 | 13.0 | 13.5 | 2.8 | 2.5 | | 74.4 |
| 8 | Armenia | 3 072 | -1.3 | 57 | 44 | 10.5 | 13.1 | 2.2 | 1.2 | | 70.0 |
| 9 | Australia | 19 544 | 1.2 | 50 | 48 | 15.6 | 16.7 | 1.9 | 1.7 | | 80.4 |
| 10 | Austria | 8 111 | 0.3 | 48 | 47 | 19.9 | 21.3 | 1.5 | 1.3 | | 79.4 |
| 11 | Azerbaijan | 8 297 | 1.1 | 63 | 57 | 7.6 | 9.2 | 2.8 | 2.1 | | 65.8 |
| 12 | Bahamas | 310 | 1.5 | 58 | 53 | 6.8 | 8.5 | 2.6 | 2.3 | | 72.6 |
| 13 | Bahrain | 709 | 3.0 | 51 | 47 | 3.7 | 4.0 | 3.5 | 2.7 | | 73.2 |
| 14 | Bangladesh | 143 809 | 2.3 | 81 | 71 | 4.8 | 5.1 | 4.4 | 3.5 | | 62.6 |
| 15 | Barbados | 269 | 0.4 | 55 | 43 | 15.0 | 13.1 | 1.6 | 1.5 | | 74.3 |
| 16 | Belarus | 9 940 | -0.4 | 52 | 46 | 17.4 | 19.3 | 1.7 | 1.2 | | 68.3 |
| 17 | Belgium | 10 296 | 0.3 | 50 | 53 | 20.9 | 22.2 | 1.6 | 1.7 | | 78.4 |
| 18 | Belize | 251 | 2.5 | 91 | 73 | 6.0 | 5.9 | 4.4 | 3.2 | | 69.7 |
| 19 | Benin | 6 558 | 2.8 | 105 | 93 | 4.6 | 4.1 | 6.5 | 5.7 | | 51.2 |
| 20 | Bhutan | 2 190 | 2.3 | 88 | 86 | 6.1 | 6.5 | 5.8 | 5.1 | | 61.3 |
| 21 | Bolivia | 8 645 | 2.2 | 81 | 77 | 6.1 | 6.6 | 4.8 | 3.9 | | 63.2 |
| 22 | Bosnia and Herzegovina | 4 126 | 0.4 | 43 | 40 | 11.1 | 15.3 | 1.6 | 1.3 | | 72.8 |
| 23 | Botswana | 1 770 | 2.1 | 89 | 74 | 3.7 | 4.4 | 4.5 | 3.7 | | 40.4 |
| 24 | Brazil | 176 257 | 1.4 | 63 | 51 | 6.8 | 8.1 | 2.6 | 2.2 | | 68.9 |
| 25 | Brunei Darussalam | 350 | 2.6 | 57 | 51 | 4.1 | 4.5 | 3.1 | 2.5 | | 76.1 |
| 26 | Bulgaria | 7 965 | -0.8 | 50 | 45 | 19.9 | 21.7 | 1.5 | 1.1 | | 72.2 |
| 27 | Burkina Faso | 12 624 | 2.9 | 108 | 106 | 4.5 | 4.0 | 7.1 | 6.7 | | 41.7 |
| 28 | Burundi | 6 602 | 1.3 | 97 | 99 | 4.6 | 4.4 | 6.8 | 6.8 | | 40.8 |
| 29 | Cambodia | 13 810 | 2.8 | 98 | 81 | 4.4 | 4.6 | 5.5 | 4.8 | | 54.6 |
| 30 | Cameroon | 15 729 | 2.4 | 94 | 86 | 5.5 | 5.6 | 5.7 | 4.7 | | 48.1 |
| 31 | Canada | 31 271 | 1.0 | 47 | 45 | 15.8 | 17.1 | 1.7 | 1.5 | | 79.8 |
| 32 | Cape Verde | 454 | 2.2 | 103 | 80 | 6.6 | 6.3 | 4.8 | 3.4 | | 70.1 |
| 33 | Central African Republic | 3 819 | 2.1 | 89 | 89 | 6.1 | 6.1 | 5.6 | 5.0 | | 42.9 |
| 34 | Chad | 8 348 | 3.1 | 96 | 99 | 5.2 | 4.9 | 6.7 | 6.7 | | 47.7 |
| 35 | Chile | 15 613 | 1.4 | 57 | 54 | 9.2 | 10.7 | 2.5 | 2.4 | | 76.7 |
| 36 | China | 1 302 307 | 0.9 | 49 | 44 | 8.6 | 10.0 | 2.0 | 1.8 | | 71.1 |
| 37 | Colombia | 43 526 | 1.8 | 66 | 59 | 6.4 | 7.1 | 3.0 | 2.6 | | 71.8 |
| 38 | Comoros | 747 | 3.0 | 95 | 82 | 4.0 | 4.2 | 5.9 | 4.9 | | 63.3 |
| 39 | Congo | 3 633 | 3.2 | 96 | 99 | 4.8 | 4.6 | 6.3 | 6.3 | | 53.1 |
| 40 | Cook Islands | 18 | -0.2 | 71 | 65 | 6.2 | 7.2 | 4.0 | 3.2 | | 71.6 |
| 41 | Costa Rica | 4 094 | 2.4 | 68 | 56 | 7.1 | 7.9 | 3.0 | 2.3 | | 77.1 |
| 42 | Côte d'Ivoire | 16 365 | 2.1 | 94 | 82 | 4.4 | 5.2 | 6.1 | 4.8 | | 45.3 |
| 43 | Croatia | 4 439 | -0.6 | 46 | 49 | 18.3 | 21.7 | 1.6 | 1.6 | | 74.8 |
| 44 | Cuba | 11 271 | 0.4 | 45 | 44 | 11.9 | 14.5 | 1.6 | 1.6 | | 77.1 |
| 45 | Cyprus | 796 | 1.2 | 58 | 51 | 14.8 | 16.1 | 2.3 | 1.9 | | 77.3 |
| 46 | Czech Republic | 10 246 | -0.1 | 50 | 42 | 17.8 | 18.8 | 1.7 | 1.2 | | 75.8 |
| 47 | Democratic People's Republic of Korea | 22 541 | 0.9 | 47 | 48 | 8.0 | 10.6 | 2.3 | 2.0 | | 65.8 |
| 48 | Democratic Republic of the Congo | 51 201 | 2.4 | 100 | 98 | 4.4 | 4.2 | 6.7 | 6.7 | | 43.5 |
| 49 | Denmark | 5 351 | 0.3 | 48 | 50 | 20.2 | 20.4 | 1.7 | 1.8 | | 77.2 |
| 50 | Djibouti | 693 | 2.3 | 85 | 86 | 4.6 | 5.1 | 6.3 | 5.7 | | 49.6 |
| 51 | Dominica | 78 | 0.7 | 63 | 56 | 9.2 | 10.5 | 2.0 | 1.8 | | 73.3 |
| 52 | Dominican Republic | 8 616 | 1.7 | 70 | 59 | 5.6 | 6.9 | 3.2 | 2.7 | | 68.0 |
| 53 | Ecuador | 12 810 | 1.8 | 73 | 62 | 6.3 | 7.3 | 3.6 | 2.8 | | 70.6 |
| 54 | Egypt | 70 507 | 1.9 | 80 | 66 | 6.3 | 6.9 | 4.1 | 3.3 | | 67.1 |
| 55 | El Salvador | 6 415 | 1.9 | 78 | 68 | 6.6 | 7.5 | 3.6 | 2.9 | | 69.7 |

| | LIFE EXPECTANCY AT BIRTH (YEARS) | | | | PROBABILITY OF DYING (PER 1000) | | | | | | | |
|---|---|---|---|---|---|---|---|---|---|---|---|---|
| | | | | | Under age 5 years | | | | Between ages 15 and 60 years | | | |
| | Males | | Females | | Males | | Females | | Males | | Females | |
| | 2002 | Uncertainty | 2002 | Uncertainty | 2002 | Uncertainty | 2002 | Uncertainty | 2002 | Uncertainty | 2002 | Uncertainty |
| 1 | 41.9 | 32.0 - 49.5 | 43.4 | 31.3 - 53.2 | 258 | 208 - 310 | 256 | 205 - 306 | 494 | 335 - 731 | 413 | 192 - 705 |
| 2 | 67.3 | 65.9 - 68.7 | 74.1 | 73.0 - 75.0 | 27 | 13 - 41 | 23 | 11 - 34 | 167 | 137 - 199 | 94 | 79 - 111 |
| 3 | 67.5 | 66.2 - 69.1 | 71.2 | 69.8 - 72.5 | 54 | 43 - 64 | 43 | 35 - 52 | 170 | 152 - 187 | 128 | 112 - 146 |
| 4 | 76.8 | 76.0 - 77.8 | 83.7 | 83.0 - 84.3 | 5 | 5 - 6 | 4 | 4 - 5 | 113 | 101 - 125 | 43 | 39 - 48 |
| 5 | 37.9 | 29.5 - 44.1 | 42.0 | 32.8 - 50.6 | 279 | 248 - 312 | 247 | 219 - 275 | 594 | 425 - 824 | 481 | 255 - 726 |
| 6 | 69.0 | 67.5 - 70.5 | 73.9 | 72.3 - 75.4 | 22 | 11 - 33 | 18 | 9 - 28 | 195 | 173 - 216 | 125 | 111 - 141 |
| 7 | 70.8 | 70.4 - 71.2 | 78.1 | 77.9 - 78.3 | 20 | 18 - 21 | 16 | 15 - 17 | 177 | 170 - 184 | 90 | 88 - 93 |
| 8 | 67.0 | 66.2 - 67.9 | 73.0 | 72.1 - 73.8 | 39 | 22 - 56 | 35 | 19 - 46 | 204 | 184 - 225 | 98 | 85 - 115 |
| 9 | 77.9 | 77.6 - 78.1 | 83.0 | 82.7 - 83.2 | 6 | 6 - 7 | 5 | 5 - 6 | 91 | 89 - 94 | 52 | 50 - 54 |
| 10 | 76.4 | 76.1 - 76.7 | 82.2 | 81.8 - 82.4 | 6 | 5 - 7 | 4 | 4 - 5 | 117 | 113 - 121 | 59 | 56 - 63 |
| 11 | 63.0 | 61.7 - 64.2 | 68.6 | 67.5 - 69.8 | 80 | 64 - 98 | 70 | 56 - 83 | 231 | 199 - 261 | 122 | 103 - 144 |
| 12 | 69.4 | 68.7 - 70.2 | 75.7 | 75.2 - 76.3 | 18 | 15 - 21 | 14 | 12 - 16 | 265 | 249 - 282 | 148 | 141 - 155 |
| 13 | 72.1 | 70.7 - 73.6 | 74.5 | 73.2 - 75.8 | 13 | 8 - 22 | 10 | 6 - 15 | 113 | 96 - 130 | 82 | 68 - 98 |
| 14 | 62.6 | 61.3 - 63.9 | 62.6 | 61.4 - 63.7 | 71 | 68 - 75 | 73 | 70 - 77 | 251 | 223 - 282 | 258 | 232 - 284 |
| 15 | 70.5 | 69.6 - 71.4 | 77.9 | 76.8 - 79.0 | 17 | 13 - 22 | 15 | 9 - 23 | 189 | 171 - 206 | 103 | 91 - 115 |
| 16 | 62.6 | 62.0 - 63.2 | 74.3 | 73.7 - 74.9 | 14 | 11 - 16 | 10 | 8 - 13 | 371 | 347 - 397 | 134 | 120 - 148 |
| 17 | 75.2 | 74.9 - 75.5 | 81.5 | 81.3 - 81.8 | 6 | 5 - 7 | 5 | 4 - 6 | 126 | 122 - 130 | 67 | 64 - 69 |
| 18 | 67.4 | 66.0 - 68.7 | 72.4 | 71.4 - 73.4 | 44 | 33 - 56 | 34 | 25 - 42 | 189 | 172 - 211 | 123 | 117 - 129 |
| 19 | 50.1 | 42.9 - 56.5 | 52.4 | 43.0 - 60.1 | 166 | 163 - 170 | 158 | 155 - 161 | 424 | 253 - 634 | 360 | 176 - 611 |
| 20 | 60.2 | 52.3 - 67.6 | 62.4 | 53.5 - 69.0 | 93 | 74 - 111 | 92 | 73 - 111 | 272 | 111 - 474 | 226 | 102 - 428 |
| 21 | 61.8 | 54.6 - 69.3 | 64.7 | 56.2 - 70.9 | 78 | 74 - 82 | 73 | 70 - 77 | 260 | 101 - 445 | 209 | 91 - 402 |
| 22 | 69.3 | 67.9 - 71.0 | 76.4 | 75.2 - 77.6 | 20 | 15 - 25 | 15 | 11 - 19 | 192 | 162 - 220 | 90 | 76 - 105 |
| 23 | 40.2 | 37.3 - 43.3 | 40.6 | 37.7 - 44.1 | 104 | 89 - 121 | 102 | 86 - 118 | 786 | 718 - 842 | 745 | 676 - 801 |
| 24 | 65.7 | 65.2 - 66.2 | 72.3 | 71.8 - 72.7 | 42 | 36 - 49 | 34 | 29 - 40 | 246 | 235 - 257 | 136 | 128 - 145 |
| 25 | 74.8 | 73.5 - 76.3 | 77.4 | 76.6 - 78.2 | 14 | 12 - 16 | 12 | 11 - 14 | 112 | 94 - 128 | 85 | 73 - 98 |
| 26 | 68.8 | 68.7 - 69.0 | 75.6 | 75.5 - 75.8 | 17 | 16 - 19 | 15 | 13 - 16 | 218 | 214 - 221 | 94 | 91 - 96 |
| 27 | 40.6 | 34.3 - 46.6 | 42.6 | 34.7 - 49.8 | 232 | 211 - 251 | 217 | 197 - 235 | 597 | 417 - 793 | 522 | 334 - 736 |
| 28 | 38.7 | 33.0 - 44.5 | 43.0 | 36.0 - 50.2 | 189 | 152 - 224 | 177 | 142 - 216 | 692 | 541 - 834 | 563 | 393 - 750 |
| 29 | 51.9 | 44.8 - 57.4 | 57.1 | 49.1 - 63.4 | 149 | 138 - 159 | 124 | 115 - 132 | 400 | 261 - 604 | 298 | 165 - 487 |
| 30 | 47.2 | 41.1 - 53.9 | 49.0 | 41.4 - 56.7 | 162 | 151 - 174 | 158 | 147 - 169 | 519 | 344 - 697 | 454 | 273 - 658 |
| 31 | 77.2 | 77.0 - 77.4 | 82.3 | 82.1 - 82.4 | 6 | 6 - 6 | 5 | 5 - 5 | 95 | 93 - 97 | 58 | 57 - 60 |
| 32 | 66.6 | 62.4 - 71.0 | 72.9 | 69.6 - 75.8 | 42 | 33 - 50 | 30 | 24 - 36 | 210 | 125 - 312 | 120 | 76 - 178 |
| 33 | 42.1 | 36.2 - 48.4 | 43.7 | 36.7 - 50.2 | 187 | 156 - 219 | 173 | 142 - 201 | 620 | 474 - 780 | 566 | 418 - 740 |
| 34 | 46.1 | 38.3 - 53.1 | 49.3 | 40.9 - 57.6 | 202 | 168 - 235 | 180 | 149 - 210 | 477 | 305 - 684 | 402 | 203 - 618 |
| 35 | 73.4 | 72.7 - 74.0 | 80.0 | 79.7 - 80.3 | 16 | 14 - 18 | 13 | 12 - 14 | 134 | 124 - 144 | 67 | 64 - 70 |
| 36 | 69.6 | 69.0 - 70.3 | 72.7 | 72.0 - 73.5 | 31 | 29 - 33 | 41 | 38 - 44 | 165 | 154 - 175 | 104 | 93 - 112 |
| 37 | 67.5 | 66.8 - 68.2 | 76.3 | 75.4 - 77.1 | 27 | 24 - 29 | 19 | 17 - 21 | 236 | 220 - 251 | 99 | 87 - 113 |
| 38 | 61.6 | 53.7 - 68.9 | 64.9 | 56.4 - 71.3 | 80 | 64 - 96 | 72 | 57 - 86 | 260 | 100 - 464 | 207 | 91 - 405 |
| 39 | 51.6 | 44.6 - 58.9 | 54.5 | 46.7 - 61.6 | 109 | 82 - 135 | 101 | 75 - 125 | 474 | 309 - 651 | 410 | 263 - 611 |
| 40 | 69.2 | 68.2 - 70.3 | 74.2 | 73.4 - 75.0 | 21 | 10 - 31 | 19 | 10 - 27 | 173 | 150 - 193 | 109 | 98 - 123 |
| 41 | 74.8 | 74.5 - 75.0 | 79.5 | 79.3 - 79.8 | 12 | 11 - 13 | 10 | 9 - 11 | 127 | 122 - 131 | 74 | 70 - 78 |
| 42 | 43.1 | 36.4 - 50.1 | 48.0 | 40.8 - 54.7 | 192 | 154 - 232 | 143 | 114 - 169 | 577 | 400 - 757 | 502 | 353 - 694 |
| 43 | 71.0 | 70.6 - 71.4 | 78.6 | 78.1 - 79.0 | 8 | 7 - 10 | 7 | 7 - 8 | 178 | 169 - 187 | 72 | 67 - 77 |
| 44 | 75.0 | 74.6 - 75.4 | 79.3 | 79.1 - 79.5 | 8 | 7 - 10 | 7 | 6 - 7 | 138 | 132 - 145 | 89 | 86 - 91 |
| 45 | 75.5 | 74.8 - 76.2 | 79.1 | 77.2 - 80.9 | 7 | 6 - 9 | 7 | 6 - 9 | 102 | 93 - 111 | 48 | 38 - 63 |
| 46 | 72.4 | 72.1 - 72.8 | 79.0 | 78.7 - 79.3 | 5 | 4 - 6 | 4 | 4 - 5 | 163 | 157 - 170 | 72 | 69 - 76 |
| 47 | 64.4 | 56.5 - 72.3 | 67.1 | 57.9 - 75.2 | 56 | 29 - 83 | 54 | 30 - 80 | 236 | 83 - 416 | 191 | 70 - 386 |
| 48 | 41.0 | 34.7 - 47.1 | 46.1 | 38.0 - 52.8 | 221 | 190 - 252 | 198 | 169 - 225 | 585 | 432 - 749 | 449 | 298 - 655 |
| 49 | 74.8 | 74.6 - 75.0 | 79.5 | 79.4 - 79.7 | 6 | 5 - 7 | 5 | 4 - 6 | 123 | 120 - 127 | 76 | 73 - 78 |
| 50 | 48.6 | 42.4 - 56.1 | 50.7 | 43.0 - 58.2 | 156 | 132 - 179 | 144 | 121 - 166 | 481 | 290 - 657 | 431 | 259 - 639 |
| 51 | 71.0 | 69.7 - 72.2 | 75.8 | 74.2 - 77.2 | 13 | 11 - 15 | 14 | 10 - 18 | 206 | 182 - 235 | 120 | 94 - 155 |
| 52 | 64.9 | 63.9 - 65.9 | 71.5 | 70.5 - 72.4 | 37 | 32 - 41 | 30 | 26 - 35 | 256 | 231 - 279 | 150 | 132 - 171 |
| 53 | 67.9 | 67.3 - 68.5 | 73.5 | 72.9 - 74.2 | 34 | 28 - 39 | 30 | 25 - 34 | 216 | 204 - 229 | 132 | 120 - 143 |
| 54 | 65.3 | 65.0 - 65.6 | 69.0 | 68.7 - 69.3 | 38 | 34 - 42 | 39 | 35 - 43 | 240 | 231 - 248 | 157 | 151 - 164 |
| 55 | 66.5 | 65.4 - 67.8 | 72.8 | 72.1 - 73.5 | 36 | 31 - 42 | 34 | 28 - 39 | 257 | 227 - 289 | 142 | 129 - 155 |

## Annex Table 1 Basic indicators for all WHO Member States

Figures computed by WHO to assure comparability;[a] they are not necessarily the official statistics of Member States, which may use alternative rigorous methods.

| | | Total population (000) | Annual growth rate (%) | Dependency ratio (per 100) | | Percentage of population aged 60+ years | | Total fertility rate | | LIFE EXPECTANCY AT BIRTH (YEARS) Both sexes |
|---|---|---|---|---|---|---|---|---|---|---|
| | Member State | 2002 | 1992–2002 | 1992 | 2002 | 1992 | 2002 | 1992 | 2002 | 2002 |
| 56 | Equatorial Guinea | 481 | 2.6 | 87 | 91 | 6.4 | 5.9 | 5.9 | 5.9 | 53.4 |
| 57 | Eritrea | 3 991 | 2.4 | 93 | 91 | 3.6 | 3.6 | 6.2 | 5.5 | 57.6 |
| 58 | Estonia | 1 338 | -1.4 | 51 | 48 | 17.8 | 21.5 | 1.7 | 1.2 | 71.1 |
| 59 | Ethiopia | 68 961 | 2.8 | 94 | 94 | 4.4 | 4.6 | 6.8 | 6.2 | 48.0 |
| 60 | Fiji | 831 | 1.2 | 67 | 57 | 5.0 | 6.0 | 3.4 | 2.9 | 67.3 |
| 61 | Finland | 5 197 | 0.3 | 49 | 49 | 18.7 | 20.3 | 1.8 | 1.7 | 78.2 |
| 62 | France | 59 850 | 0.4 | 52 | 53 | 19.5 | 20.5 | 1.7 | 1.9 | 79.8 |
| 63 | Gabon | 1 306 | 2.6 | 92 | 83 | 7.4 | 6.2 | 5.2 | 4.0 | 59.2 |
| 64 | Gambia | 1 388 | 3.3 | 84 | 80 | 5.1 | 5.8 | 5.7 | 4.8 | 57.1 |
| 65 | Georgia | 5 177 | -0.5 | 52 | 49 | 15.6 | 18.9 | 1.9 | 1.4 | 71.7 |
| 66 | Germany | 82 414 | 0.2 | 46 | 48 | 20.5 | 24.0 | 1.3 | 1.3 | 78.7 |
| 67 | Ghana | 20 471 | 2.4 | 92 | 77 | 4.6 | 5.2 | 5.4 | 4.2 | 57.6 |
| 68 | Greece | 10 970 | 0.7 | 48 | 49 | 20.7 | 23.8 | 1.4 | 1.3 | 78.4 |
| 69 | Grenada | 80 | -0.5 | 63 | 56 | 9.2 | 10.5 | 4.0 | 3.5 | 67.4 |
| 70 | Guatemala | 12 036 | 2.7 | 96 | 87 | 5.2 | 5.3 | 5.4 | 4.5 | 65.9 |
| 71 | Guinea | 8 359 | 2.4 | 93 | 88 | 4.4 | 4.5 | 6.4 | 5.9 | 52.3 |
| 72 | Guinea-Bissau | 1 449 | 3.0 | 95 | 101 | 5.4 | 4.9 | 7.1 | 7.1 | 47.2 |
| 73 | Guyana | 764 | 0.4 | 67 | 54 | 6.8 | 7.0 | 2.6 | 2.3 | 64.3 |
| 74 | Haiti | 8 218 | 1.4 | 91 | 76 | 5.7 | 5.9 | 4.9 | 4.0 | 50.1 |
| 75 | Honduras | 6 781 | 2.8 | 91 | 80 | 4.6 | 5.4 | 5.0 | 3.8 | 67.2 |
| 76 | Hungary | 9 923 | -0.4 | 49 | 45 | 19.2 | 20.0 | 1.7 | 1.2 | 72.6 |
| 77 | Iceland | 287 | 1.0 | 55 | 53 | 14.8 | 15.3 | 2.2 | 2.0 | 80.1 |
| 78 | India | 1 049 549 | 1.8 | 68 | 62 | 6.9 | 7.7 | 3.8 | 3.1 | 61.0 |
| 79 | Indonesia | 217 131 | 1.4 | 64 | 54 | 6.4 | 7.9 | 3.1 | 2.4 | 66.4 |
| 80 | Iran, Islamic Republic of | 68 070 | 1.4 | 93 | 59 | 5.9 | 6.4 | 4.5 | 2.4 | 68.9 |
| 81 | Iraq | 24 510 | 2.9 | 88 | 79 | 4.4 | 4.6 | 5.7 | 4.8 | 61.0 |
| 82 | Ireland | 3 911 | 1.0 | 60 | 47 | 15.3 | 15.3 | 2.0 | 1.9 | 77.1 |
| 83 | Israel | 6 304 | 2.7 | 66 | 61 | 12.6 | 13.1 | 2.9 | 2.7 | 79.4 |
| 84 | Italy | 57 482 | 0.1 | 45 | 49 | 21.7 | 24.5 | 1.3 | 1.2 | 79.7 |
| 85 | Jamaica | 2 627 | 0.9 | 73 | 61 | 9.9 | 9.6 | 2.8 | 2.4 | 72.8 |
| 86 | Japan | 127 478 | 0.2 | 43 | 48 | 18.6 | 24.4 | 1.5 | 1.3 | 81.9 |
| 87 | Jordan | 5 329 | 3.9 | 91 | 69 | 4.4 | 4.8 | 5.0 | 3.6 | 70.8 |
| 88 | Kazakhstan | 15 469 | -0.9 | 59 | 51 | 9.4 | 11.5 | 2.5 | 2.0 | 63.6 |
| 89 | Kenya | 31 540 | 2.3 | 104 | 82 | 4.1 | 4.2 | 5.5 | 4.1 | 50.9 |
| 90 | Kiribati | 87 | 1.5 | 70 | 68 | 6.2 | 7.0 | 4.7 | 4.1 | 64.1 |
| 91 | Kuwait | 2 443 | 2.1 | 56 | 38 | 2.1 | 2.7 | 3.3 | 2.7 | 76.4 |
| 92 | Kyrgyzstan | 5 067 | 1.3 | 75 | 64 | 8.4 | 8.7 | 3.5 | 2.7 | 64.5 |
| 93 | Lao People's Democratic Republic | 5 529 | 2.4 | 91 | 84 | 5.9 | 5.5 | 5.9 | 4.8 | 55.1 |
| 94 | Latvia | 2 329 | -1.3 | 51 | 48 | 18.4 | 21.8 | 1.7 | 1.1 | 70.3 |
| 95 | Lebanon | 3 596 | 2.3 | 65 | 56 | 8.3 | 8.6 | 2.9 | 2.2 | 69.8 |
| 96 | Lesotho | 1 800 | 1.1 | 94 | 81 | 6.7 | 6.9 | 4.8 | 3.9 | 35.7 |
| 97 | Liberia | 3 239 | 4.6 | 97 | 96 | 3.9 | 3.7 | 6.9 | 6.8 | 41.8 |
| 98 | Libyan Arab Jamahiriya | 5 445 | 2.0 | 81 | 54 | 4.5 | 6.0 | 4.3 | 3.1 | 72.6 |
| 99 | Lithuania | 3 465 | -0.6 | 51 | 51 | 16.9 | 19.7 | 1.8 | 1.3 | 71.9 |
| 100 | Luxembourg | 447 | 1.5 | 44 | 49 | 18.1 | 18.3 | 1.6 | 1.7 | 78.8 |
| 101 | Madagascar | 16 916 | 2.9 | 92 | 91 | 4.8 | 4.7 | 6.2 | 5.7 | 56.3 |
| 102 | Malawi | 11 871 | 1.9 | 94 | 99 | 4.8 | 5.2 | 6.8 | 6.1 | 40.2 |
| 103 | Malaysia | 23 965 | 2.4 | 67 | 60 | 5.8 | 6.7 | 3.7 | 2.9 | 72.0 |
| 104 | Maldives | 309 | 3.0 | 99 | 86 | 5.4 | 5.2 | 6.2 | 5.4 | 66.1 |
| 105 | Mali | 12 623 | 2.8 | 103 | 107 | 3.9 | 3.8 | 7.0 | 7.0 | 44.8 |
| 106 | Malta | 393 | 0.7 | 51 | 47 | 15.1 | 17.5 | 2.0 | 1.8 | 78.7 |
| 107 | Marshall Islands | 52 | 1.3 | 70 | 68 | 6.2 | 7.0 | 6.3 | 5.5 | 62.7 |
| 108 | Mauritania | 2 807 | 2.8 | 89 | 87 | 5.3 | 5.3 | 6.1 | 5.8 | 52.1 |
| 109 | Mauritius | 1 210 | 1.1 | 52 | 46 | 8.4 | 9.0 | 2.3 | 2.0 | 71.9 |
| 110 | Mexico | 101 965 | 1.7 | 71 | 61 | 6.0 | 7.2 | 3.2 | 2.5 | 74.3 |

| | LIFE EXPECTANCY AT BIRTH (YEARS) | | | | PROBABILITY OF DYING (PER 1000) | | | | | | | |
|---|---|---|---|---|---|---|---|---|---|---|---|---|
| | | | | | Under age 5 years | | | | Between ages 15 and 60 years | | | |
| | Males | | Females | | Males | | Females | | Males | | Females | |
| | 2002 | Uncertainty | 2002 | Uncertainty | 2002 | Uncertainty | 2002 | Uncertainty | 2002 | Uncertainty | 2002 | Uncertainty |
| 56 | 51.9 | 44.4 - 58.8 | 54.8 | 46.0 - 61.7 | 157 | 132 - 181 | 144 | 125 - 166 | 383 | 217 - 596 | 318 | 152 - 548 |
| 57 | 55.8 | 47.2 - 65.8 | 59.3 | 51.0 - 66.8 | 117 | 107 - 127 | 102 | 93 - 111 | 350 | 176 - 496 | 286 | 137 - 484 |
| 58 | 65.1 | 64.8 - 65.5 | 77.1 | 76.8 - 77.4 | 10 | 7 - 12 | 6 | 4 - 7 | 322 | 313 - 331 | 112 | 105 - 118 |
| 59 | 46.8 | 39.3 - 54.0 | 49.4 | 41.3 - 57.2 | 185 | 148 - 220 | 168 | 138 - 196 | 487 | 316 - 693 | 422 | 244 - 628 |
| 60 | 64.6 | 63.7 - 65.7 | 70.3 | 69.3 - 71.4 | 30 | 27 - 33 | 27 | 24 - 29 | 281 | 260 - 301 | 176 | 159 - 193 |
| 61 | 74.8 | 74.5 - 75.0 | 81.5 | 81.2 - 81.8 | 4 | 4 - 5 | 3 | 3 - 3 | 135 | 131 - 140 | 60 | 56 - 64 |
| 62 | 76.0 | 75.7 - 76.2 | 83.6 | 83.3 - 83.8 | 6 | 5 - 6 | 4 | 4 - 5 | 135 | 131 - 139 | 60 | 58 - 62 |
| 63 | 57.3 | 49.9 - 64.6 | 61.4 | 52.9 - 68.9 | 100 | 91 - 108 | 79 | 72 - 86 | 342 | 171 - 557 | 281 | 133 - 499 |
| 64 | 55.4 | 47.5 - 62.3 | 58.9 | 50.2 - 66.7 | 132 | 112 - 152 | 117 | 99 - 135 | 330 | 159 - 552 | 265 | 110 - 467 |
| 65 | 68.4 | 67.2 - 69.6 | 75.0 | 73.1 - 76.7 | 26 | 23 - 28 | 20 | 18 - 22 | 207 | 181 - 237 | 86 | 67 - 109 |
| 66 | 75.6 | 75.2 - 75.9 | 81.6 | 81.4 - 81.7 | 5 | 5 - 6 | 4 | 4 - 4 | 118 | 114 - 123 | 60 | 59 - 62 |
| 67 | 56.3 | 49.0 - 64.4 | 58.8 | 50.1 - 66.0 | 106 | 92 - 123 | 99 | 87 - 112 | 354 | 171 - 557 | 303 | 153 - 529 |
| 68 | 75.8 | 75.6 - 76.0 | 81.1 | 80.7 - 81.5 | 7 | 6 - 7 | 5 | 4 - 6 | 118 | 115 - 120 | 48 | 45 - 51 |
| 69 | 65.9 | 64.8 - 67.1 | 68.8 | 67.8 - 70.0 | 25 | 18 - 30 | 21 | 15 - 27 | 261 | 238 - 283 | 222 | 204 - 239 |
| 70 | 63.1 | 61.9 - 64.3 | 69.0 | 67.7 - 70.1 | 57 | 52 - 63 | 50 | 45 - 55 | 283 | 247 - 324 | 162 | 131 - 199 |
| 71 | 50.9 | 44.0 - 57.5 | 53.7 | 45.0 - 61.0 | 163 | 148 - 179 | 153 | 138 - 168 | 401 | 232 - 596 | 332 | 159 - 559 |
| 72 | 45.7 | 37.9 - 51.6 | 48.7 | 39.8 - 56.8 | 215 | 194 - 237 | 198 | 179 - 217 | 462 | 311 - 681 | 383 | 186 - 615 |
| 73 | 61.5 | 58.9 - 64.5 | 66.9 | 63.8 - 70.0 | 61 | 30 - 90 | 50 | 26 - 76 | 299 | 268 - 328 | 202 | 170 - 233 |
| 74 | 49.1 | 42.8 - 55.5 | 51.1 | 42.9 - 57.3 | 138 | 119 - 157 | 128 | 111 - 145 | 493 | 345 - 660 | 438 | 309 - 615 |
| 75 | 64.2 | 60.3 - 67.8 | 70.4 | 67.2 - 73.2 | 44 | 42 - 46 | 42 | 40 - 44 | 269 | 195 - 362 | 150 | 102 - 214 |
| 76 | 68.4 | 68.2 - 68.5 | 76.8 | 76.7 - 77.0 | 9 | 8 - 10 | 8 | 8 - 9 | 259 | 256 - 262 | 110 | 108 - 112 |
| 77 | 78.4 | 77.8 - 79.0 | 81.8 | 81.4 - 82.2 | 4 | 4 - 5 | 3 | 3 - 3 | 85 | 79 - 92 | 55 | 51 - 60 |
| 78 | 60.1 | 59.4 - 60.8 | 62.0 | 61.1 - 62.8 | 87 | 81 - 92 | 95 | 86 - 106 | 291 | 268 - 314 | 220 | 197 - 243 |
| 79 | 64.9 | 64.1 - 65.8 | 67.9 | 67.1 - 68.8 | 45 | 40 - 50 | 36 | 33 - 40 | 244 | 226 - 261 | 208 | 194 - 224 |
| 80 | 66.5 | 65.4 - 67.8 | 71.7 | 70.5 - 72.8 | 42 | 33 - 50 | 36 | 29 - 43 | 213 | 194 - 230 | 132 | 121 - 145 |
| 81 | 59.1 | 57.1 - 60.9 | 63.1 | 61.3 - 64.9 | 119 | 101 - 139 | 110 | 94 - 127 | 252 | 228 - 278 | 176 | 155 - 197 |
| 82 | 74.4 | 73.8 - 75.0 | 79.8 | 79.3 - 80.1 | 8 | 7 - 9 | 6 | 5 - 7 | 113 | 105 - 121 | 66 | 62 - 71 |
| 83 | 77.3 | 77.1 - 77.5 | 81.4 | 81.2 - 81.5 | 7 | 6 - 8 | 6 | 6 - 7 | 98 | 95 - 101 | 53 | 50 - 56 |
| 84 | 76.8 | 76.4 - 77.1 | 82.5 | 82.2 - 82.8 | 5 | 5 - 6 | 5 | 4 - 5 | 96 | 92 - 100 | 49 | 46 - 51 |
| 85 | 71.1 | 69.9 - 72.5 | 74.6 | 73.6 - 75.6 | 16 | 13 - 19 | 14 | 11 - 17 | 162 | 137 - 184 | 121 | 107 - 134 |
| 86 | 78.4 | 78.4 - 78.4 | 85.3 | 85.2 - 85.3 | 4 | 4 - 4 | 4 | 4 - 4 | 95 | 95 - 96 | 46 | 45 - 46 |
| 87 | 68.6 | 67.7 - 69.8 | 73.3 | 72.6 - 74.0 | 28 | 23 - 32 | 26 | 22 - 30 | 191 | 171 - 210 | 121 | 113 - 130 |
| 88 | 58.7 | 58.0 - 59.4 | 68.9 | 68.1 - 69.7 | 38 | 29 - 48 | 28 | 21 - 36 | 426 | 385 - 462 | 195 | 177 - 213 |
| 89 | 49.8 | 43.8 - 57.4 | 51.9 | 44.8 - 59.3 | 119 | 108 - 129 | 113 | 104 - 122 | 509 | 328 - 684 | 448 | 285 - 642 |
| 90 | 61.8 | 60.8 - 62.8 | 66.7 | 65.6 - 67.6 | 80 | 74 - 88 | 69 | 60 - 79 | 293 | 260 - 327 | 190 | 167 - 215 |
| 91 | 75.4 | 74.9 - 75.9 | 77.7 | 77.1 - 78.2 | 14 | 13 - 15 | 12 | 11 - 13 | 77 | 72 - 82 | 63 | 57 - 70 |
| 92 | 60.4 | 59.5 - 61.4 | 68.9 | 68.1 - 69.8 | 63 | 50 - 76 | 55 | 44 - 66 | 345 | 314 - 371 | 163 | 146 - 180 |
| 93 | 54.1 | 51.4 - 56.7 | 56.2 | 53.5 - 58.8 | 146 | 120 - 174 | 131 | 106 - 158 | 338 | 303 - 373 | 306 | 278 - 333 |
| 94 | 64.6 | 64.3 - 64.9 | 75.8 | 75.6 - 76.1 | 15 | 12 - 17 | 12 | 10 - 14 | 327 | 320 - 334 | 118 | 113 - 122 |
| 95 | 67.6 | 66.4 - 68.8 | 72.0 | 71.1 - 73.1 | 35 | 31 - 39 | 29 | 26 - 32 | 201 | 177 - 225 | 139 | 123 - 154 |
| 96 | 32.9 | 29.3 - 38.5 | 38.2 | 33.0 - 44.9 | 166 | 133 - 201 | 160 | 128 - 191 | 902 | 791 - 965 | 742 | 599 - 853 |
| 97 | 40.1 | 32.2 - 47.0 | 43.7 | 34.8 - 51.7 | 242 | 197 - 293 | 222 | 178 - 262 | 582 | 435 - 773 | 471 | 283 - 690 |
| 98 | 70.4 | 66.3 - 73.8 | 75.5 | 73.0 - 77.8 | 19 | 16 - 21 | 17 | 15 - 20 | 173 | 110 - 263 | 99 | 65 - 142 |
| 99 | 66.2 | 65.2 - 67.0 | 77.6 | 77.0 - 78.2 | 11 | 9 - 13 | 9 | 7 - 11 | 303 | 272 - 341 | 103 | 94 - 112 |
| 00 | 75.7 | 75.3 - 76.2 | 81.7 | 81.1 - 82.3 | 5 | 4 - 7 | 5 | 4 - 6 | 119 | 113 - 125 | 64 | 58 - 70 |
| 01 | 54.4 | 46.8 - 61.0 | 58.4 | 49.5 - 65.0 | 145 | 126 - 164 | 125 | 110 - 141 | 333 | 177 - 543 | 262 | 123 - 474 |
| 02 | 39.8 | 35.0 - 45.2 | 40.6 | 35.0 - 47.1 | 197 | 183 - 210 | 190 | 178 - 203 | 657 | 509 - 803 | 610 | 449 - 769 |
| 03 | 69.6 | 69.1 - 70.1 | 74.7 | 74.4 - 75.1 | 10 | 8 - 11 | 8 | 7 - 10 | 192 | 181 - 202 | 106 | 100 - 111 |
| 04 | 66.5 | 65.7 - 67.4 | 65.6 | 64.9 - 66.5 | 38 | 33 - 42 | 43 | 38 - 49 | 205 | 179 - 231 | 202 | 174 - 229 |
| 05 | 43.9 | 35.8 - 49.7 | 45.7 | 36.8 - 54.0 | 233 | 211 - 256 | 224 | 200 - 244 | 487 | 328 - 718 | 417 | 210 - 662 |
| 06 | 76.1 | 75.5 - 76.7 | 81.2 | 80.6 - 81.7 | 7 | 6 - 8 | 6 | 4 - 7 | 86 | 80 - 91 | 50 | 46 - 54 |
| 07 | 61.1 | 59.5 - 62.9 | 64.6 | 63.2 - 66.2 | 46 | 34 - 57 | 36 | 27 - 45 | 340 | 310 - 368 | 286 | 264 - 307 |
| 08 | 49.8 | 41.7 - 56.1 | 54.5 | 44.7 - 61.3 | 186 | 158 - 214 | 155 | 132 - 178 | 393 | 245 - 603 | 304 | 156 - 536 |
| 09 | 68.4 | 67.6 - 69.2 | 75.5 | 75.0 - 76.0 | 20 | 16 - 25 | 14 | 11 - 19 | 222 | 202 - 243 | 116 | 109 - 123 |
| 10 | 71.7 | 71.6 - 71.7 | 76.9 | 76.8 - 76.9 | 30 | 30 - 30 | 24 | 24 - 24 | 168 | 167 - 169 | 97 | 96 - 98 |

## Annex Table 1 Basic indicators for all WHO Member States

Figures computed by WHO to assure comparability;[a] they are not necessarily the official statistics of Member States, which may use alternative rigorous methods.

| | | POPULATION ESTIMATES | | | | | | | | | LIFE EXPECTANCY |
| | | Total population (000) | Annual growth rate (%) | Dependency ratio (per 100) | | Percentage of population aged 60+ years | | Total fertility rate | | AT BIRTH (YEARS) Both sexes |
| | Member State | 2002 | 1992–2002 | 1992 | 2002 | 1992 | 2002 | 1992 | 2002 | 2002 |
|---|---|---|---|---|---|---|---|---|---|---|
| 111 | Micronesia, Federated States of | 108 | 0.7 | 92 | 74 | 5.5 | 5.1 | 4.8 | 3.8 | 66.5 |
| 112 | Monaco | 34 | 1.1 | 52 | 53 | 19.5 | 20.5 | 1.7 | 1.8 | 81.2 |
| 113 | Mongolia | 2 559 | 1.1 | 81 | 59 | 5.9 | 5.6 | 3.5 | 2.4 | 62.9 |
| 114 | Morocco | 30 072 | 1.7 | 73 | 57 | 6.0 | 6.6 | 3.6 | 2.8 | 70.8 |
| 115 | Mozambique | 18 537 | 2.6 | 96 | 89 | 5.2 | 5.1 | 6.2 | 5.7 | 42.6 |
| 116 | Myanmar | 48 852 | 1.5 | 69 | 59 | 6.8 | 6.9 | 3.8 | 2.9 | 58.9 |
| 117 | Namibia | 1 961 | 2.7 | 87 | 88 | 5.4 | 5.6 | 5.6 | 4.6 | 49.3 |
| 118 | Nauru | 13 | 2.5 | 70 | 68 | 6.2 | 7.0 | 4.5 | 3.9 | 62.7 |
| 119 | Nepal | 24 609 | 2.3 | 81 | 78 | 5.6 | 5.8 | 5.0 | 4.3 | 60.1 |
| 120 | Netherlands | 16 067 | 0.6 | 45 | 48 | 17.5 | 18.5 | 1.6 | 1.7 | 78.6 |
| 121 | New Zealand | 3 846 | 1.1 | 53 | 53 | 15.3 | 15.9 | 2.1 | 2.0 | 78.9 |
| 122 | Nicaragua | 5 335 | 2.8 | 95 | 82 | 4.4 | 4.7 | 4.8 | 3.8 | 70.1 |
| 123 | Niger | 11 544 | 3.5 | 108 | 108 | 3.6 | 3.3 | 8.0 | 8.0 | 42.6 |
| 124 | Nigeria | 120 911 | 2.8 | 96 | 91 | 4.7 | 4.8 | 6.4 | 5.5 | 48.8 |
| 125 | Niue | 2 | -1.2 | 71 | 65 | 6.2 | 7.2 | 3.6 | 2.9 | 70.3 |
| 126 | Norway | 4 514 | 0.5 | 55 | 54 | 20.6 | 19.6 | 1.9 | 1.8 | 79.1 |
| 127 | Oman | 2 768 | 3.3 | 82 | 65 | 3.0 | 3.5 | 6.5 | 5.0 | 73.1 |
| 128 | Pakistan | 149 911 | 2.5 | 86 | 82 | 5.5 | 5.7 | 5.9 | 5.1 | 61.4 |
| 129 | Palau | 20 | 2.3 | 70 | 68 | 6.2 | 7.0 | 2.8 | 2.4 | 68.5 |
| 130 | Panama | 3 064 | 2.0 | 65 | 59 | 7.3 | 8.3 | 2.9 | 2.7 | 75.4 |
| 131 | Papua New Guinea | 5 586 | 2.6 | 79 | 77 | 4.2 | 4.0 | 5.1 | 4.1 | 59.8 |
| 132 | Paraguay | 5 740 | 2.5 | 84 | 74 | 5.3 | 5.5 | 4.6 | 3.9 | 71.7 |
| 133 | Peru | 26 767 | 1.7 | 71 | 63 | 6.2 | 7.4 | 3.7 | 2.9 | 69.7 |
| 134 | Philippines | 78 580 | 2.1 | 77 | 67 | 5.0 | 5.7 | 4.2 | 3.2 | 68.3 |
| 135 | Poland | 38 622 | 0.1 | 54 | 44 | 15.2 | 16.6 | 1.9 | 1.3 | 74.7 |
| 136 | Portugal | 10 049 | 0.2 | 49 | 48 | 19.5 | 21.1 | 1.5 | 1.5 | 77.1 |
| 137 | Qatar | 601 | 2.0 | 39 | 39 | 2.1 | 3.1 | 4.2 | 3.3 | 74.3 |
| 138 | Republic of Korea | 47 430 | 0.8 | 43 | 39 | 8.2 | 11.8 | 1.7 | 1.4 | 75.5 |
| 139 | Republic of Moldova | 4 270 | -0.2 | 57 | 45 | 12.9 | 13.8 | 2.2 | 1.4 | 67.8 |
| 140 | Romania | 22 387 | -0.3 | 50 | 45 | 16.3 | 18.9 | 1.6 | 1.3 | 71.4 |
| 141 | Russian Federation | 144 082 | -0.3 | 50 | 42 | 16.3 | 18.3 | 1.6 | 1.2 | 64.6 |
| 142 | Rwanda | 8 272 | 3.2 | 98 | 91 | 3.8 | 4.0 | 6.7 | 5.8 | 44.4 |
| 143 | Saint Kitts and Nevis | 42 | 0.0 | 63 | 56 | 9.2 | 10.5 | 2.7 | 2.4 | 70.4 |
| 144 | Saint Lucia | 148 | 0.9 | 75 | 57 | 8.6 | 7.8 | 3.2 | 2.3 | 72.2 |
| 145 | Saint Vincent and the Grenadines | 119 | 0.6 | 79 | 61 | 8.7 | 9.2 | 2.9 | 2.2 | 69.8 |
| 146 | Samoa | 176 | 0.8 | 81 | 81 | 6.3 | 6.5 | 4.7 | 4.2 | 68.2 |
| 147 | San Marino | 27 | 1.4 | 45 | 49 | 21.7 | 24.5 | 1.3 | 1.2 | 80.6 |
| 148 | Sao Tome and Principe | 157 | 2.6 | 104 | 83 | 6.6 | 6.4 | 5.0 | 4.0 | 62.7 |
| 149 | Saudi Arabia | 23 520 | 3.0 | 80 | 72 | 3.4 | 4.3 | 5.8 | 4.6 | 70.8 |
| 150 | Senegal | 9 855 | 2.4 | 95 | 85 | 4.1 | 4.0 | 6.1 | 5.0 | 55.8 |
| 151 | Serbia and Montenegro | 10 535 | 0.2 | 50 | 49 | 16.0 | 18.4 | 2.0 | 1.7 | 72.3 |
| 152 | Seychelles | 80 | 1.0 | 52 | 46 | 8.4 | 9.0 | 2.1 | 1.8 | 71.5 |
| 153 | Sierra Leone | 4 764 | 1.5 | 87 | 89 | 5.0 | 4.7 | 6.5 | 6.5 | 34.0 |
| 154 | Singapore | 4 183 | 2.8 | 38 | 40 | 8.7 | 11.1 | 1.8 | 1.4 | 79.6 |
| 155 | Slovakia | 5 398 | 0.2 | 54 | 43 | 15.0 | 15.5 | 1.9 | 1.3 | 74.0 |
| 156 | Slovenia | 1 986 | 0.2 | 44 | 42 | 17.4 | 19.8 | 1.4 | 1.2 | 76.7 |
| 157 | Solomon Islands | 463 | 3.2 | 93 | 84 | 4.4 | 4.4 | 5.6 | 4.5 | 65.4 |
| 158 | Somalia | 9 480 | 2.8 | 102 | 101 | 4.2 | 3.8 | 7.3 | 7.3 | 44.3 |
| 159 | South Africa | 44 759 | 1.5 | 70 | 59 | 5.2 | 6.1 | 3.4 | 2.6 | 50.7 |
| 160 | Spain | 40 977 | 0.4 | 48 | 46 | 20.0 | 21.6 | 1.3 | 1.2 | 79.6 |
| 161 | Sri Lanka | 18 910 | 0.9 | 58 | 47 | 8.8 | 10.2 | 2.4 | 2.0 | 70.3 |
| 162 | Sudan | 32 878 | 2.3 | 81 | 76 | 5.1 | 5.6 | 5.3 | 4.4 | 57.1 |
| 163 | Suriname | 432 | 0.7 | 66 | 58 | 7.1 | 8.0 | 2.5 | 2.5 | 67.6 |
| 164 | Swaziland | 1 069 | 1.9 | 97 | 89 | 4.5 | 5.1 | 5.7 | 4.6 | 38.8 |
| 165 | Sweden | 8 867 | 0.2 | 56 | 55 | 22.4 | 22.9 | 2.0 | 1.6 | 80.4 |

| | LIFE EXPECTANCY AT BIRTH (YEARS) | | | | PROBABILITY OF DYING (PER 1000) | | | | | | | |
| --- | --- | --- | --- | --- | --- | --- | --- | --- | --- | --- | --- | --- |
| | | | | | Under age 5 years | | | | Between ages 15 and 60 years | | | |
| | Males | | Females | | Males | | Females | | Males | | Females | |
| | 2002 | Uncertainty | 2002 | Uncertainty | 2002 | Uncertainty | 2002 | Uncertainty | 2002 | Uncertainty | 2002 | Uncertainty |
| 111 | 64.9 | 63.0 - 67.1 | 68.1 | 66.1 - 70.2 | 63 | 44 - 81 | 51 | 35 - 67 | 211 | 184 - 236 | 176 | 151 - 202 |
| 112 | 77.8 | 77.6 - 77.9 | 84.5 | 84.0 - 85.0 | 5 | 4 - 5 | 3 | 3 - 4 | 109 | 108 - 111 | 47 | 44 - 50 |
| 113 | 60.1 | 59.8 - 60.5 | 65.9 | 65.5 - 66.3 | 75 | 73 - 78 | 66 | 64 - 68 | 319 | 310 - 327 | 219 | 210 - 227 |
| 114 | 68.8 | 67.4 - 70.3 | 72.8 | 71.6 - 74.1 | 43 | 36 - 49 | 41 | 35 - 47 | 160 | 138 - 185 | 104 | 88 - 120 |
| 115 | 41.2 | 35.3 - 47.5 | 43.9 | 36.8 - 51.3 | 212 | 185 - 240 | 201 | 176 - 226 | 613 | 479 - 741 | 519 | 375 - 665 |
| 116 | 56.2 | 48.4 - 64.0 | 61.8 | 52.6 - 69.6 | 118 | 88 - 151 | 94 | 66 - 122 | 335 | 175 - 539 | 236 | 107 - 444 |
| 117 | 48.1 | 43.3 - 54.3 | 50.5 | 44.0 - 56.8 | 97 | 86 - 107 | 93 | 83 - 103 | 605 | 479 - 733 | 529 | 404 - 691 |
| 118 | 59.7 | 55.6 - 64.0 | 66.5 | 63.1 - 70.3 | 18 | 14 - 21 | 12 | 10 - 15 | 448 | 326 - 564 | 303 | 211 - 389 |
| 119 | 59.9 | 58.9 - 61.0 | 60.2 | 59.2 - 61.1 | 81 | 77 - 85 | 87 | 83 - 91 | 301 | 277 - 325 | 290 | 271 - 310 |
| 120 | 76.0 | 75.7 - 76.3 | 81.1 | 80.8 - 81.3 | 6 | 6 - 7 | 5 | 5 - 6 | 94 | 91 - 97 | 65 | 63 - 68 |
| 121 | 76.6 | 76.2 - 77.1 | 81.2 | 80.8 - 81.6 | 7 | 6 - 8 | 6 | 4 - 7 | 98 | 94 - 104 | 63 | 59 - 67 |
| 122 | 67.9 | 67.2 - 68.6 | 72.4 | 71.6 - 73.2 | 38 | 31 - 45 | 32 | 27 - 38 | 213 | 199 - 226 | 143 | 126 - 163 |
| 123 | 42.6 | 31.9 - 50.6 | 42.7 | 30.9 - 51.6 | 249 | 199 - 299 | 256 | 206 - 307 | 497 | 327 - 755 | 443 | 232 - 744 |
| 124 | 48.0 | 41.2 - 54.6 | 49.6 | 40.7 - 57.1 | 183 | 162 - 205 | 181 | 159 - 202 | 453 | 287 - 632 | 392 | 217 - 612 |
| 125 | 67.6 | 63.9 - 70.8 | 73.3 | 70.4 - 76.1 | 38 | 14 - 91 | 24 | 12 - 48 | 191 | 124 - 261 | 132 | 89 - 182 |
| 126 | 76.4 | 75.8 - 76.9 | 81.7 | 81.4 - 81.9 | 5 | 4 - 6 | 4 | 4 - 4 | 100 | 93 - 106 | 60 | 57 - 63 |
| 127 | 71.0 | 67.1 - 74.5 | 76.3 | 73.8 - 78.7 | 15 | 13 - 18 | 14 | 12 - 16 | 165 | 105 - 249 | 93 | 60 - 136 |
| 128 | 61.1 | 59.3 - 62.9 | 61.6 | 59.7 - 63.7 | 105 | 89 - 120 | 115 | 98 - 134 | 227 | 201 - 254 | 201 | 176 - 225 |
| 129 | 66.4 | 65.9 - 66.9 | 70.9 | 70.0 - 71.9 | 24 | 17 - 30 | 22 | 16 - 27 | 236 | 224 - 246 | 202 | 184 - 223 |
| 130 | 72.8 | 72.0 - 73.8 | 78.2 | 77.4 - 78.9 | 25 | 23 - 28 | 21 | 19 - 23 | 146 | 132 - 159 | 84 | 76 - 94 |
| 131 | 58.4 | 56.5 - 60.4 | 61.5 | 59.7 - 63.4 | 98 | 78 - 117 | 92 | 73 - 108 | 311 | 284 - 337 | 249 | 227 - 272 |
| 132 | 68.7 | 67.9 - 69.7 | 74.7 | 74.0 - 75.4 | 37 | 31 - 42 | 26 | 22 - 31 | 171 | 155 - 189 | 120 | 109 - 132 |
| 133 | 67.5 | 66.4 - 68.5 | 72.0 | 71.1 - 72.9 | 38 | 33 - 44 | 34 | 29 - 39 | 205 | 182 - 229 | 144 | 127 - 163 |
| 134 | 65.1 | 64.3 - 65.8 | 71.7 | 70.9 - 72.5 | 39 | 33 - 45 | 33 | 28 - 38 | 258 | 238 - 279 | 133 | 118 - 151 |
| 135 | 70.6 | 70.2 - 71.0 | 78.7 | 78.4 - 79.0 | 9 | 8 - 10 | 8 | 7 - 9 | 204 | 194 - 215 | 82 | 78 - 86 |
| 136 | 73.6 | 73.1 - 74.0 | 80.5 | 80.3 - 80.8 | 7 | 6 - 7 | 5 | 5 - 6 | 154 | 147 - 163 | 65 | 62 - 68 |
| 137 | 74.8 | 73.9 - 75.8 | 73.8 | 71.8 - 75.5 | 14 | 11 - 18 | 12 | 10 - 14 | 93 | 84 - 101 | 77 | 61 - 98 |
| 138 | 71.8 | 71.3 - 72.3 | 79.4 | 79.2 - 79.6 | 8 | 7 - 9 | 7 | 7 - 8 | 166 | 156 - 176 | 61 | 59 - 63 |
| 139 | 64.0 | 63.3 - 64.8 | 71.6 | 71.1 - 72.2 | 31 | 23 - 39 | 23 | 17 - 29 | 294 | 274 - 316 | 144 | 132 - 156 |
| 140 | 68.0 | 67.2 - 68.9 | 75.0 | 74.2 - 75.7 | 22 | 21 - 24 | 19 | 17 - 20 | 235 | 212 - 259 | 108 | 96 - 121 |
| 141 | 58.3 | 58.0 - 58.5 | 71.8 | 71.6 - 71.9 | 19 | 19 - 20 | 15 | 14 - 15 | 469 | 463 - 475 | 173 | 169 - 176 |
| 142 | 41.9 | 36.5 - 48.1 | 46.8 | 39.7 - 53.9 | 186 | 170 - 203 | 170 | 157 - 184 | 605 | 431 - 774 | 474 | 283 - 695 |
| 143 | 68.7 | 67.8 - 69.5 | 72.2 | 71.0 - 73.3 | 20 | 17 - 23 | 24 | 18 - 30 | 206 | 188 - 225 | 148 | 123 - 175 |
| 144 | 69.8 | 68.7 - 70.9 | 74.4 | 73.0 - 75.7 | 14 | 11 - 17 | 15 | 12 - 20 | 211 | 185 - 238 | 145 | 114 - 177 |
| 145 | 67.8 | 66.5 - 69.1 | 71.9 | 70.6 - 73.2 | 25 | 21 - 30 | 20 | 13 - 30 | 238 | 207 - 272 | 184 | 160 - 207 |
| 146 | 66.8 | 66.0 - 67.7 | 69.7 | 68.6 - 70.8 | 27 | 22 - 31 | 21 | 16 - 26 | 235 | 219 - 251 | 203 | 186 - 221 |
| 147 | 77.2 | 75.8 - 78.6 | 84.0 | 82.5 - 85.7 | 5 | 4 - 9 | 3 | 3 - 3 | 85 | 72 - 99 | 31 | 25 - 37 |
| 148 | 61.7 | 54.2 - 68.8 | 63.6 | 54.5 - 70.6 | 80 | 62 - 98 | 82 | 60 - 104 | 259 | 108 - 454 | 217 | 95 - 414 |
| 149 | 68.4 | 64.0 - 72.3 | 73.9 | 70.9 - 76.5 | 30 | 23 - 37 | 25 | 19 - 31 | 192 | 120 - 298 | 112 | 74 - 163 |
| 150 | 54.3 | 46.7 - 60.6 | 57.3 | 48.3 - 64.5 | 139 | 122 - 157 | 129 | 112 - 145 | 349 | 187 - 560 | 284 | 131 - 512 |
| 151 | 69.7 | 69.3 - 70.1 | 74.9 | 74.5 - 75.2 | 17 | 16 - 19 | 13 | 12 - 15 | 186 | 177 - 195 | 98 | 93 - 103 |
| 152 | 67.0 | 66.1 - 67.9 | 77.2 | 76.1 - 78.3 | 15 | 11 - 18 | 10 | 8 - 13 | 243 | 219 - 268 | 113 | 91 - 138 |
| 153 | 32.4 | 22.7 - 39.9 | 35.7 | 25.0 - 45.4 | 332 | 286 - 380 | 303 | 255 - 351 | 682 | 497 - 898 | 569 | 323 - 836 |
| 154 | 77.4 | 76.4 - 78.4 | 81.7 | 81.3 - 82.1 | 4 | 4 - 4 | 3 | 3 - 3 | 90 | 80 - 101 | 53 | 49 - 56 |
| 155 | 69.8 | 69.2 - 70.3 | 78.3 | 77.9 - 78.7 | 9 | 8 - 11 | 7 | 6 - 9 | 206 | 195 - 219 | 79 | 73 - 84 |
| 156 | 72.8 | 72.3 - 73.2 | 80.5 | 80.2 - 80.8 | 5 | 4 - 6 | 4 | 4 - 5 | 163 | 154 - 172 | 71 | 67 - 76 |
| 157 | 63.6 | 61.5 - 66.2 | 67.4 | 65.7 - 69.0 | 86 | 73 - 99 | 75 | 64 - 86 | 199 | 160 - 238 | 147 | 127 - 168 |
| 158 | 43.0 | 35.9 - 48.5 | 45.7 | 35.3 - 53.0 | 218 | 198 - 239 | 223 | 199 - 245 | 534 | 388 - 738 | 418 | 232 - 676 |
| 159 | 48.8 | 45.5 - 52.0 | 52.6 | 50.0 - 55.0 | 86 | 61 - 108 | 81 | 55 - 105 | 598 | 404 - 818 | 482 | 321 - 653 |
| 160 | 76.1 | 75.6 - 76.7 | 83.0 | 82.8 - 83.3 | 5 | 5 - 6 | 5 | 4 - 5 | 120 | 111 - 128 | 47 | 45 - 49 |
| 161 | 67.2 | 65.1 - 69.6 | 74.3 | 73.3 - 75.4 | 20 | 17 - 23 | 16 | 14 - 19 | 238 | 186 - 286 | 121 | 106 - 136 |
| 162 | 54.9 | 48.3 - 62.5 | 59.3 | 50.6 - 65.6 | 111 | 104 - 120 | 106 | 97 - 113 | 379 | 202 - 559 | 278 | 148 - 495 |
| 163 | 64.4 | 63.0 - 65.9 | 70.8 | 69.6 - 72.3 | 33 | 29 - 37 | 28 | 24 - 31 | 281 | 247 - 313 | 164 | 137 - 187 |
| 164 | 36.9 | 34.2 - 40.7 | 40.4 | 35.8 - 44.5 | 150 | 132 - 169 | 142 | 124 - 159 | 818 | 743 - 877 | 707 | 627 - 804 |
| 165 | 78.0 | 77.7 - 78.3 | 82.6 | 82.4 - 82.9 | 4 | 4 - 5 | 3 | 3 - 3 | 83 | 80 - 85 | 53 | 51 - 55 |

## Annex Table 1 Basic indicators for all WHO Member States

Figures computed by WHO to assure comparability;[a] they are not necessarily the official statistics of Member States, which may use alternative rigorous methods.

| | Member State | POPULATION ESTIMATES | | | | | | | | | LIFE EXPECTANCY AT BIRTH (YEARS) |
| | | Total population (000) | Annual growth rate (%) | Dependency ratio (per 100) | | Percentage of population aged 60+ years | | Total fertility rate | | Both sexes |
| | | 2002 | 1992–2002 | 1992 | 2002 | 1992 | 2002 | 1992 | 2002 | 2002 |
|---|---|---|---|---|---|---|---|---|---|---|
| 166 | Switzerland | 7 171 | 0.3 | 46 | 49 | 19.4 | 22.1 | 1.5 | 1.4 | 80.6 |
| 167 | Syrian Arab Republic | 17 381 | 2.6 | 98 | 70 | 4.2 | 4.6 | 4.8 | 3.4 | 71.2 |
| 168 | Tajikistan | 6 195 | 1.2 | 89 | 73 | 6.3 | 6.7 | 4.5 | 3.1 | 63.7 |
| 169 | Thailand | 62 193 | 1.1 | 53 | 46 | 6.7 | 8.8 | 2.1 | 1.9 | 69.3 |
| 170 | The former Yugoslav Republic of Macedonia | 2 046 | 0.6 | 50 | 48 | 12.2 | 14.7 | 1.8 | 1.9 | 72.0 |
| 171 | Timor-Leste | 739 | -0.7 | 77 | 73 | 3.6 | 5.2 | 4.8 | 3.9 | 57.5 |
| 172 | Togo | 4 801 | 2.9 | 94 | 89 | 4.8 | 4.9 | 6.2 | 5.4 | 51.7 |
| 173 | Tonga | 103 | 0.3 | 78 | 74 | 7.4 | 8.2 | 4.5 | 3.8 | 70.7 |
| 174 | Trinidad and Tobago | 1 298 | 0.5 | 64 | 43 | 8.8 | 10.0 | 2.2 | 1.6 | 69.9 |
| 175 | Tunisia | 9 728 | 1.3 | 71 | 52 | 7.4 | 8.4 | 3.2 | 2.0 | 71.6 |
| 176 | Turkey | 70 318 | 1.6 | 67 | 57 | 7.2 | 8.2 | 3.2 | 2.5 | 70.0 |
| 177 | Turkmenistan | 4 794 | 2.1 | 79 | 64 | 6.2 | 6.5 | 4.1 | 2.7 | 62.7 |
| 178 | Tuvalu | 10 | 1.4 | 71 | 65 | 6.2 | 7.2 | 3.5 | 2.9 | 60.6 |
| 179 | Uganda | 25 004 | 3.0 | 105 | 111 | 4.1 | 3.9 | 7.1 | 7.1 | 49.3 |
| 180 | Ukraine | 48 902 | -0.6 | 51 | 45 | 18.5 | 20.8 | 1.7 | 1.2 | 67.2 |
| 181 | United Arab Emirates | 2 937 | 2.8 | 42 | 37 | 1.8 | 2.4 | 3.9 | 2.9 | 72.5 |
| 182 | United Kingdom | 59 068 | 0.3 | 54 | 53 | 21.1 | 20.8 | 1.8 | 1.6 | 78.2 |
| 183 | United Republic of Tanzania | 36 276 | 2.6 | 96 | 91 | 3.7 | 3.9 | 6.1 | 5.2 | 46.5 |
| 184 | United States of America | 291 038 | 1.1 | 52 | 51 | 16.4 | 16.2 | 2.0 | 2.1 | 77.3 |
| 185 | Uruguay | 3 391 | 0.7 | 60 | 61 | 16.7 | 17.3 | 2.5 | 2.3 | 75.2 |
| 186 | Uzbekistan | 25 705 | 1.8 | 81 | 65 | 6.5 | 7.0 | 3.7 | 2.5 | 68.2 |
| 187 | Vanuatu | 207 | 2.7 | 90 | 80 | 5.3 | 4.9 | 4.9 | 4.2 | 67.7 |
| 188 | Venezuela, Bolivarian Republic of | 25 226 | 2.1 | 70 | 60 | 5.9 | 6.9 | 3.3 | 2.7 | 73.9 |
| 189 | Viet Nam | 80 278 | 1.5 | 76 | 59 | 7.3 | 7.4 | 3.4 | 2.3 | 69.6 |
| 190 | Yemen | 19 315 | 3.9 | 114 | 104 | 3.5 | 3.6 | 7.9 | 7.0 | 60.4 |
| 191 | Zambia | 10 698 | 2.1 | 94 | 98 | 4.4 | 4.7 | 6.3 | 5.7 | 39.7 |
| 192 | Zimbabwe | 12 835 | 1.5 | 96 | 87 | 4.5 | 5.1 | 5.2 | 4.0 | 37.9 |

[a] See explanatory notes for sources and methods.

| | LIFE EXPECTANCY AT BIRTH (YEARS) | | | | PROBABILITY OF DYING (PER 1000) | | | | | | | |
| | | | | | Under age 5 years | | | | Between ages 15 and 60 years | | | |
| | Males | | Females | | Males | | Females | | Males | | Females | |
| | 2002 | Uncertainty | 2002 | Uncertainty | 2002 | Uncertainty | 2002 | Uncertainty | 2002 | Uncertainty | 2002 | Uncertainty |
|---|---|---|---|---|---|---|---|---|---|---|---|---|
| 166 | 77.7 | 77.2 - 78.2 | 83.3 | 83.1 - 83.6 | 6 | 5 - 7 | 5 | 4 - 6 | 92 | 87 - 98 | 51 | 49 - 53 |
| 167 | 68.8 | 68.0 - 69.7 | 73.6 | 73.0 - 74.3 | 26 | 24 - 29 | 20 | 18 - 22 | 190 | 175 - 205 | 127 | 117 - 137 |
| 168 | 61.0 | 59.2 - 62.7 | 66.5 | 64.8 - 68.0 | 68 | 47 - 90 | 57 | 40 - 72 | 283 | 231 - 339 | 172 | 137 - 216 |
| 169 | 66.0 | 64.8 - 67.1 | 72.7 | 71.7 - 73.8 | 32 | 28 - 37 | 26 | 22 - 30 | 279 | 250 - 311 | 153 | 131 - 178 |
| 170 | 69.0 | 68.3 - 69.7 | 75.1 | 74.4 - 75.8 | 17 | 16 - 19 | 15 | 13 - 16 | 195 | 180 - 212 | 89 | 81 - 99 |
| 171 | 54.8 | 46.4 - 62.1 | 60.5 | 50.5 - 67.7 | 142 | 108 - 178 | 108 | 81 - 134 | 326 | 162 - 533 | 242 | 111 - 463 |
| 172 | 50.0 | 43.4 - 55.7 | 53.3 | 46.0 - 59.8 | 149 | 131 - 166 | 127 | 110 - 143 | 459 | 316 - 636 | 394 | 265 - 569 |
| 173 | 70.0 | 69.5 - 70.5 | 71.4 | 70.8 - 72.0 | 23 | 20 - 27 | 15 | 12 - 18 | 171 | 166 - 177 | 181 | 174 - 188 |
| 174 | 67.1 | 66.1 - 68.1 | 72.8 | 72.2 - 73.4 | 24 | 20 - 28 | 18 | 15 - 21 | 246 | 221 - 272 | 153 | 138 - 169 |
| 175 | 69.5 | 68.7 - 70.3 | 73.9 | 73.0 - 74.7 | 31 | 28 - 34 | 24 | 21 - 26 | 167 | 154 - 180 | 115 | 102 - 128 |
| 176 | 67.9 | 67.1 - 68.8 | 72.2 | 71.1 - 73.4 | 44 | 40 - 48 | 42 | 38 - 46 | 177 | 162 - 192 | 112 | 94 - 130 |
| 177 | 58.8 | 58.3 - 59.3 | 66.9 | 66.1 - 67.7 | 63 | 56 - 69 | 47 | 42 - 52 | 369 | 349 - 385 | 193 | 172 - 215 |
| 178 | 60.0 | 58.4 - 61.8 | 61.4 | 59.7 - 62.9 | 72 | 54 - 91 | 56 | 43 - 69 | 298 | 247 - 345 | 280 | 234 - 342 |
| 179 | 47.9 | 42.3 - 53.2 | 50.8 | 43.6 - 56.5 | 148 | 142 - 154 | 136 | 130 - 142 | 505 | 370 - 661 | 431 | 306 - 606 |
| 180 | 61.7 | 61.0 - 62.4 | 72.9 | 72.0 - 73.8 | 22 | 19 - 24 | 16 | 15 - 18 | 378 | 343 - 417 | 139 | 120 - 161 |
| 181 | 71.3 | 71.0 - 71.5 | 75.1 | 74.9 - 75.3 | 10 | 9 - 11 | 10 | 9 - 10 | 169 | 165 - 174 | 122 | 120 - 125 |
| 182 | 75.8 | 75.3 - 76.3 | 80.5 | 79.9 - 81.0 | 7 | 6 - 8 | 6 | 5 - 6 | 107 | 101 - 113 | 67 | 61 - 72 |
| 183 | 45.5 | 44.3 - 46.9 | 47.5 | 46.2 - 49.0 | 163 | 149 - 177 | 144 | 132 - 156 | 561 | 534 - 585 | 512 | 484 - 536 |
| 184 | 74.6 | 74.2 - 75.1 | 79.8 | 79.7 - 80.0 | 9 | 8 - 9 | 7 | 7 - 7 | 140 | 134 - 148 | 83 | 81 - 84 |
| 185 | 71.0 | 70.5 - 71.6 | 79.3 | 79.0 - 79.7 | 18 | 15 - 21 | 13 | 12 - 14 | 182 | 172 - 192 | 88 | 84 - 92 |
| 186 | 65.6 | 64.8 - 66.3 | 70.8 | 70.1 - 71.6 | 37 | 36 - 39 | 26 | 25 - 28 | 243 | 224 - 263 | 152 | 136 - 169 |
| 187 | 66.4 | 64.7 - 68.5 | 69.1 | 67.4 - 70.9 | 40 | 30 - 51 | 40 | 30 - 50 | 217 | 185 - 245 | 175 | 150 - 200 |
| 188 | 71.0 | 70.2 - 71.8 | 76.8 | 76.5 - 77.2 | 23 | 21 - 26 | 19 | 17 - 21 | 182 | 168 - 197 | 97 | 92 - 103 |
| 189 | 67.1 | 66.3 - 68.1 | 72.2 | 71.4 - 73.1 | 41 | 36 - 46 | 33 | 28 - 37 | 200 | 184 - 215 | 129 | 117 - 140 |
| 190 | 58.7 | 51.1 - 65.5 | 62.2 | 53.8 - 68.7 | 106 | 93 - 119 | 94 | 82 - 106 | 286 | 130 - 498 | 228 | 103 - 421 |
| 191 | 39.1 | 34.5 - 43.6 | 40.2 | 35.2 - 45.4 | 191 | 170 - 214 | 176 | 155 - 195 | 700 | 590 - 810 | 654 | 546 - 768 |
| 192 | 37.7 | 35.7 - 40.2 | 38.0 | 35.8 - 40.8 | 115 | 104 - 125 | 107 | 97 - 116 | 821 | 776 - 856 | 789 | 739 - 828 |

## Annex Table 2 Deaths by cause, sex and mortality stratum in WHO regions,[a] estimates for 2002

Figures computed by WHO to assure comparability;[b] they are not necessarily the official statistics of Member States, which may use alternative rigorous methods.

| Cause[d] | SEX[c] Both sexes (000) | % total | Males (000) | % total | Females (000) | % total | AFRICA High child, high adult (000) | AFRICA High child, very high adult (000) | THE AMERICAS Very low child, very low adult (000) | THE AMERICAS Low child, low adult (000) | THE AMERICAS High child, high adult (000) |
|---|---|---|---|---|---|---|---|---|---|---|---|
| Population (000) | 6 224 985 | | 3 131 052 | | 3 093 933 | | 311 273 | 360 965 | 333 580 | 445 161 | 73 810 |
| TOTAL Deaths | 57 029 | 100 | 29 891 | 100 | 27 138 | 100 | 4 657 | 6 007 | 2 720 | 2 701 | 541 |
| I. Communicable diseases, maternal and perinatal conditions and nutritional deficiencies | 18 324 | 32.1 | 9 365 | 31.3 | 8 959 | 33 | 3 245 | 4 426 | 167 | 482 | 227 |
| Infectious and parasitic diseases | 10 904 | 19.1 | 5 795 | 19.4 | 5 109 | 18.8 | 2 211 | 3 414 | 69 | 195 | 133 |
| Tuberculosis | 1 566 | 2.7 | 1 030 | 3.4 | 536 | 2.0 | 143 | 205 | 1 | 26 | 19 |
| STIs excluding HIV | 180 | 0.3 | 91 | 0.3 | 89 | 0.3 | 41 | 52 | 0 | 1 | 1 |
| Syphilis | 157 | 0.3 | 84 | 0.3 | 72 | 0.3 | 39 | 50 | 0 | 1 | 0 |
| Chlamydia | 9 | 0.0 | 0 | 0.0 | 9 | 0.0 | 1 | 0 | 0 | 0 | 0 |
| Gonorrhoea | 1 | 0.0 | 0 | 0.0 | 1 | 0.0 | 0 | 0 | 0 | 0 | 0 |
| HIV/AIDS | 2 777 | 4.9 | 1 447 | 4.8 | 1 330 | 4.9 | 479 | 1 616 | 14 | 50 | 39 |
| Diarrhoeal diseases | 1 798 | 3.2 | 939 | 3.1 | 859 | 3.2 | 351 | 356 | 2 | 34 | 21 |
| Childhood diseases | 1 124 | 2.0 | 563 | 1.9 | 562 | 2.1 | 308 | 219 | 0 | 1 | 4 |
| Pertussis | 294 | 0.5 | 147 | 0.5 | 147 | 0.5 | 78 | 53 | 0 | 0 | 3 |
| Poliomyelitis[e] | 1 | 0.0 | 0 | 0.0 | 0 | 0.0 | 0 | 0 | 0 | 0 | 0 |
| Diphtheria | 5 | 0.0 | 3 | 0.0 | 3 | 0.0 | 1 | 1 | 0 | 0 | 0 |
| Measles | 611 | 1.1 | 306 | 1.0 | 305 | 1.1 | 180 | 131 | 0 | 0 | 0 |
| Tetanus | 214 | 0.4 | 107 | 0.4 | 107 | 0.4 | 49 | 35 | 0 | 0 | 0 |
| Meningitis | 173 | 0.3 | 90 | 0.3 | 83 | 0.3 | 8 | 12 | 1 | 8 | 9 |
| Hepatitis B[f] | 103 | 0.2 | 71 | 0.2 | 32 | 0.1 | 10 | 10 | 1 | 3 | 2 |
| Hepatitis C[f] | 54 | 0.1 | 35 | 0.1 | 18 | 0.1 | 4 | 4 | 5 | 2 | 0 |
| Malaria | 1 272 | 2.2 | 607 | 2.0 | 665 | 2.5 | 557 | 579 | 0 | 1 | 0 |
| Tropical diseases | 129 | 0.2 | 79 | 0.3 | 50 | 0.2 | 28 | 28 | 0 | 12 | 4 |
| Trypanosomiasis | 48 | 0.1 | 31 | 0.1 | 17 | 0.1 | 24 | 23 | 0 | 0 | 0 |
| Chagas disease | 14 | 0.0 | 8 | 0.0 | 7 | 0.0 | 0 | 0 | 0 | 11 | 4 |
| Schistosomiasis | 15 | 0.0 | 10 | 0.0 | 5 | 0.0 | 1 | 1 | 0 | 1 | 0 |
| Leishmaniasis | 51 | 0.1 | 30 | 0.1 | 21 | 0.1 | 4 | 4 | 0 | 0 | 0 |
| Lymphatic filariasis | 0 | 0.0 | 0 | 0.0 | 0 | 0.0 | 0 | 0 | 0 | 0 | 0 |
| Onchocerciasis | 0 | 0.0 | 0 | 0.0 | 0 | 0.0 | 0 | 0 | 0 | 0 | 0 |
| Leprosy | 6 | 0.0 | 4 | 0.0 | 2 | 0.0 | 0 | 0 | 0 | 1 | 0 |
| Dengue | 19 | 0.0 | 8 | 0.0 | 10 | 0.0 | 0 | 0 | 0 | 1 | 1 |
| Japanese encephalitis | 14 | 0.0 | 7 | 0.0 | 7 | 0.0 | 0 | 0 | 0 | 0 | 0 |
| Trachoma | 0 | 0.0 | 0 | 0.0 | 0 | 0.0 | 0 | 0 | 0 | 0 | 0 |
| Intestinal nematode infections | 12 | 0.0 | 6 | 0.0 | 6 | 0.0 | 1 | 2 | 0 | 0 | 1 |
| Ascariasis | 3 | 0.0 | 1 | 0.0 | 2 | 0.0 | 0 | 1 | 0 | 0 | 0 |
| Trichuriasis | 3 | 0.0 | 2 | 0.0 | 1 | 0.0 | 0 | 0 | 0 | 0 | 0 |
| Hookworm disease | 3 | 0.0 | 2 | 0.0 | 1 | 0.0 | 1 | 1 | 0 | 0 | 0 |
| Respiratory infections | 3 963 | 6.9 | 1 989 | 6.7 | 1 974 | 7.3 | 580 | 538 | 72 | 107 | 47 |
| Lower respiratory infections | 3 884 | 6.8 | 1 948 | 6.5 | 1 936 | 7.1 | 573 | 531 | 72 | 106 | 45 |
| Upper respiratory infections | 75 | 0.1 | 38 | 0.1 | 37 | 0.1 | 7 | 6 | 0 | 1 | 2 |
| Otitis media | 4 | 0.0 | 3 | 0.0 | 1 | 0.0 | 1 | 1 | 0 | 0 | 0 |
| Maternal conditions | 510 | 0.9 | … | … | 510 | 1.9 | 102 | 129 | 1 | 9 | 7 |
| Perinatal conditions[g] | 2 462 | 4.3 | 1 367 | 4.6 | 1 095 | 4.0 | 284 | 270 | 17 | 132 | 26 |
| Nutritional deficiencies | 485 | 0.9 | 215 | 0.7 | 270 | 1.0 | 67 | 76 | 8 | 39 | 14 |
| Protein-energy malnutrition | 260 | 0.5 | 130 | 0.4 | 131 | 0.5 | 50 | 54 | 5 | 29 | 9 |
| Iodine deficiency | 7 | 0.0 | 3 | 0.0 | 3 | 0.0 | 0 | 2 | 0 | 0 | 0 |
| Vitamin A deficiency | 23 | 0.0 | 11 | 0.0 | 12 | 0.0 | 10 | 7 | 0 | 0 | 0 |
| Iron-deficiency anaemia | 137 | 0.2 | 47 | 0.2 | 90 | 0.3 | 6 | 11 | 3 | 7 | 5 |

| Cause[d] | SOUTH-EAST ASIA Mortality stratum | | EUROPE Mortality stratum | | | EASTERN MEDITERRANEAN Mortality stratum | | WESTERN PACIFIC Mortality stratum | |
|---|---|---|---|---|---|---|---|---|---|
| | Low child, low adult | High child, high adult | Very low child, very low adult | Low child, low adult | Low child, high adult | Low child, low adult | High child, high adult | Very low child, very low adult | Low child, low adult |
| Population (000) | 298 234 | 1 292 598 | 415 323 | 222 846 | 239 717 | 142 528 | 360 296 | 155 400 | 1 562 136 |
| | (000) | (000) | (000) | (000) | (000) | (000) | (000) | (000) | (000) |
| TOTAL Deaths | 2 191 | 12 466 | 3 920 | 1 865 | 3 779 | 706 | 3 446 | 1 146 | 10 794 |
| I. Communicable diseases, maternal and perinatal conditions and nutritional deficiencies | 625 | 5 143 | 241 | 166 | 156 | 92 | 1637 | 125 | 1 573 |
| Infectious and parasitic diseases | 380 | 2 542 | 50 | 60 | 85 | 37 | 916 | 23 | 781 |
| Tuberculosis | 138 | 461 | 5 | 19 | 45 | 5 | 133 | 5 | 361 |
| STIs excluding HIV | 3 | 55 | 0 | 0 | 0 | 0 | 23 | 0 | 2 |
| Syphilis | 1 | 42 | 0 | 0 | 0 | 0 | 21 | 0 | 1 |
| Chlamydia | 1 | 7 | 0 | 0 | 0 | 0 | 1 | 0 | 0 |
| Gonorrhoea | 0 | 0 | 0 | 0 | 0 | 0 | 0 | 0 | 0 |
| HIV/AIDS | 59 | 377 | 6 | 1 | 29 | 1 | 43 | 0 | 61 |
| Diarrhoeal diseases | 41 | 563 | 2 | 13 | 1 | 15 | 244 | 1 | 153 |
| Childhood diseases | 39 | 352 | 0 | 6 | 0 | 0 | 153 | 0 | 41 |
| Pertussis | 0 | 111 | 0 | 0 | 0 | 0 | 46 | 0 | 2 |
| Poliomyelitis[e] | 0 | 0 | 0 | 0 | 0 | 0 | 0 | 0 | 0 |
| Diphtheria | 0 | 3 | 0 | 0 | 0 | 0 | 0 | 0 | 0 |
| Measles | 31 | 165 | 0 | 6 | 0 | 0 | 70 | 0 | 28 |
| Tetanus | 8 | 74 | 0 | 0 | 0 | 0 | 36 | 0 | 11 |
| Meningitis | 9 | 64 | 2 | 10 | 3 | 2 | 23 | 0 | 20 |
| Hepatitis B[f] | 7 | 30 | 2 | 2 | 1 | 1 | 9 | 1 | 25 |
| Hepatitis C[f] | 3 | 11 | 3 | 1 | 0 | 1 | 4 | 4 | 10 |
| Malaria | 12 | 53 | 0 | 0 | 0 | 2 | 57 | 0 | 11 |
| Tropical diseases | 0 | 36 | 0 | 0 | 0 | 0 | 15 | 0 | 5 |
| Trypanosomiasis | 0 | 0 | 0 | 0 | 0 | 0 | 1 | 0 | 0 |
| Chagas disease | 0 | 0 | 0 | 0 | 0 | 0 | 0 | 0 | 0 |
| Schistosomiasis | 0 | 0 | 0 | 0 | 0 | 0 | 9 | 0 | 4 |
| Leishmaniasis | 0 | 36 | 0 | 0 | 0 | 0 | 5 | 0 | 2 |
| Lymphatic filariasis | 0 | 0 | 0 | 0 | 0 | 0 | 0 | 0 | 0 |
| Onchocerciasis | 0 | 0 | 0 | 0 | 0 | 0 | 0 | 0 | 0 |
| Leprosy | 1 | 2 | 0 | 0 | 0 | 0 | 1 | 0 | 1 |
| Dengue | 3 | 9 | 0 | 0 | 0 | 0 | 1 | 0 | 4 |
| Japanese encephalitis | 0 | 8 | 0 | 0 | 0 | 0 | 2 | 0 | 3 |
| Trachoma | 0 | 0 | 0 | 0 | 0 | 0 | 0 | 0 | 0 |
| Intestinal nematode infections | 1 | 4 | 0 | 0 | 0 | 0 | 1 | 0 | 1 |
| Ascariasis | 0 | 1 | 0 | 0 | 0 | 0 | 0 | 0 | 1 |
| Trichuriasis | 0 | 2 | 0 | 0 | 0 | 0 | 0 | 0 | 0 |
| Hookworm disease | 1 | 0 | 0 | 0 | 0 | 0 | 0 | 0 | 0 |
| Respiratory infections | 126 | 1 348 | 174 | 62 | 52 | 21 | 333 | 98 | 400 |
| Lower respiratory infections | 123 | 1 330 | 171 | 60 | 49 | 21 | 327 | 97 | 374 |
| Upper respiratory infections | 3 | 17 | 3 | 2 | 2 | 0 | 6 | 0 | 26 |
| Otitis media | 0 | 1 | 0 | 0 | 0 | 0 | 0 | 0 | 0 |
| Maternal conditions | 11 | 160 | 0 | 2 | 1 | 3 | 65 | 0 | 21 |
| Perinatal conditions[g] | 82 | 930 | 10 | 39 | 16 | 28 | 275 | 1 | 348 |
| Nutritional deficiencies | 26 | 163 | 7 | 3 | 2 | 4 | 49 | 3 | 24 |
| Protein-energy malnutrition | 10 | 58 | 3 | 1 | 1 | 2 | 24 | 1 | 13 |
| Iodine deficiency | 0 | 1 | 0 | 0 | 0 | 0 | 2 | 0 | 0 |
| Vitamin A deficiency | 0 | 2 | 0 | 0 | 0 | 0 | 3 | 0 | 0 |
| Iron-deficiency anaemia | 13 | 67 | 3 | 2 | 1 | 1 | 9 | 1 | 8 |

## Annex Table 2 Deaths by cause, sex and mortality stratum in WHO regions,[a] estimates for 2002

Figures computed by WHO to assure comparability;[b] they are not necessarily the official statistics of Member States, which may use alternative rigorous methods.

| Cause[d] | SEX[c] | | | | | | AFRICA | | THE AMERICAS | | |
| --- | --- | --- | --- | --- | --- | --- | --- | --- | --- | --- | --- |
| | | | | | | | Mortality stratum | | Mortality stratum | | |
| | Both sexes | | Males | | Females | | High child, high adult | High child, very high adult | Very low child, very low adult | Low child, low adult | High child, high adult |
| Population (000) | 6 224 985 | | 3 131 052 | | 3 093 933 | | 311 273 | 360 965 | 333 580 | 445 161 | 73 810 |
| | (000) | % total | (000) | % total | (000) | % total | (000) | (000) | (000) | (000) | (000) |
| II. Noncommunicable conditions | 33 537 | 58.8 | 17 062 | 57.1 | 16 474 | 60.7 | 1 068 | 1 184 | 2 380 | 1 898 | 268 |
| Malignant neoplasms | 7 121 | 12.5 | 3 974 | 13.3 | 3 147 | 11.6 | 194 | 216 | 641 | 409 | 66 |
| Mouth and oropharynx cancers | 318 | 0.6 | 221 | 0.7 | 97 | 0.4 | 8 | 10 | 10 | 12 | 2 |
| Oesophagus cancer | 446 | 0.8 | 285 | 1.0 | 161 | 0.6 | 5 | 17 | 16 | 15 | 1 |
| Stomach cancer | 850 | 1.5 | 524 | 1.8 | 326 | 1.2 | 16 | 18 | 17 | 44 | 13 |
| Colon/rectum cancer | 622 | 1.1 | 323 | 1.1 | 300 | 1.1 | 10 | 10 | 74 | 31 | 4 |
| Liver cancer | 618 | 1.1 | 427 | 1.4 | 191 | 0.7 | 22 | 23 | 17 | 17 | 3 |
| Pancreas cancer | 231 | 0.4 | 122 | 0.4 | 109 | 0.4 | 3 | 5 | 33 | 17 | 2 |
| Trachea/bronchus/lung cancers | 1 243 | 2.2 | 890 | 3.0 | 353 | 1.3 | 7 | 10 | 179 | 49 | 3 |
| Melanoma and other skin cancers | 66 | 0.1 | 35 | 0.1 | 31 | 0.1 | 4 | 4 | 12 | 6 | 1 |
| Breast cancer | 477 | 0.8 | 3 | 0.0 | 474 | 1.7 | 21 | 14 | 52 | 33 | 4 |
| Cervix uteri cancer | 239 | 0.4 | … | … | 239 | 0.9 | 15 | 23 | 5 | 19 | 7 |
| Corpus uteri cancer | 71 | 0.1 | … | … | 71 | 0.3 | 1 | 1 | 9 | 10 | 1 |
| Ovary cancer | 135 | 0.2 | … | … | 135 | 0.5 | 3 | 5 | 16 | 7 | 1 |
| Prostate cancer | 269 | 0.5 | 269 | 0.9 | … | … | 24 | 17 | 42 | 31 | 5 |
| Bladder cancer | 179 | 0.3 | 125 | 0.4 | 54 | 0.2 | 6 | 5 | 16 | 8 | 1 |
| Lymphomas, multiple myeloma | 334 | 0.6 | 169 | 0.6 | 166 | 0.6 | 17 | 16 | 45 | 18 | 5 |
| Leukaemia | 264 | 0.5 | 147 | 0.5 | 117 | 0.4 | 7 | 6 | 27 | 18 | 3 |
| Other neoplasms | 149 | 0.3 | 75 | 0.2 | 74 | 0.3 | 4 | 5 | 17 | 11 | 1 |
| Diabetes mellitus | 988 | 1.7 | 441 | 1.5 | 547 | 2.0 | 35 | 45 | 86 | 151 | 16 |
| Nutritional/endocrine disorders | 243 | 0.4 | 108 | 0.4 | 135 | 0.5 | 12 | 14 | 33 | 25 | 4 |
| Neuropsychiatric disorders | 1 112 | 1.9 | 575 | 1.9 | 536 | 2.0 | 43 | 47 | 174 | 56 | 10 |
| Unipolar depressive disorders | 13 | 0.0 | 6 | 0.0 | 7 | 0.0 | 0 | 0 | 1 | 0 | 0 |
| Bipolar affective disorder | 1 | 0.0 | 0 | 0.0 | 1 | 0.0 | 0 | 0 | 0 | 0 | 0 |
| Schizophrenia | 23 | 0.0 | 11 | 0.0 | 12 | 0.0 | 0 | 0 | 1 | 0 | 0 |
| Epilepsy | 125 | 0.2 | 70 | 0.2 | 55 | 0.2 | 18 | 20 | 2 | 6 | 2 |
| Alcohol use disorders | 91 | 0.2 | 77 | 0.3 | 13 | 0.0 | 3 | 4 | 8 | 14 | 2 |
| Alzheimer and other dementias | 397 | 0.7 | 147 | 0.5 | 250 | 0.9 | 3 | 4 | 106 | 11 | 1 |
| Parkinson disease | 98 | 0.2 | 50 | 0.2 | 48 | 0.2 | 2 | 3 | 19 | 4 | 1 |
| Multiple sclerosis | 16 | 0.0 | 6 | 0.0 | 10 | 0.0 | 0 | 0 | 4 | 1 | 0 |
| Drug use disorders | 86 | 0.2 | 70 | 0.2 | 16 | 0.1 | 2 | 0 | 5 | 2 | 0 |
| Post-traumatic stress disorder | 0 | 0.0 | 0 | 0.0 | 0 | 0.0 | 0 | 0 | 0 | 0 | 0 |
| Obsessive-compulsive disorder | 0 | 0.0 | 0 | 0.0 | 0 | 0.0 | 0 | 0 | 0 | 0 | 0 |
| Panic disorder | 0 | 0.0 | 0 | 0.0 | 0 | 0.0 | 0 | 0 | 0 | 0 | 0 |
| Insomnia (primary) | 0 | 0.0 | 0 | 0.0 | 0 | 0.0 | 0 | 0 | 0 | 0 | 0 |
| Migraine | 0 | 0.0 | 0 | 0.0 | 0 | 0.0 | 0 | 0 | 0 | 0 | 0 |
| Sense organ disorders | 3 | 0.0 | 2 | 0.0 | 2 | 0.0 | 0 | 0 | 0 | 0 | 0 |
| Glaucoma | 0 | 0.0 | 0 | 0.0 | 0 | 0.0 | 0 | 0 | 0 | 0 | 0 |
| Cataracts | 0 | 0.0 | 0 | 0.0 | 0 | 0.0 | 0 | 0 | 0 | 0 | 0 |
| Vision loss, age-related and other | 0 | 0.0 | 0 | 0.0 | 0 | 0.0 | 0 | 0 | 0 | 0 | 0 |
| Hearing loss, adult onset | 0 | 0.0 | 0 | 0.0 | 0 | 0.0 | 0 | 0 | 0 | 0 | 0 |
| Cardiovascular diseases | 16 733 | 29.3 | 8 120 | 27.2 | 8 613 | 31.7 | 496 | 540 | 1 031 | 804 | 93 |
| Rheumatic heart disease | 327 | 0.6 | 138 | 0.5 | 189 | 0.7 | 12 | 8 | 4 | 6 | 0 |
| Hypertensive heart disease | 911 | 1.6 | 419 | 1.4 | 492 | 1.8 | 27 | 33 | 47 | 73 | 15 |
| Ischaemic heart disease | 7 208 | 12.6 | 3 802 | 12.7 | 3 406 | 12.5 | 160 | 172 | 574 | 319 | 28 |
| Cerebrovascular disease | 5 509 | 9.7 | 2 550 | 8.5 | 2 959 | 10.9 | 172 | 187 | 187 | 239 | 26 |
| Inflammatory heart disease | 404 | 0.7 | 211 | 0.7 | 193 | 0.7 | 20 | 22 | 35 | 31 | 1 |

| Cause[d] | SOUTH-EAST ASIA Mortality stratum | | EUROPE Mortality stratum | | | EASTERN MEDITERRANEAN Mortality stratum | | WESTERN PACIFIC Mortality stratum | |
|---|---|---|---|---|---|---|---|---|---|
| | Low child, low adult | High child, high adult | Very low child, very low adult | Low child, low adult | Low child, high adult | Low child, low adult | High child, high adult | Very low child, very low adult | Low child, low adult |
| Population (000) | 298 234 | 1 292 598 | 415 323 | 222 846 | 239 717 | 142 528 | 360 296 | 155 400 | 1 562 136 |
| | (000) | (000) | (000) | (000) | (000) | (000) | (000) | (000) | (000) |
| II. Noncommunicable conditions | 1 341 | 6 082 | 3 489 | 1 590 | 3 131 | 501 | 1 529 | 937 | 8 076 |
| Malignant neoplasms | 267 | 893 | 1 038 | 291 | 504 | 76 | 196 | 357 | 1 961 |
| Mouth and oropharynx cancers | 16 | 133 | 24 | 9 | 18 | 2 | 18 | 7 | 50 |
| Oesophagus cancer | 4 | 78 | 28 | 7 | 13 | 4 | 12 | 12 | 233 |
| Stomach cancer | 12 | 51 | 61 | 28 | 68 | 12 | 9 | 53 | 447 |
| Colon/rectum cancer | 28 | 35 | 137 | 29 | 62 | 5 | 10 | 47 | 139 |
| Liver cancer | 31 | 30 | 40 | 12 | 14 | 6 | 9 | 36 | 358 |
| Pancreas cancer | 6 | 13 | 53 | 12 | 23 | 2 | 3 | 23 | 35 |
| Trachea/bronchus/lung cancers | 43 | 131 | 207 | 61 | 98 | 10 | 17 | 66 | 361 |
| Melanoma and other skin cancers | 1 | 2 | 15 | 4 | 6 | 1 | 1 | 3 | 4 |
| Breast cancer | 25 | 68 | 89 | 21 | 40 | 4 | 23 | 14 | 68 |
| Cervix uteri cancer | 14 | 87 | 8 | 7 | 11 | 1 | 6 | 3 | 31 |
| Corpus uteri cancer | 3 | 3 | 15 | 5 | 11 | 1 | 1 | 3 | 6 |
| Ovary cancer | 8 | 19 | 25 | 7 | 14 | 1 | 5 | 5 | 17 |
| Prostate cancer | 8 | 19 | 68 | 11 | 14 | 3 | 5 | 12 | 9 |
| Bladder cancer | 6 | 27 | 37 | 10 | 14 | 2 | 17 | 6 | 24 |
| Lymphomas, multiple myeloma | 17 | 79 | 54 | 11 | 10 | 5 | 15 | 16 | 26 |
| Leukaemia | 13 | 33 | 36 | 11 | 15 | 7 | 13 | 9 | 65 |
| Other neoplasms | 3 | 16 | 30 | 4 | 5 | 9 | 15 | 11 | 18 |
| Diabetes mellitus | 72 | 191 | 92 | 29 | 21 | 15 | 40 | 18 | 174 |
| Nutritional/endocrine disorders | 16 | 23 | 28 | 3 | 3 | 5 | 24 | 9 | 43 |
| Neuropsychiatric disorders | 53 | 214 | 185 | 24 | 47 | 22 | 67 | 24 | 143 |
| Unipolar depressive disorders | 1 | 8 | 2 | 0 | 0 | 0 | 1 | 0 | 0 |
| Bipolar affective disorder | 0 | 0 | 0 | 0 | 0 | 0 | 0 | 0 | 0 |
| Schizophrenia | 1 | 13 | 1 | 0 | 1 | 0 | 1 | 0 | 4 |
| Epilepsy | 5 | 29 | 6 | 4 | 5 | 2 | 8 | 1 | 18 |
| Alcohol use disorders | 3 | 12 | 13 | 4 | 11 | 2 | 2 | 1 | 11 |
| Alzheimer and other dementias | 9 | 79 | 95 | 3 | 7 | 2 | 9 | 10 | 56 |
| Parkinson disease | 1 | 9 | 22 | 2 | 2 | 2 | 2 | 4 | 26 |
| Multiple sclerosis | 0 | 1 | 4 | 1 | 2 | 0 | 0 | 0 | 1 |
| Drug use disorders | 3 | 20 | 7 | 2 | 9 | 7 | 24 | 1 | 3 |
| Post-traumatic stress disorder | 0 | 0 | 0 | 0 | 0 | 0 | 0 | 0 | 0 |
| Obsessive-compulsive disorder | 0 | 0 | 0 | 0 | 0 | 0 | 0 | 0 | 0 |
| Panic disorder | 0 | 0 | 0 | 0 | 0 | 0 | 0 | 0 | 0 |
| Insomnia (primary) | 0 | 0 | 0 | 0 | 0 | 0 | 0 | 0 | 0 |
| Migraine | 0 | 0 | 0 | 0 | 0 | 0 | 0 | 0 | 0 |
| Sense organ disorders | 0 | 1 | 0 | 0 | 0 | 0 | 1 | 0 | 0 |
| Glaucoma | 0 | 0 | 0 | 0 | 0 | 0 | 0 | 0 | 0 |
| Cataracts | 0 | 0 | 0 | 0 | 0 | 0 | 0 | 0 | 0 |
| Vision loss, age-related and other | 0 | 0 | 0 | 0 | 0 | 0 | 0 | 0 | 0 |
| Hearing loss, adult onset | 0 | 0 | 0 | 0 | 0 | 0 | 0 | 0 | 0 |
| Cardiovascular diseases | 600 | 3 311 | 1 612 | 1 052 | 2 263 | 283 | 796 | 377 | 3 448 |
| Rheumatic heart disease | 12 | 121 | 10 | 7 | 13 | 4 | 20 | 3 | 107 |
| Hypertensive heart disease | 56 | 96 | 66 | 68 | 45 | 30 | 67 | 8 | 276 |
| Ischaemic heart disease | 265 | 1 774 | 672 | 464 | 1 237 | 142 | 396 | 129 | 864 |
| Cerebrovascular disease | 162 | 897 | 414 | 284 | 749 | 55 | 172 | 150 | 1 807 |
| Inflammatory heart disease | 10 | 66 | 28 | 30 | 43 | 11 | 26 | 8 | 73 |

## Annex Table 2 Deaths by cause, sex and mortality stratum in WHO regions,[a] estimates for 2002

Figures computed by WHO to assure comparability;[b] they are not necessarily the official statistics of Member States, which may use alternative rigorous methods.

| Cause[d] | SEX[c] | | | | | | AFRICA | | THE AMERICAS | | |
|---|---|---|---|---|---|---|---|---|---|---|---|
| | | | | | | | Mortality stratum | | Mortality stratum | | |
| | Both sexes | | Males | | Females | | High child, high adult | High child, very high adult | Very low child, very low adult | Low child, low adult | High child, high adult |
| | (000) | % total | (000) | % total | (000) | % total | (000) | (000) | (000) | (000) | (000) |
| Population (000) | 6 224 985 | | 3 131 052 | | 3 093 933 | | 311 273 | 360 965 | 333 580 | 445 161 | 73 810 |
| Respiratory diseases | 3 702 | 6.5 | 1 912 | 6.4 | 1 790 | 6.6 | 124 | 133 | 199 | 176 | 23 |
| Chronic obstructive pulmonary disease | 2 748 | 4.8 | 1 413 | 4.7 | 1 335 | 4.9 | 52 | 65 | 141 | 90 | 10 |
| Asthma | 240 | 0.4 | 122 | 0.4 | 118 | 0.4 | 12 | 14 | 6 | 10 | 2 |
| Digestive diseases | 1 968 | 3.5 | 1 094 | 3.7 | 874 | 3.2 | 75 | 82 | 99 | 154 | 31 |
| Peptic ulcer disease | 264 | 0.5 | 155 | 0.5 | 109 | 0.4 | 7 | 8 | 6 | 11 | 3 |
| Cirrhosis of the liver | 786 | 1.4 | 503 | 1.7 | 283 | 1.0 | 26 | 28 | 31 | 61 | 13 |
| Appendicitis | 21 | 0.0 | 12 | 0.0 | 10 | 0.0 | 1 | 1 | 1 | 2 | 1 |
| Diseases of the genitourinary system | 848 | 1.5 | 442 | 1.5 | 406 | 1.5 | 51 | 55 | 66 | 55 | 15 |
| Nephritis/nephrosis | 677 | 1.2 | 345 | 1.2 | 332 | 1.2 | 47 | 52 | 47 | 43 | 12 |
| Benign prostatic hypertrophy | 32 | 0.1 | 32 | 0.1 | … | … | 1 | 1 | 1 | 2 | 0 |
| Skin diseases | 69 | 0.1 | 26 | 0.1 | 43 | 0.2 | 10 | 9 | 5 | 6 | 2 |
| Musculoskeletal diseases | 106 | 0.2 | 38 | 0.1 | 69 | 0.3 | 4 | 3 | 17 | 10 | 2 |
| Rheumatoid arthritis | 25 | 0.0 | 7 | 0.0 | 18 | 0.1 | 1 | 0 | 3 | 2 | 1 |
| Osteoarthritis | 5 | 0.0 | 2 | 0.0 | 3 | 0.0 | 0 | 0 | 1 | 1 | 0 |
| Congenital abnormalities | 493 | 0.9 | 255 | 0.9 | 238 | 0.9 | 21 | 35 | 13 | 40 | 5 |
| Oral diseases | 2 | 0.0 | 1 | 0.0 | 1 | 0.0 | 0 | 0 | 0 | 0 | 0 |
| Dental caries | 0 | 0.0 | 0 | 0.0 | 0 | 0.0 | 0 | 0 | 0 | 0 | 0 |
| Periodontal disease | 0 | 0.0 | 0 | 0.0 | 0 | 0.0 | 0 | 0 | 0 | 0 | 0 |
| Edentulism | 0 | 0.0 | 0 | 0.0 | 0 | 0.0 | 0 | 0 | 0 | 0 | 0 |
| III. Injuries | 5 168 | 9.1 | 3 464 | 11.6 | 1 705 | 6.3 | 344 | 397 | 173 | 321 | 46 |
| Unintentional | 3 551 | 6.2 | 2 307 | 7.7 | 1 244 | 4.6 | 258 | 230 | 120 | 168 | 33 |
| Road traffic accidents | 1 192 | 2.1 | 869 | 2.9 | 323 | 1.2 | 96 | 99 | 49 | 76 | 10 |
| Poisoning | 350 | 0.6 | 225 | 0.8 | 125 | 0.5 | 21 | 18 | 14 | 2 | 1 |
| Falls | 392 | 0.7 | 236 | 0.8 | 156 | 0.6 | 11 | 9 | 18 | 12 | 1 |
| Fires | 312 | 0.5 | 120 | 0.4 | 192 | 0.7 | 24 | 20 | 4 | 3 | 1 |
| Drowning | 382 | 0.7 | 262 | 0.9 | 120 | 0.4 | 36 | 29 | 4 | 15 | 3 |
| Other unintentional injuries | 923 | 1.6 | 595 | 2.0 | 328 | 1.2 | 71 | 56 | 30 | 58 | 18 |
| Intentional | 1 618 | 2.8 | 1 157 | 3.9 | 461 | 1.7 | 86 | 167 | 53 | 154 | 13 |
| Self-inflicted | 873 | 1.5 | 546 | 1.8 | 327 | 1.2 | 15 | 19 | 35 | 26 | 2 |
| Violence | 559 | 1.0 | 445 | 1.5 | 114 | 0.4 | 57 | 77 | 17 | 119 | 10 |
| War | 172 | 0.3 | 155 | 0.5 | 17 | 0.1 | 14 | 71 | 0 | 8 | 0 |

[a] See list of Member States by WHO region and mortality stratum.

[b] See explanatory notes for sources and methods.

[c] World totals for males and females include residual populations living outside WHO Member States.

[d] Estimates for specific causes may not sum to broader cause groupings owing to omission of residual categories.

[e] For WHO Regions of the Americas, Europe and the Western Pacific, these figures include only late effects of poliomyelitis cases with onset prior to regional certification of polio eradication in 1994, 2000 and 2002, respectively. For all other regions, except where vital registration reports late effects of polio cases, these deaths are from acute poliomyelitis.

[f] Does not include liver cancer and cirrhosis deaths resulting from chronic hepatitis virus infection.

[g] This category includes deaths from causes originating in the perinatal period as defined in Chapter XVI of the International Classification of Diseases, principally low birthweight, prematurity, birth asphyxia and birth trauma, and does not include all deaths occurring in the early neonatal period.

… Data not applicable.

| Cause[d] | SOUTH-EAST ASIA | | EUROPE | | | EASTERN MEDITERRANEAN | | WESTERN PACIFIC | |
|---|---|---|---|---|---|---|---|---|---|
| | Mortality stratum | | Mortality stratum | | | Mortality stratum | | Mortality stratum | |
| | Low child, low adult | High child, high adult | Very low child, very low adult | Low child, low adult | Low child, high adult | Low child, low adult | High child, high adult | Very low child, very low adult | Low child, low adult |
| Population (000) | 298 234 | 1 292 598 | 415 323 | 222 846 | 239 717 | 142 528 | 360 296 | 155 400 | 1 562 136 |
| | (000) | (000) | (000) | (000) | (000) | (000) | (000) | (000) | (000) |
| Respiratory diseases | 153 | 721 | 220 | 72 | 112 | 27 | 128 | 59 | 1 550 |
| Chronic obstructive pulmonary disease | 100 | 556 | 140 | 45 | 76 | 15 | 80 | 21 | 1 354 |
| Asthma | 20 | 77 | 12 | 9 | 22 | 2 | 14 | 5 | 37 |
| Digestive diseases | 87 | 415 | 182 | 76 | 131 | 22 | 130 | 45 | 435 |
| Peptic ulcer disease | 15 | 84 | 17 | 9 | 13 | 2 | 10 | 4 | 75 |
| Cirrhosis of the liver | 34 | 170 | 65 | 39 | 67 | 8 | 59 | 14 | 171 |
| Appendicitis | 1 | 7 | 1 | 0 | 1 | 0 | 1 | 0 | 5 |
| Diseases of the genitourinary system | 57 | 149 | 62 | 25 | 25 | 21 | 62 | 28 | 175 |
| Nephritis/nephrosis | 45 | 124 | 42 | 20 | 14 | 9 | 56 | 24 | 141 |
| Benign prostatic hypertrophy | 2 | 11 | 1 | 1 | 3 | 1 | 2 | 0 | 6 |
| Skin diseases | 5 | 10 | 9 | 0 | 3 | 1 | 4 | 1 | 3 |
| Musculoskeletal diseases | 7 | 10 | 20 | 2 | 4 | 1 | 2 | 6 | 20 |
| Rheumatoid arthritis | 1 | 3 | 4 | 1 | 1 | 0 | 0 | 2 | 5 |
| Osteoarthritis | 0 | 0 | 1 | 0 | 0 | 0 | 0 | 0 | 0 |
| Congenital abnormalities | 20 | 129 | 11 | 13 | 14 | 19 | 64 | 4 | 104 |
| Oral diseases | 0 | 0 | 0 | 0 | 0 | 0 | 0 | 0 | 0 |
| Dental caries | 0 | 0 | 0 | 0 | 0 | 0 | 0 | 0 | 0 |
| Periodontal disease | 0 | 0 | 0 | 0 | 0 | 0 | 0 | 0 | 0 |
| Edentulism | 0 | 0 | 0 | 0 | 0 | 0 | 0 | 0 | 0 |
| III. Injuries | 225 | 1 242 | 190 | 110 | 492 | 113 | 279 | 84 | 1 145 |
| Unintentional | 149 | 931 | 137 | 76 | 321 | 98 | 196 | 48 | 779 |
| Road traffic accidents | 72 | 224 | 46 | 22 | 59 | 58 | 75 | 14 | 290 |
| Poisoning | 8 | 87 | 6 | 6 | 99 | 3 | 12 | 1 | 74 |
| Falls | 15 | 106 | 47 | 9 | 24 | 6 | 17 | 7 | 108 |
| Fires | 14 | 170 | 3 | 3 | 18 | 8 | 24 | 2 | 18 |
| Drowning | 14 | 84 | 4 | 6 | 28 | 5 | 21 | 6 | 126 |
| Other unintentional injuries | 26 | 261 | 32 | 31 | 94 | 18 | 47 | 18 | 162 |
| Intentional | 76 | 310 | 53 | 33 | 170 | 15 | 83 | 36 | 366 |
| Self-inflicted | 37 | 209 | 48 | 23 | 92 | 9 | 25 | 35 | 296 |
| Violence | 28 | 85 | 4 | 8 | 61 | 4 | 22 | 1 | 65 |
| War | 10 | 11 | 0 | 2 | 17 | 0 | 35 | 0 | 3 |

## Annex Table 3 Burden of disease in DALYs by cause, sex and mortality stratum in WHO regions,[a] estimates for 2002

Figures computed by WHO to assure comparability;[b] they are not necessarily the official statistics of Member States, which may use alternative rigorous methods.

| Cause[d] | Both sexes (000) | Both sexes % total | Males (000) | Males % total | Females (000) | Females % total | AFRICA High child, high adult (000) | AFRICA High child, very high adult (000) | THE AMERICAS Very low child, very low adult (000) | THE AMERICAS Low child, low adult (000) | THE AMERICAS High child, high adult (000) |
|---|---|---|---|---|---|---|---|---|---|---|---|
| **Population (000)** | *6 224 985* | | *3 131 052* | | *3 093 933* | | *311 273* | *360 965* | *333 580* | *445 161* | *73 810* |
| TOTAL DALYs | 1 490 126 | 100 | 772 912 | 100 | 717 213 | 100 | 160 415 | 200 961 | 46 868 | 81 589 | 17 130 |
| **I. Communicable diseases, maternal and perinatal conditions and nutritional deficiencies** | 610 319 | 41.0 | 296 796 | 38.4 | 313 523 | 43.7 | 115 317 | 150 405 | 3 106 | 16 334 | 7 210 |
| Infectious and parasitic diseases | 350 333 | 23.5 | 179 307 | 23.2 | 171 025 | 23.8 | 75 966 | 111 483 | 1 228 | 6 719 | 3 944 |
| Tuberculosis | 34 736 | 2.3 | 21 905 | 2.8 | 12 831 | 1.8 | 3 786 | 5 480 | 12 | 506 | 410 |
| STIs excluding HIV | 11 347 | 0.8 | 3 855 | 0.5 | 7 492 | 1.0 | 1 930 | 2 444 | 75 | 487 | 69 |
| Syphilis | 4 200 | 0.3 | 1 970 | 0.3 | 2 230 | 0.3 | 1 028 | 1 417 | 2 | 56 | 20 |
| Chlamydia | 3 571 | 0.2 | 302 | 0.0 | 3 269 | 0.5 | 364 | 428 | 55 | 241 | 15 |
| Gonorrhoea | 3 365 | 0.2 | 1 473 | 0.2 | 1 892 | 0.3 | 520 | 573 | 16 | 183 | 31 |
| HIV/AIDS | 84 458 | 5.7 | 42 663 | 5.5 | 41 795 | 5.8 | 14 620 | 49 343 | 454 | 1 594 | 1 163 |
| Diarrhoeal diseases | 61 966 | 4.2 | 32 353 | 4.2 | 29 614 | 4.1 | 11 548 | 11 689 | 106 | 1 494 | 750 |
| Childhood diseases | 41 480 | 2.8 | 20 713 | 2.7 | 20 767 | 2.9 | 11 061 | 7 934 | 54 | 177 | 162 |
| Pertussis | 12 595 | 0.8 | 6 283 | 0.8 | 6 312 | 0.9 | 3 078 | 2 165 | 52 | 163 | 146 |
| Poliomyelitis[e] | 151 | 0.0 | 76 | 0.0 | 74 | 0.0 | 11 | 4 | 3 | 6 | 1 |
| Diphtheria | 185 | 0.0 | 96 | 0.0 | 89 | 0.0 | 24 | 24 | 0 | 2 | 7 |
| Measles | 21 475 | 1.4 | 10 727 | 1.4 | 10 748 | 1.5 | 6 328 | 4 587 | 0 | 0 | 0 |
| Tetanus | 7 074 | 0.5 | 3 530 | 0.5 | 3 543 | 0.5 | 1 620 | 1 155 | 0 | 6 | 8 |
| Meningitis | 6 192 | 0.4 | 3 082 | 0.4 | 3 110 | 0.4 | 394 | 497 | 43 | 356 | 280 |
| Hepatitis B[f] | 2 170 | 0.1 | 1 459 | 0.2 | 711 | 0.1 | 302 | 280 | 20 | 56 | 38 |
| Hepatitis C[f] | 1 004 | 0.1 | 668 | 0.1 | 336 | 0.0 | 120 | 122 | 77 | 29 | 1 |
| Malaria | 46 486 | 3.1 | 22 243 | 2.9 | 24 242 | 3.4 | 20 070 | 20 785 | 0 | 86 | 25 |
| Tropical diseases | 12 245 | 0.8 | 8 273 | 1.1 | 3 973 | 0.6 | 2 939 | 2 743 | 9 | 604 | 178 |
| Trypanosomiasis | 1 525 | 0.1 | 966 | 0.1 | 559 | 0.1 | 744 | 740 | 0 | 0 | 0 |
| Chagas disease | 667 | 0.0 | 343 | 0.0 | 324 | 0.0 | 0 | 0 | 8 | 483 | 171 |
| Schistosomiasis | 1 702 | 0.1 | 1 020 | 0.1 | 681 | 0.1 | 621 | 713 | 0 | 74 | 0 |
| Leishmaniasis | 2 090 | 0.1 | 1 249 | 0.2 | 840 | 0.1 | 208 | 175 | 1 | 38 | 5 |
| Lymphatic filariasis | 5 777 | 0.4 | 4 413 | 0.6 | 1 364 | 0.2 | 976 | 1 035 | 0 | 9 | 1 |
| Onchocerciasis | 484 | 0.0 | 280 | 0.0 | 204 | 0.0 | 390 | 80 | 0 | 1 | 1 |
| Leprosy | 199 | 0.0 | 117 | 0.0 | 82 | 0.0 | 12 | 11 | 0 | 18 | 0 |
| Dengue | 616 | 0.0 | 279 | 0.0 | 337 | 0.0 | 1 | 4 | 0 | 31 | 38 |
| Japanese encephalitis | 709 | 0.0 | 338 | 0.0 | 371 | 0.1 | 0 | 0 | 0 | 0 | 0 |
| Trachoma | 2 329 | 0.2 | 597 | 0.1 | 1 732 | 0.2 | 486 | 726 | 0 | 162 | 2 |
| Intestinal nematode infections | 2 951 | 0.2 | 1 490 | 0.2 | 1 461 | 0.2 | 809 | 329 | 1 | 66 | 101 |
| Ascariasis | 1 817 | 0.1 | 910 | 0.1 | 907 | 0.1 | 714 | 144 | 0 | 23 | 39 |
| Trichuriasis | 1 006 | 0.1 | 519 | 0.1 | 488 | 0.1 | 78 | 155 | 1 | 42 | 29 |
| Hookworm disease | 59 | 0.0 | 31 | 0.0 | 27 | 0.0 | 17 | 29 | 0 | 0 | 0 |
| Respiratory infections | 94 603 | 6.3 | 48 177 | 6.2 | 46 427 | 6.5 | 18 976 | 16 619 | 390 | 1 876 | 1 050 |
| Lower respiratory infections | 91 374 | 6.1 | 46 548 | 6.0 | 44 826 | 6.3 | 18 625 | 16 286 | 337 | 1 721 | 986 |
| Upper respiratory infections | 1 795 | 0.1 | 874 | 0.1 | 921 | 0.1 | 229 | 191 | 14 | 43 | 41 |
| Otitis media | 1 435 | 0.1 | 755 | 0.1 | 680 | 0.1 | 122 | 141 | 38 | 112 | 24 |
| Maternal conditions | 33 632 | 2.3 | ... | ... | 33 632 | 4.7 | 5 200 | 6 549 | 215 | 1 154 | 544 |
| Perinatal conditions[g] | 97 335 | 6.5 | 53 212 | 6.9 | 44 123 | 6.2 | 10 869 | 10 485 | 781 | 5 528 | 1 098 |
| Nutritional deficiencies | 34 417 | 2.3 | 16 100 | 2.1 | 18 316 | 2.6 | 4 305 | 5 269 | 493 | 1 057 | 575 |
| Protein-energy malnutrition | 16 910 | 1.1 | 8 580 | 1.1 | 8 330 | 1.2 | 2 705 | 3 044 | 36 | 651 | 264 |
| Iodine deficiency | 3 519 | 0.2 | 1 759 | 0.2 | 1 760 | 0.2 | 261 | 868 | 7 | 97 | 33 |
| Vitamin A deficiency | 793 | 0.1 | 364 | 0.0 | 428 | 0.1 | 347 | 248 | 0 | 0 | 1 |
| Iron-deficiency anaemia | 12 224 | 0.8 | 4 998 | 0.6 | 7 226 | 1.0 | 975 | 1 089 | 446 | 274 | 268 |

| Cause[d] | SOUTH-EAST ASIA | | EUROPE | | | EASTERN MEDITERRANEAN | | WESTERN PACIFIC | |
|---|---|---|---|---|---|---|---|---|---|
| | Mortality stratum | | Mortality stratum | | | Mortality stratum | | Mortality stratum | |
| | Low child, low adult | High child, high adult | Very low child, very low adult | Low child, low adult | Low child, high adult | Low child, low adult | High child, high adult | Very low child, very low adult | Low child, low adult |
| *Population (000)* | *298 234* | *1 292 598* | *415 323* | *222 846* | *239 717* | *142 528* | *360 296* | *155 400* | *1 562 136* |
| | (000) | (000) | (000) | (000) | (000) | (000) | (000) | (000) | (000) |
| TOTAL DALYs | 62 463 | 364 110 | 51 725 | 37 697 | 60 900 | 24 074 | 115 005 | 16 384 | 248 495 |
| I. Communicable diseases, maternal and perinatal conditions and nutritional deficiencies | 18 533 | 166 116 | 2 552 | 6 198 | 5 287 | 4 444 | 59 929 | 929 | 53 358 |
| Infectious and parasitic diseases | 10 598 | 78 355 | 891 | 2 040 | 2 734 | 1 529 | 30 881 | 322 | 23 349 |
| Tuberculosis | 3 167 | 10 764 | 47 | 437 | 1 031 | 112 | 2 928 | 37 | 5 993 |
| STIs excluding HIV | 479 | 3 475 | 79 | 149 | 125 | 144 | 1 327 | 34 | 515 |
| Syphilis | 35 | 860 | 3 | 7 | 4 | 3 | 706 | 1 | 54 |
| Chlamydia | 262 | 1 251 | 61 | 95 | 79 | 100 | 309 | 25 | 281 |
| Gonorrhoea | 164 | 1 261 | 15 | 43 | 39 | 39 | 296 | 7 | 172 |
| HIV/AIDS | 1 501 | 10 628 | 201 | 39 | 1 149 | 51 | 1 351 | 8 | 2 295 |
| Diarrhoeal diseases | 1 482 | 18 817 | 110 | 485 | 97 | 568 | 8 093 | 46 | 6 641 |
| Childhood diseases | 1 502 | 12 722 | 66 | 259 | 29 | 55 | 5 568 | 34 | 1 834 |
| Pertussis | 126 | 4 336 | 64 | 59 | 25 | 37 | 1 878 | 33 | 425 |
| Poliomyelitis[e] | 9 | 56 | 1 | 1 | 0 | 4 | 13 | 0 | 43 |
| Diphtheria | 7 | 96 | 0 | 1 | 2 | 0 | 16 | 0 | 6 |
| Measles | 1 111 | 5 772 | 1 | 195 | 2 | 9 | 2 470 | 0 | 988 |
| Tetanus | 249 | 2 462 | 0 | 2 | 0 | 4 | 1 192 | 0 | 371 |
| Meningitis | 219 | 1 906 | 67 | 325 | 85 | 85 | 1 134 | 11 | 781 |
| Hepatitis B[f] | 143 | 576 | 17 | 53 | 19 | 24 | 166 | 16 | 459 |
| Hepatitis C[f] | 67 | 212 | 36 | 19 | 9 | 12 | 69 | 39 | 189 |
| Malaria | 502 | 2 275 | 1 | 20 | 0 | 92 | 2 158 | 0 | 441 |
| Tropical diseases | 251 | 4 334 | 0 | 7 | 0 | 45 | 601 | 0 | 516 |
| Trypanosomiasis | 0 | 0 | 0 | 0 | 0 | 0 | 39 | 0 | 0 |
| Chagas disease | 0 | 0 | 0 | 0 | 0 | 0 | 0 | 0 | 0 |
| Schistosomiasis | 3 | 4 | 0 | 0 | 0 | 29 | 197 | 0 | 55 |
| Leishmaniasis | 6 | 1 352 | 0 | 6 | 0 | 16 | 232 | 0 | 50 |
| Lymphatic filariasis | 242 | 2 977 | 0 | 1 | 0 | 0 | 122 | 0 | 411 |
| Onchocerciasis | 0 | 0 | 0 | 0 | 0 | 0 | 10 | 0 | 0 |
| Leprosy | 13 | 105 | 0 | 0 | 0 | 0 | 25 | 0 | 13 |
| Dengue | 89 | 292 | 0 | 0 | 0 | 10 | 20 | 0 | 131 |
| Japanese encephalitis | 29 | 277 | 0 | 0 | 0 | 0 | 83 | 0 | 320 |
| Trachoma | 0 | 168 | 0 | 0 | 0 | 91 | 283 | 0 | 400 |
| Intestinal nematode infections | 135 | 669 | 0 | 1 | 0 | 1 | 225 | 2 | 611 |
| Ascariasis | 63 | 346 | 0 | 0 | 0 | 0 | 158 | 1 | 325 |
| Trichuriasis | 63 | 305 | 0 | 0 | 0 | 0 | 60 | 1 | 272 |
| Hookworm disease | 8 | 1 | 0 | 0 | 0 | 0 | 2 | 0 | 1 |
| Respiratory infections | 1 824 | 31 202 | 690 | 1 524 | 901 | 552 | 10 267 | 344 | 8 310 |
| Lower respiratory infections | 1 707 | 30 551 | 626 | 1 427 | 811 | 504 | 9 949 | 322 | 7 447 |
| Upper respiratory infections | 45 | 301 | 27 | 62 | 66 | 11 | 202 | 9 | 552 |
| Otitis media | 72 | 350 | 37 | 35 | 24 | 38 | 116 | 13 | 310 |
| Maternal conditions | 1 004 | 10 391 | 167 | 370 | 269 | 412 | 4 104 | 67 | 3 146 |
| Perinatal conditions[g] | 3 414 | 35 733 | 501 | 1 592 | 655 | 1 321 | 10 817 | 68 | 14 321 |
| Nutritional deficiencies | 1 693 | 10 435 | 303 | 671 | 729 | 631 | 3 860 | 128 | 4 232 |
| Protein-energy malnutrition | 703 | 5 392 | 24 | 109 | 54 | 174 | 1 869 | 18 | 1 850 |
| Iodine deficiency | 81 | 571 | 3 | 241 | 449 | 121 | 623 | 0 | 163 |
| Vitamin A deficiency | 1 | 100 | 0 | 1 | 0 | 0 | 90 | 0 | 5 |
| Iron-deficiency anaemia | 891 | 3 959 | 271 | 297 | 200 | 334 | 928 | 106 | 2 171 |

## Annex Table 3 Burden of disease in DALYs by cause, sex and mortality stratum in WHO regions,[a] estimates for 2002

Figures computed by WHO to assure comparability;[b] they are not necessarily the official statistics of Member States, which may use alternative rigorous methods.

| Cause[d] | SEX[c] Both sexes (000) | % total | Males (000) | % total | Females (000) | % total | AFRICA High child, high adult (000) | AFRICA High child, very high adult (000) | THE AMERICAS Very low child, very low adult (000) | THE AMERICAS Low child, low adult (000) | THE AMERICAS High child, high adult (000) |
|---|---|---|---|---|---|---|---|---|---|---|---|
| Population (000) | 6 224 985 | | 3 131 052 | | 3 093 933 | | 311 273 | 360 965 | 333 580 | 445 161 | 73 810 |
| II. Noncommunicable conditions | 697 815 | 46.8 | 356 231 | 46.1 | 341 585 | 47.6 | 30 124 | 34 727 | 39 217 | 51 825 | 8 030 |
| Malignant neoplasms | 75 545 | 5.1 | 40 536 | 5.2 | 35 009 | 4.9 | 2 238 | 2 517 | 5 830 | 4 553 | 749 |
| Mouth and oropharynx cancers | 3 566 | 0.2 | 2 568 | 0.3 | 997 | 0.1 | 83 | 111 | 97 | 135 | 16 |
| Esophagus cancer | 4 250 | 0.3 | 2 764 | 0.4 | 1 486 | 0.2 | 52 | 178 | 136 | 140 | 9 |
| Stomach cancer | 8 095 | 0.5 | 5 046 | 0.7 | 3 048 | 0.4 | 174 | 196 | 132 | 403 | 123 |
| Colon/rectum cancer | 5 818 | 0.4 | 3 121 | 0.4 | 2 697 | 0.4 | 118 | 102 | 654 | 295 | 40 |
| Liver cancer | 7 135 | 0.5 | 5 041 | 0.7 | 2 095 | 0.3 | 301 | 305 | 141 | 165 | 32 |
| Pancreas cancer | 1 975 | 0.1 | 1 112 | 0.1 | 863 | 0.1 | 34 | 56 | 247 | 149 | 17 |
| Trachea/bronchus/lung cancers | 11 228 | 0.8 | 7 955 | 1.0 | 3 273 | 0.5 | 71 | 112 | 1 398 | 453 | 28 |
| Melanoma and other skin cancers | 691 | 0.0 | 381 | 0.0 | 309 | 0.0 | 34 | 44 | 135 | 66 | 7 |
| Breast cancer | 6 171 | 0.4 | 23 | 0.0 | 6 148 | 0.9 | 258 | 164 | 687 | 439 | 55 |
| Cervix uteri cancer | 3 287 | 0.2 | … | … | 3 287 | 0.5 | 185 | 282 | 102 | 299 | 101 |
| Corpus uteri cancer | 1 121 | 0.1 | … | … | 1 121 | 0.2 | 12 | 16 | 161 | 178 | 16 |
| Ovary cancer | 1 647 | 0.1 | … | … | 1 647 | 0.2 | 44 | 68 | 156 | 102 | 18 |
| Prostate cancer | 1 629 | 0.1 | 1 629 | 0.2 | … | … | 147 | 109 | 281 | 167 | 27 |
| Bladder cancer | 1 478 | 0.1 | 1 002 | 0.1 | 476 | 0.1 | 55 | 41 | 135 | 56 | 7 |
| Lymphomas, multiple myeloma | 4 308 | 0.3 | 2 298 | 0.3 | 2 010 | 0.3 | 291 | 262 | 368 | 246 | 68 |
| Leukaemia | 4 686 | 0.3 | 2 655 | 0.3 | 2 031 | 0.3 | 104 | 109 | 251 | 362 | 76 |
| Other neoplasms | 1 749 | 0.1 | 915 | 0.1 | 834 | 0.1 | 74 | 86 | 114 | 139 | 20 |
| Diabetes mellitus | 16 194 | 1.1 | 7 608 | 1.0 | 8 587 | 1.2 | 529 | 586 | 1 455 | 1 835 | 224 |
| Nutritional/endocrine disorders | 7 961 | 0.5 | 3 568 | 0.5 | 4 393 | 0.6 | 570 | 720 | 854 | 1 162 | 224 |
| Neuropsychiatric disorders | 193 278 | 13.0 | 94 230 | 12.2 | 99 049 | 13.8 | 8 242 | 9 655 | 13 888 | 18 966 | 2 934 |
| Unipolar depressive disorders | 67 295 | 4.5 | 26 743 | 3.5 | 40 552 | 5.7 | 2 011 | 2 316 | 5 237 | 5 863 | 898 |
| Bipolar affective disorder | 13 952 | 0.9 | 7 049 | 0.9 | 6 903 | 1.0 | 795 | 936 | 531 | 1 063 | 177 |
| Schizophrenia | 16 149 | 1.1 | 8 235 | 1.1 | 7 914 | 1.1 | 777 | 899 | 537 | 1 268 | 210 |
| Epilepsy | 7 328 | 0.5 | 3 886 | 0.5 | 3 442 | 0.5 | 701 | 880 | 175 | 745 | 143 |
| Alcohol use disorders | 20 331 | 1.4 | 17 242 | 2.2 | 3 089 | 0.4 | 241 | 672 | 2 502 | 3 513 | 333 |
| Alzheimer and other dementias | 10 397 | 0.7 | 3 992 | 0.5 | 6 405 | 0.9 | 166 | 175 | 1 300 | 658 | 76 |
| Parkinson disease | 1 570 | 0.1 | 776 | 0.1 | 794 | 0.1 | 35 | 40 | 252 | 53 | 7 |
| Multiple sclerosis | 1 477 | 0.1 | 638 | 0.1 | 839 | 0.1 | 56 | 45 | 120 | 105 | 16 |
| Drug use disorders | 7 388 | 0.5 | 5 789 | 0.7 | 1 599 | 0.2 | 660 | 656 | 787 | 839 | 232 |
| Post-traumatic stress disorder | 3 335 | 0.2 | 923 | 0.1 | 2 412 | 0.3 | 149 | 173 | 184 | 209 | 32 |
| Obsessive-compulsive disorder | 4 923 | 0.3 | 2 116 | 0.3 | 2 808 | 0.4 | 393 | 459 | 227 | 558 | 87 |
| Panic disorder | 6 758 | 0.5 | 2 292 | 0.3 | 4 466 | 0.6 | 360 | 427 | 278 | 512 | 85 |
| Insomnia (primary) | 3 477 | 0.2 | 1 494 | 0.2 | 1 983 | 0.3 | 141 | 161 | 269 | 326 | 49 |
| Migraine | 7 666 | 0.5 | 2 078 | 0.3 | 5 588 | 0.8 | 193 | 254 | 508 | 754 | 150 |
| Sense organ disorders | 69 381 | 4.7 | 32 453 | 4.2 | 36 928 | 5.1 | 4 289 | 4 649 | 1 950 | 3 638 | 528 |
| Glaucoma | 3 866 | 0.3 | 1 716 | 0.2 | 2 150 | 0.3 | 451 | 481 | 35 | 219 | 11 |
| Cataracts | 25 251 | 1.7 | 11 051 | 1.4 | 14 200 | 2.0 | 2 483 | 2 670 | 123 | 1 156 | 248 |
| Vision loss, age-related and other | 14 191 | 1.0 | 6 303 | 0.8 | 7 889 | 1.1 | 437 | 440 | 414 | 1 116 | 119 |
| Hearing loss, adult onset | 26 034 | 1.7 | 13 364 | 1.7 | 12 669 | 1.8 | 918 | 1 058 | 1 377 | 1 144 | 148 |
| Cardiovascular diseases | 148 190 | 9.9 | 79 886 | 10.3 | 68 304 | 9.5 | 5 187 | 5 724 | 6 847 | 7 426 | 901 |
| Rheumatic heart disease | 5 862 | 0.4 | 2 556 | 0.3 | 3 306 | 0.5 | 300 | 207 | 40 | 107 | 11 |
| Hypertensive heart disease | 7 647 | 0.5 | 3 856 | 0.5 | 3 791 | 0.5 | 260 | 327 | 322 | 580 | 126 |
| Ischaemic heart disease | 58 645 | 3.9 | 34 338 | 4.4 | 24 307 | 3.4 | 1 461 | 1 564 | 3 304 | 2 685 | 230 |
| Cerebrovascular disease | 49 200 | 3.3 | 25 429 | 3.3 | 23 771 | 3.3 | 1 757 | 1 911 | 1 654 | 2 534 | 288 |
| Inflammatory heart disease | 5 854 | 0.4 | 3 438 | 0.4 | 2 417 | 0.3 | 400 | 467 | 382 | 437 | 27 |

| Cause[d] | SOUTH-EAST ASIA | | EUROPE | | | EASTERN MEDITERRANEAN | | WESTERN PACIFIC | |
|---|---|---|---|---|---|---|---|---|---|
| | Mortality stratum | | Mortality stratum | | | Mortality stratum | | Mortality stratum | |
| | Low child, low adult | High child, high adult | Very low child, very low adult | Low child, low adult | Low child, high adult | Low child, low adult | High child, high adult | Very low child, very low adult | Low child, low adult |
| Population (000) | 298 234 | 1 292 598 | 415 323 | 222 846 | 239 717 | 142 528 | 360 296 | 155 400 | 1 562 136 |
| | (000) | (000) | (000) | (000) | (000) | (000) | (000) | (000) | (000) |
| II. Noncommunicable conditions | 35 713 | 150 663 | 45 091 | 27 441 | 42 807 | 14 862 | 42 361 | 13 827 | 159 791 |
| Malignant neoplasms | 3 231 | 10 511 | 8 549 | 3 289 | 5 322 | 981 | 2 835 | 2 787 | 22 035 |
| Mouth and oropharynx cancers | 198 | 1 407 | 264 | 109 | 209 | 24 | 226 | 60 | 624 |
| Esophagus cancer | 34 | 764 | 233 | 72 | 123 | 34 | 133 | 96 | 2 242 |
| Stomach cancer | 114 | 516 | 421 | 283 | 648 | 118 | 124 | 366 | 4 469 |
| Colon/rectum cancer | 295 | 365 | 1 027 | 285 | 550 | 58 | 138 | 392 | 1 488 |
| Liver cancer | 347 | 431 | 282 | 113 | 137 | 63 | 113 | 265 | 4 432 |
| Pancreas cancer | 65 | 131 | 377 | 111 | 217 | 17 | 32 | 154 | 365 |
| Trachea/bronchus/lung cancers | 419 | 1 324 | 1 668 | 620 | 956 | 99 | 183 | 433 | 3 452 |
| Melanoma and other skin cancers | 12 | 28 | 147 | 46 | 73 | 10 | 21 | 25 | 40 |
| Breast cancer | 367 | 835 | 939 | 277 | 487 | 75 | 348 | 198 | 1 029 |
| Cervix uteri cancer | 226 | 1 171 | 111 | 112 | 169 | 21 | 97 | 44 | 364 |
| Corpus uteri cancer | 44 | 32 | 206 | 91 | 157 | 13 | 21 | 61 | 111 |
| Ovary cancer | 129 | 225 | 238 | 91 | 172 | 16 | 75 | 60 | 250 |
| Prostate cancer | 49 | 116 | 369 | 69 | 103 | 25 | 37 | 70 | 56 |
| Bladder cancer | 50 | 277 | 243 | 80 | 115 | 19 | 178 | 41 | 178 |
| Lymphomas, multiple myeloma | 236 | 1 161 | 428 | 167 | 138 | 76 | 326 | 116 | 416 |
| Leukaemia | 257 | 791 | 316 | 195 | 201 | 147 | 328 | 93 | 1 450 |
| Other neoplasms | 49 | 281 | 185 | 36 | 65 | 127 | 240 | 68 | 261 |
| Diabetes mellitus | 1 245 | 3 562 | 1 105 | 566 | 522 | 410 | 843 | 387 | 2 873 |
| Nutritional/endocrine disorders | 449 | 637 | 632 | 176 | 168 | 209 | 633 | 213 | 1 278 |
| Neuropsychiatric disorders | 8 340 | 39 974 | 13 732 | 7 055 | 8 562 | 4 340 | 10 680 | 3 812 | 42 722 |
| Unipolar depressive disorders | 2 897 | 17 671 | 4 117 | 2 626 | 2 598 | 1 259 | 3 754 | 1 007 | 14 926 |
| Bipolar affective disorder | 704 | 2 994 | 618 | 479 | 449 | 380 | 869 | 237 | 3 697 |
| Schizophrenia | 1 047 | 3 683 | 593 | 577 | 442 | 471 | 1 037 | 231 | 4 348 |
| Epilepsy | 367 | 1 883 | 245 | 191 | 188 | 122 | 502 | 65 | 1 105 |
| Alcohol use disorders | 325 | 1 623 | 2 227 | 636 | 1 799 | 55 | 44 | 489 | 5 836 |
| Alzheimer and other dementias | 369 | 1 213 | 1 989 | 398 | 549 | 101 | 242 | 765 | 2 374 |
| Parkinson disease | 36 | 211 | 288 | 70 | 93 | 40 | 59 | 117 | 268 |
| Multiple sclerosis | 63 | 276 | 157 | 63 | 87 | 35 | 75 | 29 | 347 |
| Drug use disorders | 159 | 827 | 774 | 192 | 489 | 562 | 812 | 57 | 322 |
| Post-traumatic stress disorder | 181 | 719 | 208 | 127 | 130 | 84 | 192 | 81 | 860 |
| Obsessive-compulsive disorder | 172 | 837 | 257 | 275 | 277 | 191 | 349 | 62 | 765 |
| Panic disorder | 363 | 1 494 | 322 | 248 | 239 | 186 | 428 | 124 | 1 680 |
| Insomnia (primary) | 118 | 861 | 348 | 119 | 158 | 35 | 161 | 130 | 595 |
| Migraine | 340 | 1 727 | 742 | 258 | 236 | 136 | 421 | 151 | 1 781 |
| Sense organ disorders | 6 151 | 16 217 | 2 465 | 1 589 | 2 167 | 2 108 | 5 016 | 809 | 17 655 |
| Glaucoma | 209 | 195 | 107 | 91 | 102 | 216 | 512 | 16 | 1 207 |
| Cataracts | 3 479 | 7 562 | 112 | 149 | 167 | 570 | 1 873 | 29 | 4 581 |
| Vision loss, age-related and other | 813 | 1 418 | 390 | 588 | 633 | 757 | 1 127 | 141 | 5 755 |
| Hearing loss, adult onset | 1 648 | 7 029 | 1 855 | 760 | 1 261 | 564 | 1 497 | 623 | 6 109 |
| Cardiovascular diseases | 6 576 | 36 411 | 8 838 | 8 175 | 17 405 | 2 945 | 9 115 | 2 545 | 29 868 |
| Rheumatic heart disease | 242 | 2 376 | 71 | 122 | 192 | 104 | 476 | 17 | 1 594 |
| Hypertensive heart disease | 518 | 1 138 | 307 | 521 | 389 | 249 | 642 | 35 | 2 209 |
| Ischaemic heart disease | 2 804 | 17 930 | 3 569 | 3 382 | 8 800 | 1 365 | 3 956 | 770 | 6 732 |
| Cerebrovascular disease | 1 681 | 8 714 | 2 654 | 2 522 | 5 618 | 577 | 1 954 | 1 228 | 16 048 |
| Inflammatory heart disease | 173 | 1 338 | 265 | 360 | 683 | 133 | 423 | 76 | 678 |

## Annex Table 3 Burden of disease in DALYs by cause, sex and mortality stratum in WHO regions,[a] estimates for 2002

Figures computed by WHO to assure comparability;[b] they are not necessarily the official statistics of Member States, which may use alternative rigorous methods.

| Cause[d] | SEX[c] Both sexes (000) | % total | Males (000) | % total | Females (000) | % total | AFRICA High child, high adult (000) | AFRICA High child, very high adult (000) | THE AMERICAS Very low child, very low adult (000) | THE AMERICAS Low child, low adult (000) | THE AMERICAS High child, high adult (000) |
|---|---|---|---|---|---|---|---|---|---|---|---|
| Population (000) | 6 224 985 | | 3 131 052 | | 3 093 933 | | 311 273 | 360 965 | 333 580 | 445 161 | 73 810 |
| Respiratory diseases | 55 153 | 3.7 | 30 247 | 3.9 | 24 907 | 3.5 | 2 505 | 2 978 | 3 239 | 4 061 | 668 |
| Chronic obstructive pulmonary disease | 27 756 | 1.9 | 15 302 | 2.0 | 12 454 | 1.7 | 514 | 668 | 1 743 | 1 419 | 195 |
| Asthma | 15 334 | 1.0 | 8 240 | 1.1 | 7 094 | 1.0 | 952 | 1 260 | 792 | 1 576 | 278 |
| Digestive diseases | 46 476 | 3.1 | 25 374 | 3.3 | 21 102 | 2.9 | 2 377 | 2 727 | 1 589 | 3 309 | 645 |
| Peptic ulcer disease | 4 630 | 0.3 | 2 926 | 0.4 | 1 704 | 0.2 | 151 | 176 | 52 | 136 | 37 |
| Cirrhosis of the liver | 13 977 | 0.9 | 8 629 | 1.1 | 5 348 | 0.7 | 447 | 510 | 485 | 1 094 | 206 |
| Appendicitis | 395 | 0.0 | 228 | 0.0 | 167 | 0.0 | 23 | 26 | 15 | 39 | 16 |
| Diseases of the genitourinary system | 15 217 | 1.0 | 8 575 | 1.1 | 6 642 | 0.9 | 986 | 1 101 | 631 | 1 091 | 244 |
| Nephritis/nephrosis | 8 394 | 0.6 | 4 443 | 0.6 | 3 951 | 0.6 | 620 | 681 | 265 | 496 | 148 |
| Benign prostatic hypertrophy | 2 466 | 0.2 | 2 466 | 0.3 | ... | ... | 113 | 126 | 88 | 210 | 29 |
| Skin diseases | 3 748 | 0.3 | 1 854 | 0.2 | 1 894 | 0.3 | 395 | 452 | 79 | 323 | 68 |
| Musculoskeletal diseases | 30 169 | 2.0 | 13 244 | 1.7 | 16 925 | 2.4 | 1 080 | 1 151 | 1 751 | 2 223 | 311 |
| Rheumatoid arthritis | 4 866 | 0.3 | 1 385 | 0.2 | 3 482 | 0.5 | 133 | 143 | 332 | 550 | 86 |
| Osteoarthritis | 14 861 | 1.0 | 5 797 | 0.7 | 9 065 | 1.3 | 595 | 641 | 860 | 857 | 102 |
| Congenital abnormalities | 27 381 | 1.8 | 14 125 | 1.8 | 13 256 | 1.8 | 1 384 | 2 072 | 682 | 2 275 | 364 |
| Oral diseases | 7 372 | 0.5 | 3 617 | 0.5 | 3 754 | 0.5 | 269 | 311 | 308 | 824 | 150 |
| Dental caries | 4 769 | 0.3 | 2 414 | 0.3 | 2 355 | 0.3 | 186 | 216 | 183 | 715 | 132 |
| Periodontal disease | 302 | 0.0 | 152 | 0.0 | 150 | 0.0 | 15 | 17 | 13 | 21 | 3 |
| Edentulism | 2 185 | 0.1 | 1 015 | 0.1 | 1 170 | 0.2 | 64 | 72 | 109 | 80 | 13 |
| III. Injuries | 181 991 | 12.2 | 119 885 | 15.5 | 62 106 | 8.7 | 14 974 | 15 829 | 4 545 | 13 430 | 1 889 |
| Unintentional | 133 112 | 8.9 | 84 118 | 10.9 | 48 993 | 6.8 | 11 621 | 9 921 | 3 133 | 6 813 | 1 451 |
| Road traffic accidents | 38 676 | 2.6 | 27 224 | 3.5 | 11 452 | 1.6 | 3 654 | 3 537 | 1 368 | 2 580 | 348 |
| Poisoning | 7 401 | 0.5 | 4 820 | 0.6 | 2 581 | 0.4 | 577 | 490 | 333 | 64 | 16 |
| Falls | 16 201 | 1.1 | 9 929 | 1.3 | 6 271 | 0.9 | 612 | 456 | 371 | 645 | 131 |
| Fires | 11 471 | 0.8 | 4 595 | 0.6 | 6 875 | 1.0 | 1 090 | 897 | 100 | 132 | 37 |
| Drowning | 10 840 | 0.7 | 7 458 | 1.0 | 3 382 | 0.5 | 1 065 | 853 | 116 | 455 | 81 |
| Other unintentional injuries | 48 523 | 3.3 | 30 091 | 3.9 | 18 432 | 2.6 | 4 623 | 3 688 | 844 | 2 937 | 838 |
| Intentional | 48 879 | 3.3 | 35 767 | 4.6 | 13 112 | 1.8 | 3 353 | 5 908 | 1 412 | 6 617 | 437 |
| Self-inflicted | 20 767 | 1.4 | 12 344 | 1.6 | 8 423 | 1.2 | 391 | 502 | 772 | 652 | 77 |
| Violence | 21 429 | 1.4 | 17 505 | 2.3 | 3 925 | 0.5 | 2 343 | 2 924 | 629 | 5 657 | 358 |
| War | 6 328 | 0.4 | 5 629 | 0.7 | 700 | 0.1 | 619 | 2 482 | 1 | 283 | 2 |

[a] See list of Member States by WHO region and mortality stratum.

[b] See explanatory notes for sources and methods.

[c] World totals for males and females include residual populations living outside WHO Member States.

[d] Estimates for specific causes may not sum to broader cause groupings owing to omission of residual categories.

[e] For WHO Regions of the Americas, Europe and the Western Pacific, these figures include only late effects of poliomyelitis cases with onset prior to regional certification of polio eradication in 1994, 2000 and 2002, respectively. For all other regions, except where vital registration reports late effects of polio cases, these deaths are from acute poliomyelitis.

[f] Does not include liver cancer and cirrhosis deaths resulting from chronic hepatitis virus infection.

[g] This category includes causes originating in the perinatal period as defined in Chapter XVI of the International Classification of Diseases, principally low birthweight, prematurity, birth asphyxia and birth trauma, and does not include all diseases and injuries occurring in the early neonatal period.

... Data not applicable.

| Cause[d] | SOUTH-EAST ASIA Mortality stratum | | EUROPE Mortality stratum | | | EASTERN MEDITERRANEAN Mortality stratum | | WESTERN PACIFIC Mortality stratum | |
|---|---|---|---|---|---|---|---|---|---|
| | Low child, low adult | High child, high adult | Very low child, very low adult | Low child, low adult | Low child, high adult | Low child, low adult | High child, high adult | Very low child, very low adult | Low child, low adult |
| Population (000) | 298 234 | 1 292 598 | 415 323 | 222 846 | 239 717 | 142 528 | 360 296 | 155 400 | 1 562 136 |
| | (000) | (000) | (000) | (000) | (000) | (000) | (000) | (000) | (000) |
| Respiratory diseases | 2 620 | 13 010 | 3 406 | 1 547 | 1 782 | 843 | 2 877 | 1 067 | 14 469 |
| Chronic obstructive pulmonary disease | 1 420 | 6 740 | 1 744 | 673 | 1 036 | 349 | 989 | 415 | 9 820 |
| Asthma | 614 | 3 821 | 700 | 358 | 301 | 280 | 1 006 | 361 | 3 007 |
| Digestive diseases | 2 534 | 11 671 | 2 414 | 1 900 | 3 082 | 679 | 3 353 | 664 | 9 448 |
| Peptic ulcer disease | 229 | 1 809 | 130 | 149 | 211 | 34 | 230 | 36 | 1 249 |
| Cirrhosis of the liver | 666 | 3 676 | 909 | 649 | 1 176 | 128 | 1 021 | 177 | 2 814 |
| Appendicitis | 18 | 94 | 16 | 10 | 22 | 6 | 16 | 5 | 89 |
| Diseases of the genitourinary system | 905 | 3 180 | 546 | 534 | 636 | 378 | 1 175 | 229 | 3 529 |
| Nephritis/nephrosis | 549 | 1 984 | 196 | 259 | 205 | 115 | 785 | 97 | 1 978 |
| Benign prostatic hypertrophy | 125 | 539 | 123 | 65 | 81 | 59 | 138 | 51 | 714 |
| Skin diseases | 332 | 745 | 90 | 66 | 173 | 66 | 270 | 21 | 659 |
| Musculoskeletal diseases | 1 593 | 5 334 | 2 197 | 1 513 | 1 924 | 518 | 1 278 | 878 | 8 359 |
| Rheumatoid arthritis | 122 | 880 | 427 | 277 | 344 | 101 | 228 | 142 | 1 090 |
| Osteoarthritis | 893 | 2 302 | 1 187 | 828 | 1 073 | 216 | 548 | 526 | 4 208 |
| Congenital abnormalities | 1 170 | 7 540 | 555 | 684 | 683 | 947 | 3 464 | 205 | 5 294 |
| Oral diseases | 517 | 1 590 | 378 | 311 | 315 | 312 | 583 | 142 | 1 341 |
| Dental caries | 253 | 1 088 | 201 | 194 | 163 | 197 | 382 | 75 | 771 |
| Periodontal disease | 15 | 100 | 17 | 11 | 13 | 5 | 19 | 6 | 47 |
| Edentulism | 239 | 376 | 157 | 105 | 138 | 106 | 174 | 59 | 488 |
| III. Injuries | 8 217 | 47 330 | 4 081 | 4 058 | 12 806 | 4 767 | 12 714 | 1 627 | 35 347 |
| Unintentional | 5 866 | 37 872 | 3 042 | 3 123 | 8 317 | 4 225 | 9 768 | 971 | 26 732 |
| Road traffic accidents | 2 415 | 7 601 | 1 233 | 641 | 1 732 | 1 856 | 2 732 | 309 | 8 595 |
| Poisoning | 156 | 1 668 | 126 | 126 | 1 885 | 73 | 266 | 37 | 1 572 |
| Falls | 669 | 5 037 | 615 | 481 | 939 | 508 | 1 212 | 179 | 4 316 |
| Fires | 459 | 6 095 | 57 | 153 | 425 | 293 | 1 091 | 27 | 603 |
| Drowning | 397 | 2 343 | 74 | 167 | 649 | 155 | 651 | 64 | 3 751 |
| Other unintentional injuries | 1 770 | 15 128 | 937 | 1 556 | 2 686 | 1 340 | 3 815 | 356 | 7 895 |
| Intentional | 2 351 | 9 459 | 1 039 | 935 | 4 489 | 543 | 2 946 | 656 | 8 614 |
| Self-inflicted | 961 | 6 230 | 890 | 532 | 1 969 | 258 | 749 | 616 | 6 152 |
| Violence | 936 | 2 644 | 134 | 255 | 1 912 | 241 | 1 031 | 37 | 2 260 |
| War | 437 | 437 | 14 | 130 | 605 | 26 | 1 115 | 2 | 139 |

## Annex Table 4 Healthy life expectancy (HALE) in all WHO Member States, estimates for 2002

Figures computed by WHO to assure comparability;[a] they are not necessarily the official statistics of Member States, which may use alternative rigorous methods.

| | Member State | Total population At birth | Males At birth | Males Uncertainty interval | Males At age 60 | Males Uncertainty interval | Females At birth | Females Uncertainty interval | Females At age 60 | Females Uncertainty interval | Expectation of lost healthy years at birth (years) Males | Females | Percentage of total life expectancy lost Males | Females |
|---|---|---|---|---|---|---|---|---|---|---|---|---|---|---|
| 1 | Afghanistan | 35.5 | 35.3 | 26.7 - 40.4 | 8.6 | 8.0 - 9.1 | 35.8 | 26.3 - 43.5 | 9.5 | 9.0 - 10.2 | 6.6 | 7.7 | 15.8 | 17.7 |
| 2 | Albania | 61.4 | 59.5 | 58.0 - 60.8 | 10.5 | 9.6 - 11.2 | 63.3 | 61.7 - 63.9 | 13.9 | 13.1 - 14.6 | 7.8 | 10.8 | 11.6 | 14.6 |
| 3 | Algeria | 60.6 | 59.7 | 58.2 - 61.1 | 12.5 | 12.2 - 12.8 | 61.6 | 60.4 - 63.2 | 13.3 | 12.9 - 13.6 | 7.9 | 9.6 | 11.7 | 13.5 |
| 4 | Andorra | 72.2 | 69.8 | 68.5 - 70.7 | 16.6 | 15.9 - 16.9 | 74.6 | 73.7 - 75.5 | 19.9 | 19.4 - 20.3 | 7.0 | 9.1 | 9.2 | 10.8 |
| 5 | Angola | 33.4 | 31.6 | 25.0 - 36.4 | 8.1 | 7.6 - 8.7 | 35.1 | 28.1 - 42.1 | 9.6 | 9.2 - 10.6 | 6.3 | 6.9 | 16.6 | 16.4 |
| 6 | Antigua and Barbuda | 61.9 | 60.1 | 58.6 - 61.7 | 11.6 | 11.3 - 12.0 | 63.6 | 62.4 - 65.3 | 13.8 | 13.4 - 14.3 | 8.9 | 10.3 | 12.8 | 13.9 |
| 7 | Argentina | 65.3 | 62.5 | 61.8 - 63.2 | 13.0 | 12.8 - 13.2 | 68.1 | 67.5 - 68.8 | 16.5 | 16.3 - 16.7 | 8.3 | 10.0 | 11.7 | 12.8 |
| 8 | Armenia | 61.0 | 59.4 | 58.3 - 60.5 | 10.9 | 10.5 - 11.3 | 62.6 | 61.1 - 63.1 | 13.3 | 12.3 - 13.8 | 7.6 | 10.4 | 11.3 | 14.2 |
| 9 | Australia | 72.6 | 70.9 | 70.2 - 71.4 | 16.9 | 16.6 - 17.1 | 74.3 | 73.7 - 75.1 | 19.5 | 19.2 - 19.8 | 7.0 | 8.7 | 9.0 | 10.4 |
| 10 | Austria | 71.4 | 69.3 | 68.6 - 70.0 | 16.2 | 16.0 - 16.5 | 73.5 | 72.9 - 74.3 | 19.3 | 19.0 - 19.6 | 7.1 | 8.6 | 9.3 | 10.5 |
| 11 | Azerbaijan | 57.2 | 55.8 | 54.5 - 57.2 | 10.6 | 10.3 - 10.9 | 58.7 | 57.0 - 59.4 | 12.4 | 11.8 - 12.9 | 7.2 | 10.0 | 11.4 | 14.6 |
| 12 | Bahamas | 63.5 | 61.0 | 60.0 - 62.0 | 14.4 | 14.2 - 14.8 | 66.0 | 65.1 - 67.0 | 16.2 | 15.6 - 16.7 | 8.4 | 9.7 | 12.1 | 12.8 |
| 13 | Bahrain | 64.3 | 64.2 | 63.2 - 65.5 | 11.5 | 10.6 - 12.7 | 64.4 | 63.6 - 65.8 | 11.6 | 11.1 - 12.6 | 7.9 | 10.1 | 10.9 | 13.6 |
| 14 | Bangladesh | 54.3 | 55.3 | 54.0 - 56.7 | 11.1 | 10.8 - 11.5 | 53.3 | 52.2 - 54.7 | 11.1 | 10.8 - 11.4 | 7.3 | 9.3 | 11.7 | 14.8 |
| 15 | Barbados | 65.6 | 62.9 | 61.9 - 64.1 | 13.1 | 12.8 - 13.5 | 68.2 | 67.0 - 69.5 | 16.6 | 16.1 - 17.2 | 7.6 | 9.8 | 10.7 | 12.5 |
| 16 | Belarus | 60.7 | 56.6 | 55.7 - 57.5 | 10.5 | 10.1 - 10.9 | 64.9 | 63.6 - 65.5 | 14.6 | 14.3 - 14.9 | 6.1 | 9.4 | 9.7 | 12.6 |
| 17 | Belgium | 71.1 | 68.9 | 68.3 - 69.5 | 15.7 | 15.4 - 15.9 | 73.3 | 72.8 - 74.1 | 19.1 | 18.9 - 19.4 | 6.3 | 8.2 | 8.3 | 10.1 |
| 18 | Belize | 60.3 | 58.4 | 57.0 - 59.8 | 11.5 | 11.2 - 11.8 | 62.2 | 61.2 - 63.4 | 13.3 | 13.0 - 13.6 | 9.0 | 10.2 | 13.3 | 14.1 |
| 19 | Benin | 44.0 | 43.4 | 37.6 - 48.5 | 9.7 | 8.8 - 10.8 | 44.5 | 37.4 - 50.9 | 10.4 | 9.5 - 11.6 | 6.6 | 7.9 | 13.3 | 15.0 |
| 20 | Bhutan | 52.9 | 52.9 | 46.3 - 58.8 | 10.8 | 9.6 - 12.6 | 52.9 | 45.5 - 57.5 | 11.3 | 10.0 - 12.3 | 7.3 | 9.5 | 12.1 | 15.2 |
| 21 | Bolivia | 54.4 | 53.6 | 47.5 - 59.2 | 10.9 | 9.5 - 12.6 | 55.2 | 47.8 - 59.6 | 12.1 | 10.6 - 13.3 | 8.2 | 9.4 | 13.2 | 14.6 |
| 22 | Bosnia and Herzegovina | 64.3 | 62.3 | 60.8 - 63.9 | 12.4 | 12.0 - 13.0 | 66.4 | 64.7 - 67.2 | 15.4 | 15.0 - 16.0 | 7.0 | 10.0 | 10.2 | 13.1 |
| 23 | Botswana | 35.7 | 36.0 | 34.4 - 40.0 | 10.9 | 10.7 - 13.0 | 35.4 | 33.9 - 39.5 | 11.9 | 11.7 - 13.5 | 4.2 | 5.2 | 10.4 | 12.9 |
| 24 | Brazil | 59.8 | 57.2 | 56.3 - 58.0 | 11.6 | 11.4 - 11.8 | 62.4 | 61.7 - 63.3 | 13.7 | 13.4 - 13.9 | 8.5 | 9.8 | 13.0 | 13.6 |
| 25 | Brunei Darussalam | 65.3 | 65.1 | 63.8 - 66.4 | 13.1 | 12.5 - 13.8 | 65.5 | 64.7 - 66.6 | 13.3 | 13.0 - 13.7 | 9.7 | 11.9 | 13.0 | 15.4 |
| 26 | Bulgaria | 64.8 | 62.6 | 61.9 - 63.3 | 12.5 | 12.2 - 12.7 | 67.1 | 66.4 - 67.8 | 15.0 | 14.8 - 15.3 | 6.2 | 8.5 | 9.1 | 11.3 |
| 27 | Burkina Faso | 35.6 | 34.9 | 30.3 - 40.3 | 8.6 | 8.1 - 9.7 | 36.3 | 30.2 - 42.4 | 9.7 | 9.2 - 10.8 | 5.6 | 6.3 | 13.9 | 14.8 |
| 28 | Burundi | 35.1 | 33.4 | 29.3 - 38.8 | 8.6 | 7.9 - 10.0 | 36.8 | 32.0 - 43.9 | 10.4 | 9.5 - 12.0 | 5.3 | 6.2 | 13.7 | 14.4 |
| 29 | Cambodia | 47.5 | 45.6 | 39.5 - 49.9 | 9.7 | 8.7 - 10.7 | 49.5 | 42.5 - 54.0 | 11.0 | 10.0 - 12.0 | 6.3 | 7.6 | 12.1 | 13.3 |
| 30 | Cameroon | 41.5 | 41.1 | 36.8 - 47.2 | 9.7 | 8.9 - 11.6 | 41.8 | 36.3 - 48.4 | 10.4 | 9.6 - 12.0 | 6.0 | 7.3 | 12.8 | 14.8 |
| 31 | Canada | 72.0 | 70.1 | 69.5 - 70.7 | 16.1 | 15.8 - 16.3 | 74.0 | 73.4 - 74.6 | 19.3 | 19.0 - 19.5 | 7.1 | 8.3 | 9.2 | 10.0 |
| 32 | Cape Verde | 60.8 | 58.8 | 55.1 - 62.6 | 11.8 | 10.7 - 13.1 | 62.9 | 60.5 - 65.5 | 13.4 | 12.5 - 14.3 | 7.9 | 10.0 | 11.8 | 13.7 |
| 33 | Central African Republic | 37.4 | 37.0 | 32.5 - 42.9 | 9.6 | 8.9 - 11.2 | 37.7 | 32.5 - 43.6 | 10.4 | 9.7 - 11.9 | 5.1 | 6.1 | 12.0 | 13.8 |
| 34 | Chad | 40.7 | 39.7 | 33.2 - 45.2 | 9.2 | 8.5 - 10.2 | 41.7 | 35.1 - 48.5 | 10.0 | 9.3 - 11.2 | 6.4 | 7.6 | 13.9 | 15.5 |
| 35 | Chile | 67.3 | 64.9 | 64.2 - 65.7 | 13.9 | 13.5 - 14.3 | 69.7 | 69.2 - 70.5 | 16.8 | 16.6 - 17.1 | 8.5 | 10.3 | 11.5 | 12.9 |
| 36 | China | 64.1 | 63.1 | 62.2 - 63.9 | 13.1 | 12.9 - 13.4 | 65.2 | 64.3 - 66.2 | 14.7 | 14.4 - 15.0 | 6.5 | 7.6 | 9.3 | 10.4 |
| 37 | Colombia | 62.0 | 57.8 | 57.7 - 59.1 | 12.6 | 12.4 - 12.8 | 66.3 | 65.6 - 67.4 | 15.4 | 15.0 - 15.8 | 9.7 | 10.0 | 14.4 | 13.1 |
| 38 | Comoros | 54.6 | 53.9 | 47.3 - 59.4 | 10.8 | 9.4 - 12.6 | 55.3 | 48.2 - 60.0 | 11.5 | 10.1 - 12.6 | 7.8 | 9.6 | 12.6 | 14.8 |
| 39 | Congo | 46.3 | 45.3 | 39.9 - 51.7 | 10.4 | 9.3 - 12.6 | 47.3 | 41.4 - 53.7 | 11.5 | 10.4 - 13.6 | 6.3 | 7.2 | 12.2 | 13.2 |
| 40 | Cook Islands | 61.6 | 60.6 | 58.9 - 61.2 | 11.5 | 11.0 - 12.0 | 62.7 | 61.7 - 63.8 | 12.6 | 12.1 - 12.7 | 8.6 | 11.5 | 12.5 | 15.5 |
| 41 | Costa Rica | 67.2 | 65.2 | 64.4 - 66.0 | 14.4 | 13.7 - 15.1 | 69.3 | 68.6 - 70.0 | 16.7 | 16.1 - 17.3 | 9.5 | 10.3 | 12.8 | 12.9 |
| 42 | Côte d'Ivoire | 39.5 | 37.6 | 32.6 - 44.2 | 9.5 | 8.8 - 11.1 | 41.3 | 36.2 - 47.7 | 10.7 | 9.9 - 12.4 | 5.4 | 6.7 | 12.6 | 13.9 |
| 43 | Croatia | 66.6 | 63.8 | 63.2 - 64.6 | 12.5 | 12.4 - 12.9 | 69.3 | 68.4 - 70.0 | 16.1 | 15.5 - 16.2 | 7.2 | 9.3 | 10.1 | 11.8 |
| 44 | Cuba | 68.3 | 67.1 | 66.1 - 67.9 | 15.2 | 14.8 - 15.4 | 69.5 | 68.8 - 70.3 | 16.7 | 16.4 - 16.9 | 7.9 | 9.8 | 10.5 | 12.4 |
| 45 | Cyprus | 67.6 | 66.7 | 65.9 - 67.5 | 14.2 | 13.8 - 14.6 | 68.5 | 67.1 - 70.0 | 15.0 | 14.1 - 16.0 | 8.8 | 10.6 | 11.7 | 13.4 |
| 46 | Czech Republic | 68.4 | 65.9 | 65.2 - 66.5 | 13.5 | 13.3 - 13.7 | 70.9 | 70.2 - 71.7 | 16.8 | 16.5 - 17.1 | 6.6 | 8.1 | 9.1 | 10.3 |
| 47 | Democratic People's Republic of Korea | 58.8 | 58.0 | 50.9 - 64.2 | 12.1 | 10.5 - 14.4 | 59.7 | 51.6 - 65.7 | 13.2 | 11.4 - 14.9 | 6.4 | 7.4 | 10.0 | 11.0 |
| 48 | Democratic Republic of the Congo | 37.1 | 35.0 | 29.6 - 39.5 | 8.6 | 7.9 - 9.4 | 39.1 | 32.6 - 44.4 | 10.2 | 9.5 - 11.1 | 6.0 | 7.0 | 14.7 | 15.1 |
| 49 | Denmark | 69.8 | 68.6 | 68.0 - 69.1 | 15.2 | 15.0 - 15.4 | 71.1 | 70.6 - 71.8 | 17.2 | 16.9 - 17.4 | 6.3 | 8.4 | 8.4 | 10.5 |
| 50 | Djibouti | 42.9 | 42.5 | 37.8 - 48.9 | 9.8 | 9.0 - 11.7 | 43.2 | 37.7 - 49.7 | 10.6 | 9.6 - 12.2 | 6.1 | 7.4 | 12.6 | 14.7 |

| | Member State | Total population At birth | Males At birth | Males Uncertainty interval | Males At age 60 | Males Uncertainty interval | Females At birth | Females Uncertainty interval | Females At age 60 | Females Uncertainty interval | Expectation of lost healthy years at birth (years) Males | Females | Percentage of total life expectancy lost Males | Females |
|---|---|---|---|---|---|---|---|---|---|---|---|---|---|---|
| | | | | Healthy life expectancy (HALE) (years) | | | | | | | | | | |
| 51 | Dominica | 63.7 | 61.9 | 60.5 - 63.1 | 13.8 | 13.4 - 14.1 | 65.6 | 64.3 - 67.2 | 15.3 | 14.9 - 15.7 | 9.1 | 10.2 | 12.9 | 13.5 |
| 52 | Dominican Republic | 59.6 | 57.2 | 54.7 - 59.7 | 11.3 | 11.1 - 11.6 | 61.9 | 60.9 - 63.1 | 13.7 | 13.4 - 13.9 | 7.7 | 9.6 | 11.9 | 13.4 |
| 53 | Ecuador | 61.9 | 59.8 | 58.9 - 60.6 | 13.2 | 13.0 - 13.5 | 64.1 | 63.3 - 65.1 | 15.2 | 14.9 - 15.4 | 8.1 | 9.4 | 11.9 | 12.8 |
| 54 | Egypt | 59.0 | 57.8 | 57.0 - 58.2 | 9.9 | 9.7 - 10.1 | 60.2 | 59.6 - 60.9 | 11.3 | 11.0 - 11.4 | 7.4 | 8.8 | 11.4 | 12.8 |
| 55 | El Salvador | 59.7 | 57.2 | 55.9 - 58.5 | 12.6 | 12.4 - 12.9 | 62.3 | 61.5 - 63.3 | 14.1 | 13.8 - 14.3 | 9.3 | 10.4 | 14.0 | 14.3 |
| 56 | Equatorial Guinea | 45.5 | 44.7 | 38.7 - 50.3 | 9.7 | 8.8 - 10.9 | 46.3 | 39.7 - 52.2 | 10.5 | 9.7 - 11.7 | 7.2 | 8.5 | 13.9 | 15.5 |
| 57 | Eritrea | 50.0 | 49.3 | 39.0 - 53.3 | 10.6 | 8.9 - 12.0 | 50.8 | 43.7 - 56.4 | 11.3 | 9.9 - 12.7 | 6.5 | 8.6 | 11.7 | 14.5 |
| 58 | Estonia | 64.1 | 59.2 | 58.6 - 59.8 | 11.9 | 11.4 - 12.2 | 69.0 | 67.5 - 70.5 | 16.5 | 16.3 - 16.9 | 6.0 | 8.1 | 9.2 | 10.5 |
| 59 | Ethiopia | 41.2 | 40.7 | 34.6 - 46.7 | 9.7 | 8.9 - 11.0 | 41.7 | 35.6 - 48.2 | 10.2 | 9.5 - 11.6 | 6.1 | 7.7 | 13.0 | 15.6 |
| 60 | Fiji | 58.8 | 56.9 | 56.4 - 58.6 | 10.4 | 10.1 - 10.7 | 60.6 | 60.1 - 62.4 | 11.9 | 11.5 - 12.4 | 7.7 | 9.7 | 12.0 | 13.8 |
| 61 | Finland | 71.1 | 68.7 | 68.0 - 69.3 | 15.7 | 15.4 - 15.9 | 73.5 | 72.7 - 74.1 | 18.9 | 18.5 - 19.1 | 6.1 | 8.0 | 8.1 | 9.9 |
| 62 | France | 72.0 | 69.3 | 68.7 - 70.0 | 16.6 | 16.3 - 16.9 | 74.7 | 74.0 - 75.4 | 20.4 | 20.1 - 20.7 | 6.7 | 8.8 | 8.8 | 10.6 |
| 63 | Gabon | 51.4 | 50.2 | 44.5 - 56.4 | 10.6 | 9.4 - 12.7 | 52.6 | 45.9 - 58.6 | 11.6 | 10.2 - 13.5 | 7.1 | 8.8 | 12.4 | 14.3 |
| 64 | Gambia | 49.5 | 48.5 | 42.0 - 54.1 | 10.4 | 9.3 - 11.7 | 50.5 | 43.1 - 56.2 | 11.2 | 10.1 - 12.4 | 6.9 | 8.4 | 12.5 | 14.2 |
| 65 | Georgia | 64.4 | 62.2 | 61.1 - 63.3 | 12.6 | 12.3 - 13.0 | 66.6 | 64.8 - 67.7 | 14.6 | 13.3 - 15.1 | 6.2 | 8.4 | 9.1 | 11.2 |
| 66 | Germany | 71.8 | 69.6 | 68.9 - 70.4 | 15.9 | 15.6 - 16.2 | 74.0 | 73.4 - 74.8 | 19.0 | 18.8 - 19.3 | 5.9 | 7.6 | 7.8 | 9.3 |
| 67 | Ghana | 49.8 | 49.2 | 43.3 - 55.8 | 10.5 | 9.3 - 12.4 | 50.3 | 43.8 - 56.3 | 11.2 | 10.0 - 12.8 | 7.2 | 8.5 | 12.7 | 14.4 |
| 68 | Greece | 71.0 | 69.1 | 68.4 - 69.7 | 16.0 | 15.8 - 16.3 | 72.9 | 72.3 - 73.8 | 18.1 | 17.7 - 18.4 | 6.7 | 8.1 | 8.9 | 10.0 |
| 69 | Grenada | 59.2 | 58.4 | 57.0 - 59.7 | 11.1 | 10.8 - 11.5 | 60.0 | 58.8 - 61.3 | 12.6 | 12.3 - 12.9 | 7.5 | 8.9 | 11.4 | 12.9 |
| 70 | Guatemala | 57.4 | 54.9 | 53.6 - 56.2 | 12.3 | 11.9 - 12.7 | 59.9 | 58.6 - 61.4 | 13.3 | 13.0 - 13.6 | 8.2 | 9.1 | 13.0 | 13.2 |
| 71 | Guinea | 44.8 | 43.9 | 38.2 - 49.0 | 9.6 | 8.7 - 10.7 | 45.6 | 38.9 - 51.7 | 10.5 | 9.6 - 11.6 | 7.0 | 8.2 | 13.7 | 15.2 |
| 72 | Guinea-Bissau | 40.5 | 39.6 | 33.1 - 44.1 | 9.2 | 8.5 - 10.0 | 41.5 | 34.3 - 48.0 | 10.1 | 9.4 - 11.0 | 6.1 | 7.2 | 13.4 | 14.7 |
| 73 | Guyana | 55.2 | 53.1 | 50.6 - 55.9 | 10.2 | 9.9 - 10.6 | 57.2 | 54.6 - 59.9 | 12.2 | 11.8 - 12.7 | 8.4 | 9.7 | 13.6 | 14.5 |
| 74 | Haiti | 43.8 | 43.5 | 38.1 - 48.7 | 10.3 | 9.2 - 11.9 | 44.1 | 37.9 - 49.1 | 11.7 | 10.5 - 12.9 | 5.6 | 6.9 | 11.4 | 13.6 |
| 75 | Honduras | 58.4 | 56.3 | 53.1 - 59.2 | 11.4 | 10.4 - 12.6 | 60.5 | 58.1 - 62.9 | 13.1 | 12.3 - 14.0 | 7.9 | 9.9 | 12.4 | 14.0 |
| 76 | Hungary | 64.9 | 61.5 | 61.0 - 62.0 | 12.1 | 12.0 - 12.3 | 68.2 | 67.6 - 68.8 | 16.0 | 15.8 - 16.2 | 6.8 | 8.6 | 10.0 | 11.2 |
| 77 | Iceland | 72.8 | 72.1 | 71.2 - 72.9 | 17.5 | 17.1 - 17.9 | 73.6 | 72.7 - 74.2 | 18.7 | 18.2 - 18.9 | 6.3 | 8.2 | 8.1 | 10.0 |
| 78 | India | 53.5 | 53.3 | 52.5 - 54.1 | 10.8 | 10.6 - 11.0 | 53.6 | 52.7 - 54.6 | 11.4 | 11.0 - 11.8 | 6.8 | 8.4 | 11.3 | 13.6 |
| 79 | Indonesia | 58.1 | 57.4 | 56.6 - 58.4 | 10.7 | 10.5 - 11.0 | 58.9 | 58.1 - 59.9 | 11.5 | 11.3 - 11.8 | 7.5 | 9.1 | 11.5 | 13.4 |
| 80 | Iran, Islamic Republic of | 57.6 | 56.1 | 54.9 - 57.3 | 10.4 | 10.2 - 10.7 | 59.1 | 58.2 - 60.5 | 11.9 | 11.6 - 12.2 | 10.4 | 12.5 | 15.7 | 17.5 |
| 81 | Iraq | 50.1 | 48.8 | 47.0 - 50.4 | 9.2 | 8.9 - 9.5 | 51.5 | 50.1 - 53.4 | 10.6 | 10.3 - 10.9 | 10.3 | 11.6 | 17.5 | 18.4 |
| 82 | Ireland | 69.8 | 68.1 | 67.3 - 68.9 | 14.8 | 14.4 - 15.2 | 71.5 | 70.8 - 72.3 | 17.5 | 17.2 - 17.8 | 6.3 | 8.2 | 8.5 | 10.3 |
| 83 | Israel | 71.4 | 70.5 | 69.4 - 71.2 | 16.8 | 16.4 - 17.2 | 72.3 | 71.6 - 73.1 | 18.2 | 17.6 - 18.8 | 6.9 | 9.0 | 8.9 | 11.1 |
| 84 | Italy | 72.7 | 70.7 | 70.0 - 71.5 | 16.4 | 16.0 - 16.7 | 74.7 | 74.0 - 75.5 | 19.4 | 19.1 - 19.8 | 6.0 | 7.8 | 7.8 | 9.5 |
| 85 | Jamaica | 65.1 | 64.2 | 62.8 - 65.6 | 13.0 | 12.6 - 13.5 | 65.9 | 64.9 - 67.2 | 14.5 | 14.1 - 14.9 | 6.9 | 8.6 | 9.7 | 11.5 |
| 86 | Japan | 75.0 | 72.3 | 71.5 - 73.1 | 17.5 | 17.2 - 17.8 | 77.7 | 76.9 - 78.1 | 21.7 | 21.4 - 22.0 | 6.1 | 7.5 | 7.8 | 8.8 |
| 87 | Jordan | 61.0 | 59.7 | 58.2 - 60.3 | 11.1 | 10.8 - 11.4 | 62.3 | 61.4 - 63.0 | 12.9 | 12.5 - 13.1 | 9.0 | 10.9 | 13.1 | 14.9 |
| 88 | Kazakhstan | 55.9 | 52.6 | 51.6 - 53.7 | 9.7 | 8.1 - 12.0 | 59.3 | 58.0 - 60.0 | 12.5 | 12.2 - 12.8 | 6.1 | 9.6 | 10.4 | 13.9 |
| 89 | Kenya | 44.4 | 44.1 | 39.8 - 51.2 | 10.7 | 9.5 - 13.2 | 44.8 | 39.9 - 51.6 | 11.5 | 10.3 - 13.5 | 5.7 | 7.1 | 11.5 | 13.7 |
| 90 | Kiribati | 54.0 | 52.3 | 51.1 - 53.4 | 11.5 | 11.2 - 11.9 | 55.6 | 54.7 - 57.0 | 11.6 | 11.3 - 11.9 | 9.5 | 11.0 | 15.4 | 16.5 |
| 91 | Kuwait | 67.1 | 67.2 | 66.4 - 67.9 | 13.8 | 13.2 - 14.4 | 67.1 | 66.7 - 67.6 | 14.2 | 13.9 - 14.5 | 8.2 | 10.6 | 10.9 | 13.6 |
| 92 | Kyrgyzstan | 55.3 | 52.2 | 51.2 - 53.3 | 9.8 | 9.4 - 10.2 | 58.4 | 56.9 - 59.1 | 12.6 | 12.3 - 12.9 | 8.2 | 10.6 | 13.5 | 15.3 |
| 93 | Lao People's Democratic Republic | 47.0 | 47.1 | 44.8 - 49.6 | 9.6 | 9.4 - 9.9 | 47.0 | 44.7 - 49.5 | 10.1 | 9.8 - 10.4 | 7.0 | 9.2 | 12.9 | 16.4 |
| 94 | Latvia | 62.8 | 58.0 | 57.2 - 59.2 | 11.3 | 10.9 - 11.7 | 67.5 | 66.7 - 68.5 | 15.7 | 15.5 - 16.1 | 6.6 | 8.3 | 10.2 | 10.9 |
| 95 | Lebanon | 60.4 | 59.2 | 57.9 - 60.4 | 11.3 | 10.9 - 11.6 | 61.6 | 60.7 - 62.9 | 12.6 | 12.3 - 13.0 | 8.4 | 10.4 | 12.5 | 14.5 |
| 96 | Lesotho | 31.4 | 29.6 | 27.1 - 35.2 | 9.9 | 9.3 - 12.9 | 33.2 | 29.9 - 40.0 | 11.0 | 10.1 - 13.4 | 3.3 | 5.0 | 10.1 | 13.1 |
| 97 | Liberia | 35.3 | 33.6 | 27.4 - 38.7 | 7.9 | 7.3 - 8.6 | 37.0 | 29.8 - 43.2 | 9.7 | 9.2 - 10.7 | 6.5 | 6.7 | 16.1 | 15.4 |
| 98 | Libyan Arab Jamahiriya | 63.7 | 62.3 | 59.1 - 65.2 | 12.0 | 10.9 - 13.3 | 65.0 | 63.2 - 67.2 | 13.8 | 13.0 - 14.7 | 8.1 | 10.5 | 11.5 | 13.9 |
| 99 | Lithuania | 63.3 | 58.9 | 58.1 - 60.1 | 12.0 | 11.8 - 12.3 | 67.7 | 67.0 - 68.6 | 16.2 | 15.9 - 16.5 | 7.2 | 9.9 | 10.9 | 12.8 |
| 100 | Luxembourg | 71.5 | 69.3 | 68.6 - 69.9 | 16.0 | 15.7 - 16.3 | 73.7 | 73.1 - 74.7 | 19.2 | 18.9 - 19.6 | 6.4 | 8.0 | 8.4 | 9.8 |

## Annex Table 4 Healthy life expectancy (HALE) in all WHO Member States, estimates for 2002

Figures computed by WHO to assure comparability;[a] they are not necessarily the official statistics of Member States, which may use alternative rigorous methods.

| | Member State | Total population At birth | Males At birth | Males Uncertainty interval | Males At age 60 | Males Uncertainty interval | Females At birth | Females Uncertainty interval | Females At age 60 | Females Uncertainty interval | Expectation of lost healthy years at birth (years) Males | Females | Percentage of total life expectancy lost Males | Females |
|---|---|---|---|---|---|---|---|---|---|---|---|---|---|---|
| 101 | Madagascar | 48.6 | 47.3 | 40.8 - 52.3 | 10.1 | 9.1 - 11.1 | 49.9 | 42.5 - 54.8 | 11.1 | 10.0 - 12.0 | 7.2 | 8.4 | 13.1 | 14.4 |
| 102 | Malawi | 34.9 | 35.0 | 31.6 - 40.5 | 9.7 | 9.0 - 11.4 | 34.8 | 30.8 - 40.7 | 10.4 | 9.7 - 11.9 | 4.8 | 5.8 | 12.1 | 14.3 |
| 103 | Malaysia | 63.2 | 61.6 | 60.8 - 62.5 | 10.9 | 10.7 - 11.1 | 64.8 | 64.1 - 65.6 | 12.0 | 11.8 - 12.3 | 8.0 | 10.0 | 11.4 | 13.3 |
| 104 | Maldives | 57.8 | 59.0 | 58.1 - 60.5 | 10.5 | 10.3 - 10.7 | 56.6 | 55.7 - 57.7 | 9.4 | 9.2 - 9.6 | 7.5 | 9.0 | 11.3 | 13.8 |
| 105 | Mali | 37.9 | 37.5 | 31.0 - 42.0 | 8.8 | 8.2 - 9.4 | 38.3 | 31.4 - 44.7 | 9.5 | 8.9 - 10.3 | 6.4 | 7.4 | 14.6 | 16.1 |
| 106 | Malta | 71.4 | 69.9 | 69.1 - 70.6 | 15.4 | 15.0 - 15.9 | 72.9 | 72.2 - 73.7 | 18.2 | 17.7 - 18.7 | 6.2 | 8.3 | 8.2 | 10.2 |
| 107 | Marshall Islands | 54.8 | 53.9 | 52.3 - 55.7 | 9.8 | 9.6 - 10.1 | 55.7 | 54.4 - 57.3 | 10.7 | 10.4 - 10.9 | 7.2 | 8.9 | 11.7 | 13.8 |
| 108 | Mauritania | 44.5 | 42.8 | 36.0 - 47.5 | 9.5 | 8.6 - 10.2 | 46.3 | 38.4 - 51.4 | 10.5 | 9.7 - 11.4 | 6.9 | 8.2 | 14.0 | 15.1 |
| 109 | Mauritius | 62.4 | 60.3 | 59.2 - 61.3 | 11.7 | 11.4 - 12.0 | 64.6 | 63.8 - 65.6 | 13.8 | 13.6 - 14.1 | 8.1 | 10.9 | 11.9 | 14.5 |
| 110 | Mexico | 65.4 | 63.3 | 62.8 - 63.9 | 14.4 | 14.2 - 14.6 | 67.6 | 67.0 - 68.2 | 16.2 | 16.0 - 16.4 | 8.3 | 9.3 | 11.6 | 12.1 |
| 111 | Micronesia, Federated States of | 57.7 | 57.0 | 55.2 - 59.0 | 10.9 | 10.6 - 11.3 | 58.4 | 56.6 - 60.4 | 11.5 | 11.2 - 11.9 | 7.9 | 9.6 | 12.2 | 14.2 |
| 112 | Monaco | 72.9 | 70.7 | 70.0 - 71.4 | 17.3 | 17.1 - 17.6 | 75.2 | 74.4 - 76.0 | 20.5 | 20.1 - 20.9 | 7.1 | 9.3 | 9.1 | 11.0 |
| 113 | Mongolia | 55.6 | 53.3 | 52.4 - 54.4 | 10.2 | 10.0 - 10.4 | 58.0 | 57.1 - 58.9 | 12.4 | 12.2 - 12.6 | 6.8 | 8.0 | 11.3 | 12.1 |
| 114 | Morocco | 60.2 | 59.5 | 58.2 - 60.7 | 11.4 | 11.0 - 11.8 | 60.9 | 59.9 - 62.2 | 12.7 | 12.3 - 13.1 | 9.4 | 11.9 | 13.6 | 16.4 |
| 115 | Mozambique | 36.9 | 36.3 | 29.5 - 39.2 | 9.8 | 9.0 - 11.1 | 37.5 | 30.1 - 41.3 | 10.4 | 9.7 - 11.7 | 4.9 | 6.4 | 11.9 | 14.5 |
| 116 | Myanmar | 51.7 | 49.9 | 43.2 - 55.9 | 10.1 | 9.1 - 11.6 | 53.5 | 45.5 - 58.8 | 11.3 | 10.0 - 12.5 | 6.3 | 8.4 | 11.2 | 13.5 |
| 117 | Namibia | 43.3 | 42.9 | 39.8 - 49.1 | 11.2 | 9.9 - 14.8 | 43.8 | 39.2 - 49.7 | 12.1 | 10.6 - 14.8 | 5.2 | 6.7 | 10.8 | 13.3 |
| 118 | Nauru | 55.1 | 52.7 | 49.6 - 56.2 | 8.7 | 8.1 - 9.6 | 57.5 | 55.0 - 60.5 | 10.5 | 10.0 - 11.4 | 6.9 | 9.0 | 11.6 | 13.5 |
| 119 | Nepal | 51.8 | 52.5 | 51.3 - 53.6 | 10.5 | 10.3 - 10.8 | 51.1 | 50.2 - 52.3 | 10.8 | 10.5 - 11.0 | 7.4 | 9.1 | 12.4 | 15.1 |
| 120 | Netherlands | 71.2 | 69.7 | 69.1 - 70.4 | 15.5 | 15.2 - 15.8 | 72.6 | 72.0 - 73.4 | 18.4 | 18.1 - 18.7 | 6.3 | 8.5 | 8.3 | 10.4 |
| 121 | New Zealand | 70.8 | 69.5 | 68.8 - 70.2 | 16.0 | 15.7 - 16.3 | 72.2 | 71.5 - 73.0 | 18.2 | 17.8 - 18.5 | 7.2 | 9.0 | 9.3 | 11.1 |
| 122 | Nicaragua | 61.4 | 59.7 | 58.4 - 60.3 | 13.0 | 12.8 - 13.3 | 63.1 | 61.9 - 64.0 | 14.5 | 14.3 - 14.9 | 8.2 | 9.3 | 12.0 | 12.9 |
| 123 | Niger | 35.5 | 35.8 | 26.8 - 41.3 | 8.5 | 7.9 - 9.2 | 35.2 | 26.2 - 42.5 | 9.3 | 8.9 - 10.0 | 6.8 | 7.5 | 15.9 | 17.5 |
| 124 | Nigeria | 41.5 | 41.3 | 35.2 - 45.6 | 9.3 | 8.5 - 10.4 | 41.8 | 34.9 - 47.7 | 10.0 | 9.3 - 11.2 | 6.8 | 7.8 | 14.1 | 15.6 |
| 125 | Niue | 60.4 | 58.9 | 55.7 - 61.4 | 11.6 | 10.5 - 12.7 | 62.0 | 59.9 - 64.3 | 12.8 | 12.0 - 13.6 | 8.6 | 11.3 | 12.8 | 15.5 |
| 126 | Norway | 72.0 | 70.4 | 69.5 - 71.3 | 16.2 | 15.7 - 16.6 | 73.6 | 72.8 - 74.4 | 18.9 | 18.5 - 19.1 | 5.9 | 8.1 | 7.8 | 9.9 |
| 127 | Oman | 64.0 | 62.7 | 59.9 - 65.3 | 11.9 | 10.7 - 13.1 | 65.3 | 63.4 - 67.1 | 13.7 | 12.3 - 14.6 | 8.3 | 11.1 | 11.8 | 14.5 |
| 128 | Pakistan | 53.3 | 54.2 | 52.5 - 56.0 | 11.4 | 11.0 - 11.7 | 52.3 | 50.7 - 54.4 | 11.4 | 11.1 - 11.7 | 6.9 | 9.3 | 11.3 | 15.0 |
| 129 | Palau | 59.6 | 58.7 | 57.9 - 59.7 | 10.2 | 10.0 - 10.4 | 60.5 | 59.6 - 61.7 | 12.0 | 11.8 - 12.4 | 7.7 | 10.4 | 11.5 | 14.7 |
| 130 | Panama | 66.2 | 64.3 | 63.2 - 65.4 | 14.9 | 14.5 - 15.4 | 68.0 | 67.2 - 69.2 | 16.8 | 16.4 - 17.2 | 8.5 | 10.2 | 11.7 | 13.0 |
| 131 | Papua New Guinea | 51.9 | 51.4 | 49.7 - 53.6 | 10.1 | 9.8 - 10.3 | 52.4 | 50.9 - 54.4 | 10.6 | 10.3 - 10.9 | 7.0 | 9.1 | 12.0 | 14.8 |
| 132 | Paraguay | 61.9 | 59.6 | 58.5 - 60.6 | 11.7 | 11.2 - 12.0 | 64.2 | 63.3 - 65.1 | 14.6 | 14.1 - 14.7 | 9.1 | 10.5 | 13.2 | 14.0 |
| 133 | Peru | 61.0 | 59.6 | 58.4 - 60.7 | 12.7 | 12.4 - 13.1 | 62.4 | 61.4 - 63.6 | 14.4 | 14.1 - 14.7 | 7.9 | 9.6 | 11.7 | 13.3 |
| 134 | Philippines | 59.3 | 57.1 | 56.2 - 58.1 | 10.6 | 10.4 - 10.8 | 61.5 | 60.6 - 62.6 | 12.1 | 11.9 - 12.4 | 8.0 | 10.2 | 12.4 | 14.3 |
| 135 | Poland | 65.8 | 63.1 | 62.4 - 63.8 | 12.8 | 12.6 - 13.0 | 68.5 | 67.9 - 69.2 | 16.1 | 15.8 - 16.3 | 7.5 | 10.2 | 10.6 | 13.0 |
| 136 | Portugal | 69.2 | 66.7 | 66.0 - 67.4 | 14.9 | 14.7 - 15.2 | 71.7 | 71.1 - 72.5 | 17.7 | 17.4 - 17.9 | 6.9 | 8.8 | 9.4 | 10.9 |
| 137 | Qatar | 65.2 | 66.7 | 65.6 - 67.6 | 13.7 | 13.1 - 14.4 | 63.8 | 62.4 - 65.4 | 11.2 | 10.2 - 12.3 | 8.2 | 10.0 | 10.9 | 13.5 |
| 138 | Republic of Korea | 67.8 | 64.8 | 64.1 - 65.6 | 13.2 | 13.0 - 13.5 | 70.8 | 70.1 - 71.6 | 17.1 | 16.8 - 17.3 | 6.9 | 8.6 | 9.7 | 10.8 |
| 139 | Republic of Moldova | 59.8 | 57.2 | 56.2 - 58.2 | 11.0 | 10.8 - 11.1 | 62.4 | 61.2 - 62.9 | 13.2 | 12.9 - 13.4 | 6.8 | 9.2 | 10.6 | 12.9 |
| 140 | Romania | 63.1 | 61.0 | 59.9 - 62.1 | 12.3 | 12.1 - 12.6 | 65.2 | 64.3 - 66.3 | 14.6 | 14.2 - 15.0 | 7.0 | 9.7 | 10.3 | 13.0 |
| 141 | Russian Federation | 58.4 | 52.8 | 51.9 - 53.6 | 9.7 | 7.0 - 12.3 | 64.1 | 63.3 - 64.8 | 14.0 | 13.8 - 14.2 | 5.5 | 7.7 | 9.4 | 10.7 |
| 142 | Rwanda | 38.3 | 36.4 | 33.0 - 42.5 | 9.0 | 8.3 - 10.4 | 40.2 | 35.6 - 47.4 | 10.5 | 9.7 - 11.8 | 5.6 | 6.6 | 13.3 | 14.1 |
| 143 | Saint Kitts and Nevis | 61.5 | 59.9 | 59.0 - 61.0 | 11.9 | 11.6 - 12.2 | 63.1 | 61.9 - 64.3 | 13.5 | 13.2 - 13.8 | 8.7 | 9.1 | 12.7 | 12.7 |
| 144 | Saint Lucia | 62.7 | 61.2 | 60.0 - 62.5 | 12.5 | 12.2 - 12.8 | 64.2 | 63.0 - 65.7 | 14.4 | 14.1 - 14.8 | 8.6 | 10.2 | 12.3 | 13.7 |
| 145 | Saint Vincent and the Grenadines | 61.0 | 59.9 | 58.6 - 61.3 | 12.6 | 12.4 - 12.9 | 62.2 | 61.0 - 63.6 | 14.2 | 13.6 - 14.8 | 7.9 | 9.8 | 11.7 | 13.6 |
| 146 | Samoa | 59.7 | 59.2 | 58.1 - 60.3 | 10.9 | 10.7 - 11.2 | 60.3 | 59.3 - 61.6 | 11.6 | 11.3 - 11.9 | 7.6 | 9.4 | 11.3 | 13.5 |
| 147 | San Marino | 73.4 | 70.9 | 69.4 - 72.3 | 16.2 | 15.3 - 17.1 | 75.9 | 75.0 - 78.0 | 19.9 | 19.5 - 21.6 | 6.3 | 8.1 | 8.2 | 9.6 |
| 148 | Sao Tome and Principe | 54.4 | 54.2 | 47.7 - 59.7 | 11.0 | 9.6 - 12.7 | 54.7 | 46.7 - 59.5 | 11.4 | 10.1 - 12.6 | 7.5 | 9.0 | 12.2 | 14.1 |
| 149 | Saudi Arabia | 61.4 | 59.8 | 56.5 - 63.1 | 11.2 | 10.2 - 12.5 | 62.9 | 60.7 - 65.2 | 13.0 | 12.2 - 13.9 | 8.6 | 11.0 | 12.6 | 14.9 |
| 150 | Senegal | 48.0 | 47.1 | 41.0 - 52.1 | 9.9 | 8.9 - 11.1 | 48.9 | 41.9 - 54.4 | 10.7 | 9.8 - 11.9 | 7.3 | 8.4 | 13.4 | 14.7 |
| 151 | Serbia and Montenegro | 63.8 | 62.7 | 62.0 - 63.5 | 12.1 | 11.8 - 12.4 | 64.9 | 63.7 - 65.3 | 13.9 | 13.7 - 14.2 | 7.0 | 10.0 | 10.1 | 13.3 |
| 152 | Seychelles | 61.2 | 57.4 | 56.4 - 58.4 | 9.9 | 9.6 - 10.1 | 64.9 | 63.8 - 66.2 | 14.0 | 13.6 - 14.5 | 9.6 | 12.3 | 14.3 | 15.9 |
| 153 | Sierra Leone | 28.6 | 27.2 | 19.4 - 32.6 | 7.8 | 7.4 - 8.3 | 29.9 | 21.7 - 37.7 | 9.2 | 8.9 - 10.0 | 5.1 | 5.8 | 15.9 | 16.2 |
| 154 | Singapore | 70.1 | 68.8 | 67.7 - 70.0 | 14.5 | 14.0 - 15.1 | 71.3 | 70.6 - 72.1 | 16.3 | 15.9 - 16.5 | 8.6 | 10.4 | 11.1 | 12.7 |
| 155 | Slovakia | 66.2 | 63.0 | 62.3 - 63.8 | 12.3 | 12.1 - 12.5 | 69.4 | 68.7 - 70.2 | 16.1 | 15.9 - 16.4 | 6.7 | 8.9 | 9.6 | 11.4 |

| | Member State | Total population At birth | Healthy life expectancy (HALE) (years) | | | | | | | | Expectation of lost healthy years at birth (years) | | Percentage of total life expectancy lost | |
|---|---|---|---|---|---|---|---|---|---|---|---|---|---|---|
| | | | Males | | | | Females | | | | Males | Females | Males | Females |
| | | At birth | At birth | Uncertainty interval | At age 60 | Uncertainty interval | At birth | Uncertainty interval | At age 60 | Uncertainty interval | | | | |
| 156 | Slovenia | 69.5 | 66.6 | 65.8 - 67.4 | 14.3 | 14.0 - 14.5 | 72.3 | 71.6 - 73.1 | 18.1 | 17.8 - 18.3 | 6.1 | 8.2 | 8.4 | 10.2 |
| 157 | Solomon Islands | 56.2 | 55.4 | 53.4 - 57.6 | 10.9 | 10.5 - 11.4 | 57.1 | 55.7 - 58.8 | 11.6 | 11.2 - 11.9 | 8.3 | 10.3 | 13.0 | 15.3 |
| 158 | Somalia | 36.8 | 36.1 | 30.5 - 40.4 | 8.3 | 7.6 - 9.0 | 37.5 | 29.6 - 43.3 | 9.4 | 8.9 - 10.2 | 6.9 | 8.1 | 16.1 | 17.7 |
| 159 | South Africa | 44.3 | 43.3 | 39.8 - 46.8 | 10.6 | 10.0 - 12.0 | 45.3 | 39.8 - 50.8 | 12.1 | 11.5 - 13.1 | 5.5 | 7.3 | 11.3 | 13.8 |
| 160 | Spain | 72.6 | 69.9 | 69.1 - 70.7 | 16.4 | 16.1 - 16.8 | 75.3 | 74.6 - 76.1 | 19.9 | 19.6 - 20.2 | 6.2 | 7.7 | 8.2 | 9.3 |
| 161 | Sri Lanka | 61.6 | 59.2 | 57.3 - 61.0 | 10.5 | 9.9 - 11.1 | 64.0 | 63.0 - 65.1 | 12.7 | 12.3 - 13.0 | 8.0 | 10.3 | 11.8 | 13.9 |
| 162 | Sudan | 48.5 | 47.2 | 41.8 - 52.7 | 9.8 | 8.7 - 11.5 | 49.9 | 43.0 - 54.6 | 10.7 | 9.5 - 11.8 | 7.8 | 9.4 | 14.1 | 15.9 |
| 163 | Suriname | 58.8 | 56.7 | 55.3 - 58.3 | 10.6 | 10.2 - 11.0 | 60.8 | 59.7 - 62.4 | 12.8 | 12.3 - 13.2 | 7.6 | 10.0 | 11.8 | 14.1 |
| 164 | Swaziland | 34.2 | 33.2 | 30.9 - 36.5 | 10.2 | 9.1 - 12.1 | 35.2 | 31.5 - 38.9 | 10.9 | 9.7 - 12.5 | 3.7 | 5.2 | 10.1 | 12.9 |
| 165 | Sweden | 73.3 | 71.9 | 71.2 - 72.5 | 17.1 | 16.8 - 17.4 | 74.8 | 74.0 - 75.5 | 19.6 | 19.3 - 19.9 | 6.2 | 7.9 | 7.9 | 9.5 |
| 166 | Switzerland | 73.2 | 71.1 | 70.3 - 71.8 | 17.1 | 16.7 - 17.5 | 75.3 | 74.5 - 76.0 | 20.4 | 20.1 - 20.7 | 6.6 | 8.1 | 8.5 | 9.7 |
| 167 | Syrian Arab Republic | 61.7 | 60.4 | 59.3 - 61.5 | 11.3 | 11.0 - 11.6 | 63.1 | 62.3 - 64.1 | 12.9 | 12.6 - 13.2 | 8.5 | 10.5 | 12.3 | 14.2 |
| 168 | Tajikistan | 54.7 | 53.1 | 51.7 - 55.0 | 9.5 | 9.3 - 9.7 | 56.4 | 54.5 - 57.6 | 11.0 | 10.7 - 11.2 | 7.9 | 10.1 | 13.0 | 15.2 |
| 169 | Thailand | 60.1 | 57.7 | 56.5 - 58.9 | 12.7 | 12.4 - 13.0 | 62.4 | 61.5 - 63.5 | 13.2 | 13.0 - 13.5 | 8.4 | 10.2 | 12.7 | 14.1 |
| 170 | The former Yugoslav Republic of Macedonia | 63.4 | 61.9 | 61.0 - 62.8 | 12.2 | 11.9 - 12.7 | 65.0 | 63.7 - 65.6 | 14.0 | 13.6 - 14.5 | 7.2 | 10.2 | 10.4 | 13.5 |
| 171 | Timor-Leste | 49.8 | 47.9 | 40.8 - 53.6 | 10.0 | 9.0 - 11.2 | 51.8 | 43.5 - 56.9 | 11.1 | 10.0 - 12.2 | 6.9 | 8.7 | 12.7 | 14.4 |
| 172 | Togo | 44.6 | 43.5 | 38.0 - 48.1 | 9.8 | 8.8 - 11.0 | 45.7 | 39.6 - 50.6 | 10.7 | 9.7 - 11.9 | 6.5 | 7.7 | 12.9 | 14.3 |
| 173 | Tonga | 61.8 | 61.9 | 61.0 - 62.7 | 11.9 | 11.7 - 12.1 | 61.8 | 61.0 - 62.7 | 12.0 | 11.8 - 12.2 | 8.2 | 9.6 | 11.7 | 13.5 |
| 174 | Trinidad and Tobago | 62.0 | 59.8 | 58.8 - 60.8 | 11.9 | 11.6 - 12.1 | 64.2 | 63.4 - 65.1 | 14.1 | 13.9 - 14.4 | 7.3 | 8.6 | 10.8 | 11.9 |
| 175 | Tunisia | 62.5 | 61.3 | 60.4 - 62.4 | 12.0 | 11.7 - 12.3 | 63.6 | 62.7 - 64.8 | 13.3 | 13.0 - 13.7 | 8.2 | 10.3 | 11.8 | 13.9 |
| 176 | Turkey | 62.0 | 61.2 | 60.3 - 62.2 | 12.8 | 12.5 - 13.0 | 62.8 | 61.7 - 64.0 | 14.2 | 13.8 - 14.6 | 6.7 | 9.3 | 9.8 | 12.9 |
| 177 | Turkmenistan | 54.4 | 51.6 | 50.8 - 52.5 | 9.2 | 8.9 - 9.5 | 57.2 | 55.9 - 57.8 | 11.5 | 11.4 - 11.8 | 7.1 | 9.7 | 12.2 | 14.5 |
| 178 | Tuvalu | 53.0 | 53.0 | 51.3 - 54.7 | 9.7 | 9.5 - 9.8 | 53.1 | 51.1 - 54.9 | 10.3 | 9.4 - 11.8 | 7.0 | 8.3 | 11.7 | 13.6 |
| 179 | Uganda | 42.7 | 41.7 | 37.1 - 46.1 | 9.8 | 8.9 - 11.1 | 43.7 | 37.5 - 48.0 | 10.9 | 9.8 - 11.9 | 6.2 | 7.2 | 12.9 | 14.1 |
| 180 | Ukraine | 59.2 | 54.9 | 54.1 - 55.9 | 10.3 | 9.7 - 11.1 | 63.6 | 62.8 - 64.7 | 13.7 | 13.4 - 14.0 | 6.8 | 9.4 | 11.0 | 12.8 |
| 181 | United Arab Emirates | 63.9 | 63.5 | 62.6 - 64.0 | 12.0 | 11.8 - 12.2 | 64.2 | 63.6 - 65.0 | 12.5 | 12.3 - 12.7 | 7.8 | 10.9 | 10.9 | 14.5 |
| 182 | United Kingdom | 70.6 | 69.1 | 68.5 - 69.9 | 15.7 | 15.4 - 16.1 | 72.1 | 71.3 - 73.0 | 18.1 | 17.7 - 18.4 | 6.7 | 8.4 | 8.8 | 10.4 |
| 183 | United Republic of Tanzania | 40.4 | 40.0 | 38.7 - 41.5 | 9.6 | 9.4 - 9.8 | 40.7 | 39.6 - 42.3 | 10.1 | 9.9 - 10.3 | 5.5 | 6.8 | 12.1 | 14.3 |
| 184 | United States of America | 69.3 | 67.2 | 66.6 - 67.8 | 15.3 | 15.0 - 15.5 | 71.3 | 70.8 - 72.0 | 17.9 | 17.7 - 18.1 | 7.4 | 8.5 | 9.9 | 10.7 |
| 185 | Uruguay | 66.2 | 63.0 | 62.1 - 63.9 | 13.0 | 12.8 - 13.3 | 69.4 | 68.6 - 70.2 | 17.1 | 16.8 - 17.4 | 8.0 | 9.9 | 11.3 | 12.5 |
| 186 | Uzbekistan | 59.4 | 57.9 | 56.9 - 58.9 | 10.8 | 10.6 - 11.1 | 60.9 | 59.4 - 61.4 | 12.6 | 12.3 - 12.9 | 7.6 | 10.0 | 11.6 | 14.1 |
| 187 | Vanuatu | 58.9 | 58.5 | 56.9 - 60.3 | 11.1 | 10.7 - 11.5 | 59.4 | 57.9 - 61.2 | 11.7 | 11.3 - 12.1 | 8.0 | 9.8 | 12.0 | 14.1 |
| 188 | Venezuela, Bolivarian Republic of | 64.2 | 61.7 | 60.8 - 62.6 | 13.9 | 13.6 - 14.2 | 66.7 | 66.0 - 67.6 | 15.7 | 15.4 - 15.9 | 9.3 | 10.1 | 13.1 | 13.1 |
| 189 | Viet Nam | 61.3 | 59.8 | 58.7 - 60.9 | 11.4 | 11.2 - 11.7 | 62.9 | 62.0 - 64.2 | 13.1 | 12.8 - 13.4 | 7.4 | 9.3 | 11.0 | 12.9 |
| 190 | Yemen | 49.3 | 48.0 | 42.3 - 52.6 | 8.7 | 7.7 - 9.9 | 50.7 | 44.2 - 55.2 | 10.4 | 9.2 - 11.4 | 10.8 | 11.5 | 18.4 | 18.5 |
| 191 | Zambia | 34.9 | 34.8 | 30.8 - 38.7 | 9.8 | 8.9 - 11.0 | 35.0 | 30.8 - 39.4 | 10.4 | 9.6 - 11.6 | 4.3 | 5.3 | 11.0 | 13.1 |
| 192 | Zimbabwe | 33.6 | 33.8 | 31.9 - 36.0 | 9.7 | 9.4 - 9.9 | 33.3 | 31.5 - 36.0 | 10.6 | 10.4 - 10.9 | 3.9 | 4.7 | 10.4 | 12.3 |

ᵃ See explanatory notes for sources and methods.

## Annex Table 5 Selected national health accounts indicators: measured levels of expenditure on health, 1997–2001

Figures computed by WHO to assure comparability;[a] they are not necessarily the official statistics of Member States, which may use alternative rigorous methods.

| | Member State | Total expenditure on health as % of GDP | | | | | General government expenditure on health as % of total expenditure on health | | | | | Private expenditure on health as % of total expenditure on health | | | | | General government expenditure on health as % of total government expenditure | | | | |
|---|---|---|---|---|---|---|---|---|---|---|---|---|---|---|---|---|---|---|---|---|---|
| | | 1997 | 1998 | 1999 | 2000 | 2001 | 1997 | 1998 | 1999 | 2000 | 2001 | 1997 | 1998 | 1999 | 2000 | 2001 | 1997 | 1998 | 1999 | 2000 | 2001 |
| 1 | Afghanistan | 5.6 | 5.5 | 5.5 | 5 | 5.2 | 50 | 52.8 | 53.1 | 53.8 | 52.6 | 50 | 47.2 | 46.9 | 46.2 | 47.4 | 14 | 14.6 | 14.8 | 13.5 | 11.8 |
| 2 | Albania | 3.8 | 3.4 | 3.6 | 3.8 | 3.7 | 61.2 | 61.9 | 62.3 | 63.9 | 64.6 | 38.8 | 38.1 | 37.7 | 36.1 | 35.4 | 7.8 | 6.9 | 6.9 | 7.7 | 7.3 |
| 3 | Algeria | 3.4 | 3.6 | 3.6 | 3.8 | 4.1 | 71.7 | 70.5 | 69.6 | 70.6 | 75 | 28.3 | 29.5 | 30.4 | 29.4 | 25 | 7.9 | 8.2 | 8.5 | 9.3 | 9.9 |
| 4 | Andorra | 5.7 | 7.8 | 5.9 | 5.5 | 5.7 | 71.5 | 78.6 | 71.6 | 70.1 | 71 | 28.5 | 21.4 | 28.4 | 29.9 | 29 | 32.5 | 39.2 | 31.8 | 32 | 26.3 |
| 5 | Angola | 3.9 | 3.5 | 3.3 | 3.5 | 4.4 | 45.2 | 39.8 | 44.3 | 55.8 | 63.1 | 54.8 | 60.2 | 55.7 | 44.2 | 36.9 | 4.6 | 2.5 | 2.4 | 3.3 | 5.5 |
| 6 | Antigua and Barbuda | 5.4 | 5.3 | 5.3 | 5.5 | 5.6 | 61.9 | 62.5 | 61.3 | 59.9 | 60.9 | 38.1 | 37.5 | 38.7 | 40.1 | 39.1 | 14.2 | 14.5 | 13.9 | 14.1 | 13 |
| 7 | Argentina | 8.1 | 8.2 | 9 | 8.9 | 9.5 | 55.5 | 55.2 | 56.2 | 55.2 | 53.4 | 44.5 | 44.8 | 43.8 | 44.8 | 46.6 | 22.9 | 22.6 | 23.3 | 22 | 21.3 |
| 8 | Armenia | 7.1 | 7.1 | 7.9 | 8 | 7.8 | 35.2 | 36.8 | 41 | 40.2 | 41.2 | 64.8 | 63.2 | 59 | 59.8 | 58.8 | 9.4 | 10.8 | 10.5 | 10.6 | 11.5 |
| 9 | Australia | 8.5 | 8.6 | 8.7 | 8.9 | 9.2 | 67.8 | 68.2 | 69.1 | 68.9 | 67.9 | 32.2 | 31.8 | 30.9 | 31.1 | 32.1 | 15.8 | 16.2 | 16.8 | 16.5 | 16.8 |
| 10 | Austria | 8 | 8 | 8 | 8 | 8 | 70.9 | 71.4 | 70 | 69.7 | 69.3 | 29.1 | 28.6 | 30 | 30.3 | 30.7 | 10.4 | 10.5 | 10.4 | 10.6 | 10.7 |
| 11 | Azerbaijan | 2.2 | 2.3 | 2 | 1.7 | 1.6 | 73.4 | 73.1 | 70.3 | 67.9 | 66.9 | 26.6 | 26.9 | 29.7 | 32.1 | 33.1 | 8.8 | 11 | 8 | 7.3 | 7.2 |
| 12 | Bahamas | 5.4 | 5.6 | 5.4 | 5.7 | 5.7 | 55.6 | 57.6 | 57.4 | 56.8 | 57 | 44.4 | 42.4 | 42.6 | 43.2 | 43 | 13.7 | 15.3 | 15 | 15.9 | 15.1 |
| 13 | Bahrain | 4.8 | 5 | 4.8 | 4.1 | 4.1 | 70.5 | 69.7 | 69.3 | 69.1 | 69 | 29.5 | 30.3 | 30.7 | 30.9 | 31 | 11.9 | 11.5 | 11.4 | 10.8 | 10.8 |
| 14 | Bangladesh | 2.9 | 2.9 | 3.1 | 3.6 | 3.5 | 33.7 | 36 | 36.9 | 45.3 | 44.2 | 66.3 | 64 | 63.1 | 54.7 | 55.8 | 5.6 | 5.9 | 6.3 | 8.6 | 8.7 |
| 15 | Barbados | 5.9 | 5.9 | 6.1 | 6.2 | 6.5 | 65.2 | 65.6 | 65.7 | 65.9 | 66.3 | 34.8 | 34.4 | 34.3 | 34.1 | 33.7 | 11.7 | 11.8 | 12 | 12 | 11.5 |
| 16 | Belarus | 6.1 | 5.7 | 5.8 | 5.4 | 5.6 | 87.2 | 86.1 | 85.5 | 85.4 | 86.7 | 12.8 | 13.9 | 14.5 | 14.6 | 13.3 | 11.6 | 11.9 | 11.7 | 13.1 | 14.2 |
| 17 | Belgium | 8.4 | 8.4 | 8.5 | 8.6 | 8.9 | 71.5 | 72 | 72.2 | 72.1 | 71.7 | 28.5 | 28 | 27.8 | 27.9 | 28.3 | 11.7 | 11.9 | 12.3 | 12.6 | 13 |
| 18 | Belize | 4.7 | 4.9 | 5.1 | 5 | 5.2 | 51 | 51.7 | 48.6 | 48 | 45.1 | 49 | 48.3 | 51.4 | 52 | 54.9 | 5.6 | 5.6 | 5.5 | 5.3 | 5 |
| 19 | Benin | 3.7 | 3.8 | 3.9 | 4.2 | 4.4 | 34 | 36.5 | 38.6 | 43.3 | 46.9 | 66 | 63.5 | 61.4 | 56.7 | 53.1 | 6.7 | 8.5 | 8.7 | 8.9 | 10.9 |
| 20 | Bhutan | 3.6 | 3.8 | 3.5 | 3.9 | 3.9 | 90.4 | 90.3 | 89.6 | 90.6 | 90.6 | 9.6 | 9.7 | 10.4 | 9.4 | 9.4 | 10.1 | 9.6 | 8.3 | 9.2 | 7.5 |
| 21 | Bolivia | 4.7 | 5 | 5.2 | 5.2 | 5.3 | 63.9 | 65.6 | 66.1 | 67 | 66.3 | 36.1 | 34.4 | 33.9 | 33 | 33.7 | 9.1 | 10 | 10.4 | 10.3 | 10.3 |
| 22 | Bosnia and Herzegovina | 6.7 | 7.9 | 7.7 | 7.7 | 7.5 | 52.4 | 40.2 | 39.4 | 39.7 | 36.8 | 47.6 | 59.8 | 60.6 | 60.3 | 63.2 | 12.6 | 11.7 | 9.4 | 9.1 | 9.6 |
| 23 | Botswana | 5.7 | 5.5 | 6 | 6 | 6.6 | 58.8 | 59.7 | 60.6 | 62 | 66.2 | 41.2 | 40.3 | 39.4 | 38 | 33.8 | 7.8 | 7.2 | 7.4 | 8.4 | 7.6 |
| 24 | Brazil | 7.4 | 7.4 | 7.8 | 7.6 | 7.6 | 43.5 | 44 | 42.8 | 40.8 | 41.6 | 56.5 | 56 | 57.2 | 59.2 | 58.4 | 9.1 | 9 | 9.3 | 8.4 | 8.8 |
| 25 | Brunei Darussalam | 2.8 | 3 | 3.2 | 3.1 | 3.1 | 79.4 | 81.3 | 79.4 | 80 | 79.4 | 20.6 | 18.7 | 20.6 | 20 | 20.6 | 4.5 | 5.1 | 5.1 | 5.2 | 5.1 |
| 26 | Bulgaria | 4.7 | 3.9 | 5 | 4.8 | 4.8 | 82.8 | 79.4 | 83.7 | 82.5 | 82.1 | 17.2 | 20.6 | 16.3 | 17.5 | 17.9 | 10 | 8.1 | 10.5 | 9.3 | 9.3 |
| 27 | Burkina Faso | 3.5 | 3.5 | 3.8 | 3.5 | 3 | 67.1 | 65.3 | 66.6 | 63.5 | 60.1 | 32.9 | 34.7 | 33.4 | 36.5 | 39.9 | 9.6 | 9.6 | 8.8 | 8.1 | 8.1 |
| 28 | Burundi | 3.1 | 3.2 | 3.2 | 3.5 | 3.6 | 50.3 | 53.8 | 55.3 | 55.6 | 59 | 49.7 | 46.2 | 44.7 | 44.4 | 41 | 7.5 | 7.7 | 8.4 | 7.1 | 8.1 |
| 29 | Cambodia | 10.9 | 10.8 | 10.8 | 11.8 | 11.8 | 10.2 | 10.1 | 10.1 | 14.2 | 14.9 | 89.8 | 89.9 | 89.9 | 85.8 | 85.1 | 12.5 | 11.8 | 11.3 | 15.7 | 16 |
| 30 | Cameroon | 3.7 | 3.4 | 3.1 | 3.1 | 3.3 | 21.2 | 19.2 | 22.8 | 33.7 | 37.1 | 78.8 | 80.8 | 77.2 | 66.3 | 62.9 | 5.2 | 4.1 | 4.4 | 7.9 | 7.8 |
| 31 | Canada | 8.9 | 9.1 | 9.1 | 9.1 | 9.5 | 70 | 70.7 | 70.4 | 70.9 | 70.8 | 30 | 29.3 | 29.6 | 29.1 | 29.2 | 13.9 | 14.4 | 15 | 15.5 | 16.2 |
| 32 | Cape Verde | 3.8 | 4.1 | 3.9 | 4.3 | 4.5 | 75.8 | 79.1 | 80.1 | 82.9 | 83.9 | 24.2 | 20.9 | 19.9 | 17.1 | 16.1 | 6.8 | 8.9 | 8.4 | 10.1 | 12.2 |
| 33 | Central African Republic | 3.6 | 4 | 4.1 | 4.3 | 4.5 | 37.9 | 44.4 | 48 | 49.2 | 51.2 | 62.1 | 55.6 | 52 | 50.8 | 48.8 | 8.4 | 9 | 10.1 | 13.9 | 18.5 |
| 34 | Chad | 2.8 | 2.3 | 2.7 | 3.1 | 2.6 | 78.1 | 72.7 | 75 | 78.7 | 76 | 21.9 | 27.3 | 25 | 21.3 | 24 | 12.5 | 10.8 | 11.2 | 12.2 | 15.2 |
| 35 | Chile | 6.6 | 6.9 | 6.8 | 6.8 | 7 | 37.8 | 39.6 | 40.8 | 42.6 | 44 | 62.2 | 60.4 | 59.2 | 57.4 | 56 | 12.1 | 12.4 | 11.8 | 11.9 | 12.7 |
| 36 | China | 4.6 | 4.8 | 5.1 | 5.3 | 5.5 | 40 | 39 | 38 | 36.6 | 37.2 | 60 | 61 | 62 | 63.4 | 62.8 | 14.2 | 13.3 | 11.8 | 10.8 | 10.2 |
| 37 | Colombia | 7.7 | 5.8 | 6.4 | 5.5 | 5.5 | 47.7 | 60.2 | 62 | 67.3 | 65.7 | 52.3 | 39.8 | 38 | 32.7 | 34.3 | 14.5 | 13 | 12.9 | 12.7 | 10.8 |
| 38 | Comoros | 3.1 | 3 | 3.1 | 3.1 | 3.1 | 60.3 | 58.6 | 59.6 | 59.7 | 60 | 39.7 | 41.4 | 40.4 | 40.3 | 40 | 5.9 | 5.1 | 5.8 | 5.7 | 5.8 |
| 39 | Congo | 3 | 3.1 | 2.6 | 2 | 2.1 | 70.3 | 76.9 | 70.6 | 73.3 | 63.8 | 29.7 | 23.1 | 29.4 | 26.7 | 36.2 | 5.7 | 5.6 | 5.7 | 5.6 | 5.7 |
| 40 | Cook Islands | 5.1 | 5.1 | 4.8 | 4.6 | 4.7 | 72.7 | 71.9 | 65.1 | 64.4 | 67.6 | 27.3 | 28.1 | 34.9 | 35.6 | 32.4 | 9.5 | 9.2 | 9.1 | 8.6 | 8.9 |
| 41 | Costa Rica | 6.7 | 6.7 | 6.5 | 6.9 | 7.2 | 70.7 | 67.6 | 68.5 | 68.5 | 68.5 | 29.3 | 32.4 | 31.5 | 31.5 | 31.5 | 20.8 | 20.5 | 20.1 | 20.4 | 19.5 |
| 42 | Côte d'Ivoire | 6.2 | 6.4 | 6.3 | 6.2 | 6.2 | 19 | 19.2 | 20 | 15.4 | 16 | 81 | 80.8 | 80 | 84.6 | 84 | 5.4 | 5.9 | 6.4 | 5.3 | 6 |
| 43 | Croatia | 8.1 | 8.8 | 8.9 | 9.4 | 9 | 80.5 | 81.8 | 82.6 | 83.2 | 81.8 | 19.5 | 18.2 | 17.4 | 16.8 | 18.2 | 13.2 | 13.7 | 13.4 | 14.4 | 12.8 |
| 44 | Cuba | 6.6 | 6.6 | 7.1 | 7.1 | 7.2 | 83.7 | 84.7 | 85.5 | 85.8 | 86.2 | 16.3 | 15.3 | 14.5 | 14.2 | 13.8 | 10 | 10.3 | 11.1 | 10.8 | 11.4 |
| 45 | Cyprus | 8.3 | 8.1 | 7.6 | 8 | 8.1 | 50.3 | 52 | 50.6 | 48.7 | 47.7 | 49.7 | 48 | 49.4 | 51.3 | 52.3 | 11.4 | 11.4 | 10.9 | 10.7 | 10.2 |
| 46 | Czech Republic | 7.1 | 7.1 | 7.1 | 7.1 | 7.4 | 91.7 | 91.9 | 91.5 | 91.4 | 91.4 | 8.3 | 8.1 | 8.5 | 8.6 | 8.6 | 14 | 13.6 | 13.9 | 13.9 | 14.1 |
| 47 | Democratic People's Republic of Korea | 2.2 | 2.8 | 2.6 | 2.4 | 2.5 | 71.4 | 76.9 | 75.3 | 73.5 | 73.4 | 28.6 | 23.1 | 24.7 | 26.5 | 26.6 | 3.5 | 3.3 | 3.2 | 2.9 | 3 |
| 48 | Democratic Republic of the Congo | 3.3 | 3 | 3.1 | 3.2 | 3.5 | 47.1 | 41.7 | 41.5 | 44.7 | 44.4 | 52.9 | 58.3 | 58.5 | 55.3 | 55.6 | 10.3 | 8.3 | 8.7 | 9.7 | 10.3 |
| 49 | Denmark | 8.2 | 8.4 | 8.5 | 8.2 | 8.4 | 82.3 | 82 | 82.2 | 82.5 | 82.4 | 17.7 | 18 | 17.8 | 17.5 | 17.6 | 11.7 | 11.9 | 12.4 | 12.6 | 12.8 |
| 50 | Djibouti | 7.3 | 7.2 | 7.1 | 7.1 | 7 | 58.1 | 58 | 58.4 | 58.4 | 58.8 | 41.9 | 42 | 41.6 | 41.6 | 41.2 | 11.8 | 12.5 | 12.4 | 12.5 | 13.7 |
| 51 | Dominica | 5.9 | 5.7 | 6.2 | 5.8 | 6 | 75 | 74.7 | 74.3 | 71.5 | 71.3 | 25 | 25.3 | 25.7 | 28.5 | 28.7 | 11.8 | 11.8 | 12.8 | 12.8 | 10.5 |
| 52 | Dominican Republic | 5.8 | 5.8 | 5.7 | 6.2 | 6.1 | 32 | 31.4 | 32.2 | 35.4 | 36.1 | 68 | 68.6 | 67.8 | 64.6 | 63.9 | 12.2 | 11.8 | 11.3 | 14.6 | 13.5 |
| 53 | Ecuador | 4.4 | 4.4 | 3.7 | 4.1 | 4.5 | 53.3 | 50.3 | 55.6 | 55.2 | 50.3 | 46.7 | 49.7 | 44.4 | 44.8 | 49.7 | 10.4 | 10.7 | 9 | 9.3 | 9.5 |
| 54 | Egypt | 3.9 | 3.9 | 3.9 | 3.8 | 3.9 | 45.9 | 46 | 46.4 | 46.1 | 48.9 | 54.1 | 54 | 53.6 | 53.9 | 51.1 | 5.9 | 6.5 | 6.2 | 6.5 | 7.4 |
| 55 | El Salvador | 8.1 | 8.2 | 8 | 8 | 8 | 38.7 | 42.5 | 43.5 | 45.1 | 46.7 | 61.3 | 57.5 | 56.5 | 54.9 | 53.3 | 22.6 | 24.2 | 25.1 | 25 | 24 |

| | Member State | External resources for health as % of total expenditure on health | | | | | Social security expenditure on health as % of general government expenditure on health | | | | | Out-of-pocket expenditure as % of private expenditure on health | | | | | Private prepaid plans as % of private expenditure on health | | | | |
|---|---|---|---|---|---|---|---|---|---|---|---|---|---|---|---|---|---|---|---|---|---|
| | | 1997 | 1998 | 1999 | 2000 | 2001 | 1997 | 1998 | 1999 | 2000 | 2001 | 1997 | 1998 | 1999 | 2000 | 2001 | 1997 | 1998 | 1999 | 2000 | 2001 |
| 1 | Afghanistan | 9.1 | 3.7 | 4.4 | 14.8 | 11.2 | 0 | 0 | 0 | 0 | 0 | 100 | 100 | 100 | 100 | 100 | 0 | 0 | 0 | 0 | 0 |
| 2 | Albania | 9.4 | 7.4 | 5.1 | 7 | 3.4 | 20.6 | 24.2 | 22.5 | 18.5 | 19.3 | 65.1 | 61.2 | 63.3 | 65 | 65.3 | 34.1 | 38 | 36 | 34.3 | 33.9 |
| 3 | Algeria | 0.2 | 0 | 0.1 | 0.1 | 0.1 | 46.9 | 45.2 | 43.5 | 39.9 | 37.4 | 91.9 | 91.6 | 92 | 91.1 | 89.9 | 4.1 | 4.2 | 4 | 4.2 | 5.1 |
| 4 | Andorra | 0 | 0 | 0 | 0 | 0 | 78.6 | 60 | 87.5 | 88.1 | 86.2 | 95.5 | 95.2 | 95.6 | 96.1 | 92.6 | n/a | n/a | n/a | n/a | n/a |
| 5 | Angola | 9.4 | 5.6 | 8.7 | 14.3 | 14.2 | 0 | 0 | 0 | 0 | 0 | 100 | 100 | 100 | 100 | 100 | 0 | 0 | 0 | 0 | 0 |
| 6 | Antigua and Barbuda | 2.4 | 3.4 | 3.2 | 3.1 | 2.9 | n/a | n/a | n/a | n/a | n/a | 100 | 100 | 100 | 100 | 100 | n/a | n/a | n/a | n/a | n/a |
| 7 | Argentina | 0.3 | 0.3 | 0.3 | 0.3 | 0.3 | 61 | 60.2 | 59 | 59.5 | 58.6 | 63.2 | 63.8 | 64 | 63.3 | 62.4 | 33.4 | 32 | 31.9 | 32.6 | 31.1 |
| 8 | Armenia | 4.5 | 5.2 | 2.2 | 2 | 3.7 | 0 | 0 | 0 | 0 | 0 | 100 | 100 | 100 | 100 | 100 | 0 | 0 | 0 | 0 | 0 |
| 9 | Australia | 0 | 0 | 0 | 0 | 0 | 0 | 0 | 0 | 0 | 0 | 53.7 | 57.6 | 59.3 | 60.4 | 59.6 | 27.8 | 24 | 21.3 | 23.4 | 24.2 |
| 10 | Austria | 0 | 0 | 0 | 0 | 0 | 59.8 | 59.8 | 60.6 | 61 | 61.7 | 59.4 | 58.7 | 60.7 | 61.3 | 61.3 | 26.6 | 25.6 | 23.8 | 23.2 | 23.3 |
| 11 | Azerbaijan | 1.5 | 1.7 | 2.5 | 4.7 | 7.7 | 0 | 0 | 0 | 0 | 0 | 100 | 100 | 100 | 90.5 | 97.7 | 0 | 0 | 0 | 0 | 2.3 |
| 12 | Bahamas | 0 | 0 | 0 | 0 | 0.3 | 0 | 0 | 0 | 0 | 0 | 100 | 100 | 100 | 100 | 100 | n/a | n/a | n/a | n/a | n/a |
| 13 | Bahrain | 0 | 0 | 0 | 0 | 0 | 0.4 | 0.4 | 0.4 | 0.4 | 0.3 | 70.7 | 70.1 | 70.1 | 70 | 69.3 | 25.4 | 26.2 | 26 | 26.3 | 27.2 |
| 14 | Bangladesh | 10 | 12.6 | 11.8 | 13.8 | 13.3 | 0 | 0 | 0 | 0 | 0 | 94 | 93 | 93.2 | 93.2 | 93.2 | 0 | 0 | 0 | 0 | 0 |
| 15 | Barbados | 4.9 | 4.5 | 4.2 | 4 | 4.6 | 0 | 0 | 0 | 0 | 0 | 75.8 | 76.3 | 77 | 77.3 | 76.6 | 24.2 | 23.7 | 23 | 22.7 | 23.4 |
| 16 | Belarus | 0.1 | 0 | 0 | 0 | 0 | 19 | 20.8 | 19.9 | 22.8 | 24.8 | 100 | 100 | 100 | 99.6 | 99.7 | 0 | 0 | 0 | 0.4 | 0.3 |
| 17 | Belgium | 0 | 0 | 0 | 0 | 0 | 89.5 | 89.3 | 86.6 | 82.2 | 77.6 | 48.8 | 50.6 | 49.6 | 58.4 | 58.8 | 7.1 | 7.4 | 7.3 | 7.1 | 6.8 |
| 18 | Belize | 5.5 | 3.6 | 3.1 | 2.9 | 6.1 | 0 | 0 | 0 | 0 | 0 | 100 | 100 | 100 | 100 | 100 | 0 | 0 | 0 | 0 | 0 |
| 19 | Benin | 20.9 | 20.1 | 20.4 | 21.3 | 21.5 | 0 | 0 | 0 | 0 | 0 | 99.9 | 99.9 | 99.9 | 99.9 | 99.9 | n/a | n/a | n/a | n/a | n/a |
| 20 | Bhutan | 32.1 | 30.6 | 29.2 | 42 | 38.2 | 0 | 0 | 0 | 0 | 0 | 100 | 100 | 100 | 100 | 100 | 0 | 0 | 0 | 0 | 0 |
| 21 | Bolivia | 6 | 5.2 | 9.6 | 12.1 | 12.2 | 65.3 | 64.8 | 62 | 66.7 | 66.3 | 85.7 | 85.7 | 85.5 | 85.4 | 85.7 | 7.8 | 7.8 | 8.1 | 7.9 | 7.7 |
| 22 | Bosnia and Herzegovina | 15 | 8 | 6.2 | 7.9 | 2.4 | 0 | 0 | 0 | 0 | 0 | 100 | 100 | 100 | 100 | 100 | 0 | 0 | 0 | 0 | 0 |
| 23 | Botswana | 1.8 | 1.4 | 1.4 | 1.3 | 0.4 | 0 | 0 | 0 | 0 | 0 | 26.3 | 28.8 | 30.3 | 30.8 | 35.3 | 24.1 | 23.8 | 22.7 | 20.8 | 20.5 |
| 24 | Brazil | 0.2 | 0.3 | 0.5 | 0.5 | 0.5 | 0 | 0 | 0 | 0 | 0 | 66.9 | 66.9 | 67.1 | 64.9 | 64.1 | 33.1 | 33.1 | 32.9 | 35.1 | 35.9 |
| 25 | Brunei Darussalam | n/a | n/a | n/a | n/a | n/a | 0 | 0 | 0 | 0 | 0 | 100 | 100 | 100 | 100 | 100 | 0 | 0 | 0 | 0 | 0 |
| 26 | Bulgaria | 0.1 | 0 | 0.2 | 2.5 | 2.1 | 9.3 | 14.3 | 9.3 | 11.8 | 36.7 | 100 | 100 | 100 | 100 | 98 | 0 | 0 | 0 | 0 | 0 |
| 27 | Burkina Faso | 32.5 | 24.7 | 26.4 | 23.9 | 25.6 | 0 | 0 | 0 | 0 | 0 | 99.6 | 97.3 | 97.4 | 97.4 | 97.4 | n/a | n/a | n/a | n/a | n/a |
| 28 | Burundi | 30.5 | 35.2 | 39.6 | 40.4 | 43.7 | 0 | 0 | 0 | 0 | 0 | 100 | 100 | 100 | 100 | 100 | 0 | 0 | 0 | 0 | 0 |
| 29 | Cambodia | 13.5 | 12 | 13.4 | 18.8 | 19.7 | 0 | 0 | 0 | 0 | 0 | 89.9 | 90.2 | 90.1 | 85.4 | 84.6 | 0 | 0 | 0 | 0 | 0 |
| 30 | Cameroon | 5.9 | 6 | 6.1 | 5.7 | 6.3 | 0 | 0 | 0 | 0 | 0 | 87 | 85.5 | 84.1 | 81.9 | 81.6 | n/a | n/a | n/a | n/a | n/a |
| 31 | Canada | 0 | 0 | 0 | 0 | 0 | 1.8 | 1.8 | 1.9 | 2 | 2 | 56 | 55.2 | 55.3 | 54.3 | 52.3 | 36.5 | 38.4 | 37.6 | 39.1 | 39.3 |
| 32 | Cape Verde | 10.5 | 11.6 | 5.6 | 7 | 16.6 | 40.3 | 34.9 | 39.7 | 34.2 | 35.7 | 100 | 100 | 100 | 100 | 100 | n/a | n/a | n/a | n/a | n/a |
| 33 | Central African Republic | 14.7 | 25.4 | 28.4 | 30.8 | 32.4 | 0 | 0 | 0 | 0 | 0 | 95.2 | 95.3 | 95.1 | 95.5 | 95.4 | 0 | 0 | 0 | 0 | 0 |
| 34 | Chad | 66.9 | 58.7 | 65.2 | 59.7 | 62.9 | 0 | 0 | 0 | 0 | 0 | 80.4 | 80.6 | 82 | 81.6 | 80.9 | n/a | n/a | n/a | n/a | n/a |
| 35 | Chile | 0.2 | 0.1 | 0.1 | 0.1 | 0.1 | 83.6 | 75.7 | 77.3 | 71.8 | 71.8 | 66.2 | 66.2 | 65.5 | 59.7 | 59.6 | 33.7 | 33.7 | 34.5 | 40.2 | 40.3 |
| 36 | China | 0.3 | 0.2 | 0.3 | 0.2 | 0.2 | 58 | 53 | 51.4 | 50.7 | 50.7 | 94.2 | 94 | 94.9 | 95.2 | 95.4 | 0.4 | 0.6 | 0.4 | 0.4 | 0.4 |
| 37 | Colombia | 0.3 | 0.5 | 0.5 | 0.4 | 0.2 | 16.7 | 22.8 | 20.2 | 19.6 | 25 | 85 | 76.2 | 73.2 | 65.1 | 65.2 | 15 | 23.8 | 26.8 | 34.8 | 34.8 |
| 38 | Comoros | 58.5 | 44 | 44.5 | 42.9 | 39.9 | 0 | 0 | 0 | 0 | 0 | 100 | 100 | 100 | 100 | 100 | 0 | 0 | 0 | 0 | 0 |
| 39 | Congo | 3.1 | 3.6 | 4.7 | 4 | 3.3 | 0 | 0 | 0 | 0 | 0 | 100 | 100 | 100 | 100 | 100 | n/a | n/a | n/a | n/a | n/a |
| 40 | Cook Islands | 0.2 | 33.4 | 26.8 | 25.4 | 23.2 | 0 | 0 | 0 | 0 | 0 | 100 | 100 | 100 | 100 | 100 | 0 | 0 | 0 | 0 | 0 |
| 41 | Costa Rica | 1.7 | 1.7 | 1.6 | 1.3 | 1.3 | 88.1 | 89.8 | 89.6 | 90.2 | 90.8 | 90.1 | 91.5 | 91.6 | 91.8 | 92.1 | 2.1 | 1.8 | 1.6 | 1.6 | 1.5 |
| 42 | Côte d'Ivoire | 2.6 | 3.1 | 6 | 2.1 | 3.2 | 0 | 0 | 0 | 0 | 0 | 87 | 88.1 | 88.1 | 89.2 | 89.7 | 13 | 11.9 | 11.9 | 10.8 | 10.3 |
| 43 | Croatia | 0.2 | 0.2 | 0.4 | 0.3 | 0.1 | 86.6 | 91.7 | 97.9 | 97.8 | 94.9 | 100 | 100 | 100 | 100 | 100 | 0 | 0 | 0 | 0 | 0 |
| 44 | Cuba | 0.1 | 0.1 | 0.2 | 0.2 | 0.2 | 0 | 0 | 0 | 0 | 0 | 72.8 | 78.5 | 76 | 75.6 | 76.8 | 0 | 0 | 0 | 0 | 0 |
| 45 | Cyprus | 0 | 0 | 0 | 0 | 2.3 | 44.7 | 44.6 | 47.3 | 48.1 | 48.2 | 98.2 | 98.8 | 98.4 | 97.9 | 98 | 1.8 | 1.2 | 1.6 | 2.1 | 2 |
| 46 | Czech Republic | 0 | 0 | 0 | 0 | 0 | 89.5 | 90.2 | 89.4 | 89.4 | 86.1 | 100 | 100 | 100 | 100 | 100 | 0 | 0 | 0 | 0 | 0 |
| 47 | Democratic People's Republic of Korea | n/a | 0.2 | 0.2 | 0.3 | 0.3 | 0 | 0 | 0 | 0 | 0 | 100 | 100 | 100 | 100 | 100 | 0 | 0 | 0 | 0 | 0 |
| 48 | Democratic Republic of the Congo | 11 | 12.6 | 5.7 | 6.6 | 18 | 0 | 0 | 0 | 0 | 0 | 100 | 100 | 100 | 100 | 100 | 0 | 0 | 0 | 0 | 0 |
| 49 | Denmark | 0 | 0 | 0 | 0 | 0 | 0 | 0 | 0 | 0 | 0 | 92.1 | 92 | 90.4 | 90.9 | 90.8 | 7.9 | 8 | 9.6 | 9.1 | 9.2 |
| 50 | Djibouti | 29.3 | 29.2 | 29.4 | 29.5 | 30 | 0 | 0 | 0 | 0 | 0 | 53.7 | 54.5 | 54.1 | 53.9 | 55.2 | 0 | 0 | 0 | 0 | 0 |
| 51 | Dominica | 3.2 | 2.3 | 2.1 | 1.3 | 0.9 | 0 | 0 | 0 | 0 | 0 | 100 | 100 | 100 | 100 | 100 | 0 | 0 | 0 | 0 | 0 |
| 52 | Dominican Republic | 1.5 | 3.2 | 3.2 | 2.5 | 1.8 | 26.8 | 21.4 | 20.3 | 22.4 | 22.6 | 88.6 | 88.4 | 88.4 | 88.4 | 88.4 | 0.1 | 0.4 | 0.4 | 0.4 | 0.4 |
| 53 | Ecuador | 2.1 | 1.8 | 3.2 | 3.2 | 1.9 | 32.8 | 36 | 37.9 | 38.7 | 45.3 | 74.3 | 74.3 | 71.6 | 72.7 | 73.8 | 7.8 | 7.8 | 9.4 | 8.3 | 9.5 |
| 54 | Egypt | 1.9 | 2.1 | 1.8 | 1.8 | 2 | 28 | 28.4 | 29.5 | 29.5 | 29.7 | 91.5 | 91.6 | 91.9 | 92 | 92.2 | 0.5 | 0.6 | 0.5 | 0.5 | 0.5 |
| 55 | El Salvador | 3.4 | 2.9 | 1.5 | 0.9 | 0.9 | 43.3 | 41.7 | 44 | 44.2 | 44.5 | 95.4 | 94 | 90.2 | 95.6 | 94.9 | 4.4 | 5.8 | 9.6 | 4.2 | 4.9 |

## Annex Table 5 Selected national health accounts indicators: measured levels of expenditure on health, 1997–2001

Figures computed by WHO to assure comparability;[a] they are not necessarily the official statistics of Member States, which may use alternative rigorous methods.

| | Member State | Total expenditure on health as % of GDP | | | | | General government expenditure on health as % of total expenditure on health | | | | | Private expenditure on health as % of total expenditure on health | | | | | General government expenditure on health as % of total government expenditure | | | | |
|---|---|---|---|---|---|---|---|---|---|---|---|---|---|---|---|---|---|---|---|---|---|
| | | 1997 | 1998 | 1999 | 2000 | 2001 | 1997 | 1998 | 1999 | 2000 | 2001 | 1997 | 1998 | 1999 | 2000 | 2001 | 1997 | 1998 | 1999 | 2000 | 2001 |
| 56 | Equatorial Guinea | 3 | 4.1 | 2.8 | 2.1 | 2 | 63.1 | 62 | 61.9 | 62.5 | 60.4 | 36.9 | 38 | 38.1 | 37.5 | 39.6 | 10.4 | 8.3 | 9.9 | 10 | 10 |
| 57 | Eritrea | 4.4 | 5 | 5.4 | 5.6 | 5.7 | 65.8 | 66.1 | 67.6 | 67.2 | 65.1 | 34.2 | 33.9 | 32.4 | 32.8 | 34.9 | 5.3 | 4.5 | 4.5 | 4.5 | 4.5 |
| 58 | Estonia | 5.5 | 6 | 6.5 | 5.9 | 5.5 | 86.7 | 86.4 | 80.4 | 76.8 | 77.8 | 13.3 | 13.6 | 19.6 | 23.2 | 22.2 | 12.6 | 13.4 | 12.7 | 12.4 | 12.1 |
| 59 | Ethiopia | 3.4 | 3.6 | 3.5 | 3.2 | 3.6 | 37.9 | 39.3 | 37.7 | 34.5 | 40.5 | 62.1 | 60.7 | 62.3 | 65.5 | 59.5 | 5.8 | 5.9 | 4.3 | 3.2 | 4.9 |
| 60 | Fiji | 3.9 | 4.1 | 3.7 | 3.9 | 4 | 66.7 | 65.4 | 65.2 | 65.2 | 67.1 | 33.3 | 34.6 | 34.8 | 34.8 | 32.9 | 7.4 | 6.9 | 7.5 | 7.2 | 6.9 |
| 61 | Finland | 7.3 | 6.9 | 6.9 | 6.6 | 7 | 76.1 | 76.3 | 75.3 | 75.1 | 75.6 | 23.9 | 23.7 | 24.7 | 24.9 | 24.4 | 9.8 | 10 | 10 | 10.3 | 10.7 |
| 62 | France | 9.4 | 9.3 | 9.3 | 9.4 | 9.6 | 76.2 | 76 | 76 | 75.8 | 76 | 23.8 | 24 | 24 | 24.2 | 24 | 13 | 13.1 | 13.2 | 13.4 | 13.7 |
| 63 | Gabon | 2.9 | 3.7 | 3.5 | 3.3 | 3.6 | 65.6 | 66.8 | 64.9 | 50.2 | 47.9 | 34.4 | 33.2 | 35.1 | 49.8 | 52.1 | 5.9 | 7.4 | 7.5 | 7.2 | 7.3 |
| 64 | Gambia | 6.1 | 7.1 | 6.7 | 6.3 | 6.4 | 47.2 | 42.9 | 46.9 | 46.8 | 49.4 | 52.8 | 57.1 | 53.1 | 53.2 | 50.6 | 11.3 | 13.2 | 13.8 | 13.3 | 13.6 |
| 65 | Georgia | 2.9 | 2.4 | 2.5 | 3.4 | 3.6 | 39.9 | 45.4 | 37.6 | 33.5 | 37.8 | 60.1 | 54.6 | 62.4 | 66.5 | 62.2 | 5.3 | 5.1 | 4.3 | 5.9 | 6.7 |
| 66 | Germany | 10.7 | 10.6 | 10.7 | 10.6 | 10.8 | 75.3 | 74.8 | 74.8 | 75 | 74.9 | 24.7 | 25.2 | 25.2 | 25 | 25.1 | 16.3 | 16.3 | 16.3 | 17.3 | 16.6 |
| 67 | Ghana | 4.1 | 4.3 | 4.2 | 4.3 | 4.7 | 47.6 | 53.8 | 53.9 | 55.9 | 59.6 | 52.4 | 46.2 | 46.1 | 44.1 | 40.4 | 9.4 | 9 | 9.2 | 8.1 | 8.6 |
| 68 | Greece | 9.4 | 9.4 | 9.6 | 9.4 | 9.4 | 52.8 | 52.1 | 53.4 | 56.1 | 56 | 47.2 | 47.9 | 46.6 | 43.9 | 44 | 10.8 | 10.5 | 11 | 10.8 | 11.2 |
| 69 | Grenada | 4.7 | 4.8 | 4.8 | 4.9 | 5.3 | 66.1 | 65.8 | 69.7 | 70.1 | 71.9 | 33.9 | 34.2 | 30.3 | 29.9 | 28.1 | 10.6 | 11.3 | 12.3 | 12.3 | 12.4 |
| 70 | Guatemala | 3.8 | 4.4 | 4.7 | 4.7 | 4.8 | 37.2 | 47.4 | 48.3 | 47.6 | 48.3 | 62.8 | 52.6 | 51.7 | 52.4 | 51.7 | 11.3 | 14 | 15.5 | 16.3 | 15.7 |
| 71 | Guinea | 3.6 | 3.3 | 3.6 | 3.4 | 3.5 | 56.3 | 51.4 | 55.3 | 53.4 | 54.1 | 43.7 | 48.6 | 44.7 | 46.6 | 45.9 | 9.3 | 9.6 | 9.4 | 10.9 | 11.3 |
| 72 | Guinea-Bissau | 5.4 | 5.5 | 5.9 | 6.1 | 5.9 | 43.2 | 44.5 | 48.5 | 55.3 | 53.8 | 56.8 | 55.5 | 51.5 | 44.7 | 46.2 | 7.3 | 9.8 | 9.1 | 7.7 | 7.4 |
| 73 | Guyana | 4.8 | 5 | 4.8 | 5.1 | 5.3 | 83.5 | 83.4 | 84 | 82.7 | 79.9 | 16.5 | 16.6 | 16 | 17.3 | 20.1 | 9.3 | 9.3 | 9.1 | 9.3 | 9.3 |
| 74 | Haiti | 4.9 | 5.1 | 4.9 | 4.8 | 5 | 51.7 | 49.9 | 51 | 50.7 | 53.4 | 48.3 | 50.1 | 49 | 49.3 | 46.6 | 12 | 11.7 | 11 | 12.3 | 14.1 |
| 75 | Honduras | 5.4 | 5.6 | 5.6 | 6 | 6.1 | 53 | 53.8 | 51.8 | 53.5 | 53.1 | 47 | 46.2 | 48.2 | 46.5 | 46.9 | 13.7 | 14.6 | 13.7 | 13.6 | 13.8 |
| 76 | Hungary | 7 | 6.9 | 6.8 | 6.7 | 6.8 | 81.3 | 79.4 | 78.1 | 75.5 | 75 | 18.7 | 20.6 | 21.9 | 24.5 | 25 | 11.4 | 10.1 | 11.4 | 11.7 | 11.5 |
| 77 | Iceland | 8.2 | 8.6 | 9.5 | 9.3 | 9.2 | 83.1 | 83 | 84 | 83.7 | 82.9 | 16.9 | 17 | 16 | 16.3 | 17.1 | 16.3 | 16.8 | 18.3 | 18 | 17.5 |
| 78 | India | 5.3 | 5 | 5.2 | 5.1 | 5.1 | 15.7 | 18.4 | 17.9 | 17.6 | 17.9 | 84.3 | 81.6 | 82.1 | 82.4 | 82.1 | 3.2 | 3.5 | 3.3 | 3.1 | 3.1 |
| 79 | Indonesia | 2.4 | 2.5 | 2.6 | 2.7 | 2.4 | 23.7 | 27.2 | 28 | 23.7 | 25.1 | 76.3 | 72.8 | 72 | 76.3 | 74.9 | 2.8 | 3.2 | 3.6 | 3.2 | 3 |
| 80 | Iran, Islamic Republic of | 5.9 | 6 | 6.5 | 6.4 | 6.3 | 45 | 43.9 | 41.9 | 41.5 | 43.5 | 55 | 56.1 | 58.1 | 58.5 | 56.5 | 10.5 | 10.8 | 11.2 | 11.8 | 12 |
| 81 | Iraq | 3.4 | 3.3 | 3.3 | 3.3 | 3.2 | 32.7 | 31.7 | 31 | 31.2 | 31.8 | 67.3 | 68.3 | 69 | 68.8 | 68.2 | 4.2 | 4.3 | 4.5 | 4.5 | 4.6 |
| 82 | Ireland | 6.4 | 6.2 | 6.2 | 6.4 | 6.5 | 74.6 | 76.5 | 72.8 | 73.3 | 76 | 25.4 | 23.5 | 27.2 | 26.7 | 24 | 12.9 | 13.6 | 13.1 | 14.6 | 14 |
| 83 | Israel | 8.1 | 8.1 | 8.2 | 8.2 | 8.7 | 74 | 72 | 71 | 69.8 | 69.2 | 26 | 28 | 29 | 30.2 | 30.8 | 12.1 | 11.4 | 11.8 | 12.1 | 11.5 |
| 84 | Italy | 7.7 | 7.7 | 7.8 | 8.2 | 8.4 | 72.2 | 71.8 | 72 | 73.4 | 75.3 | 27.8 | 28.2 | 28 | 26.6 | 24.7 | 10.9 | 11.1 | 11.5 | 12.8 | 13 |
| 85 | Jamaica | 6.5 | 6.5 | 6.1 | 6.2 | 6.8 | 56.2 | 59.5 | 50.9 | 47 | 42.1 | 43.8 | 40.5 | 49.1 | 53 | 57.9 | 7.7 | 7.7 | 5.9 | 5.3 | 4.4 |
| 86 | Japan | 6.8 | 7.1 | 7.5 | 7.7 | 8 | 77.2 | 77.4 | 78.1 | 77.7 | 77.9 | 22.8 | 22.6 | 21.9 | 22.3 | 22.1 | 14.9 | 13.2 | 15.3 | 15.5 | 16.4 |
| 87 | Jordan | 8.2 | 8.1 | 8.6 | 9.2 | 9.5 | 54.5 | 57 | 50.8 | 46.5 | 47 | 45.5 | 43 | 49.2 | 53.5 | 53 | 11.7 | 12.4 | 12.4 | 12.5 | 12.8 |
| 88 | Kazakhstan | 3.2 | 3.5 | 3.5 | 3.3 | 3.1 | 72.9 | 70 | 63.5 | 62.9 | 60.4 | 27.1 | 30 | 36.5 | 37.1 | 39.6 | 8.9 | 9.4 | 9.6 | 9 | 8 |
| 89 | Kenya | 8 | 8.4 | 7.9 | 8.7 | 7.8 | 21.7 | 24.1 | 18.7 | 23.8 | 21.4 | 78.3 | 75.9 | 81.3 | 76.2 | 78.6 | 6.1 | 7.2 | 5.1 | 8.6 | 6.2 |
| 90 | Kiribati | 8.7 | 8.3 | 7.8 | 8.3 | 8.6 | 99.1 | 99 | 98.9 | 98.8 | 98.8 | 0.9 | 1 | 1.1 | 1.2 | 1.2 | 11.2 | 10.9 | 9.7 | 10 | 9.3 |
| 91 | Kuwait | 3.7 | 4.4 | 3.9 | 3.5 | 3.9 | 79.5 | 78.8 | 78.7 | 78.7 | 78.8 | 20.5 | 21.2 | 21.3 | 21.3 | 21.2 | 8.4 | 8 | 8.2 | 8.9 | 8.1 |
| 92 | Kyrgyzstan | 5.7 | 5.6 | 5 | 4.2 | 4 | 48.4 | 49.5 | 48.3 | 48.3 | 48.7 | 51.6 | 50.5 | 51.7 | 51.7 | 51.3 | 10.5 | 10.1 | 10.2 | 9.5 | 9 |
| 93 | Lao People's Democratic Republic | 2.9 | 2.5 | 3 | 2.9 | 3.1 | 62.1 | 48.6 | 49.4 | 53.3 | 55.5 | 37.9 | 51.4 | 50.6 | 46.7 | 44.5 | 9.8 | 5.7 | 8.8 | 7.6 | 8.7 |
| 94 | Latvia | 6.8 | 6.8 | 6.9 | 6.3 | 6.4 | 56.8 | 60.7 | 59.7 | 55.8 | 52.5 | 43.2 | 39.3 | 40.3 | 44.2 | 47.5 | 10.1 | 10.6 | 10 | 8.8 | 9.1 |
| 95 | Lebanon | 11.8 | 12.4 | 12.1 | 12.6 | 12.2 | 31.1 | 27.2 | 26.7 | 29.3 | 28.1 | 68.9 | 72.8 | 73.3 | 70.7 | 71.9 | 8.6 | 9.8 | 9 | 8 | 9.5 |
| 96 | Lesotho | 5.3 | 5.9 | 6.1 | 6.1 | 5.5 | 76 | 78.3 | 80.9 | 80.8 | 78.9 | 24 | 21.7 | 19.1 | 19.2 | 21.1 | 12.4 | 11.5 | 11.9 | 12 | 12 |
| 97 | Liberia | 3.2 | 3.5 | 4 | 4.2 | 4.3 | 69.1 | 73.4 | 76.5 | 76.2 | 75.9 | 30.9 | 26.6 | 23.5 | 23.8 | 24.1 | 9.3 | 10.1 | 10.8 | 10.7 | 10.6 |
| 98 | Libyan Arab Jamahiriya | 3.4 | 3.7 | 3.5 | 2.8 | 2.9 | 47.9 | 49.6 | 49.1 | 51.5 | 56 | 52.1 | 50.4 | 50.9 | 48.5 | 44 | 6.2 | 5.3 | 5.6 | 4.9 | 5 |
| 99 | Lithuania | 6 | 6.4 | 6.3 | 6.2 | 6 | 76.2 | 75.1 | 73.5 | 70.7 | 70.5 | 23.8 | 24.9 | 26.5 | 29.3 | 29.5 | 13.6 | 14.8 | 11.7 | 13.9 | 14 |
| 100 | Luxembourg | 6 | 5.9 | 6 | 5.5 | 6 | 91.1 | 90.9 | 89.4 | 89.3 | 89.9 | 8.9 | 9.1 | 10.6 | 10.7 | 10.1 | 12.5 | 12.7 | 12.9 | 12.3 | 13.3 |
| 101 | Madagascar | 1.8 | 2.7 | 2.5 | 2.4 | 2 | 78.4 | 64.4 | 58.5 | 64.8 | 65.9 | 21.6 | 35.6 | 41.5 | 35.2 | 34.1 | 9 | 10.3 | 8.4 | 9.2 | 7.7 |
| 102 | Malawi | 8.7 | 8.5 | 8.7 | 8.2 | 7.8 | 35.6 | 35.5 | 37.8 | 36.9 | 35 | 64.4 | 64.5 | 62.2 | 63.1 | 65 | 12.2 | 12.9 | 13.9 | 12.2 | 12.3 |
| 103 | Malaysia | 2.8 | 3 | 3.1 | 3.3 | 3.8 | 53.5 | 51.6 | 52.9 | 53.1 | 53.7 | 46.5 | 48.4 | 47.1 | 46.9 | 46.3 | 6.1 | 5.1 | 6 | 6.1 | 6.5 |
| 104 | Maldives | 6.5 | 6.4 | 6.8 | 6.9 | 6.7 | 81.9 | 81.8 | 82.5 | 84 | 83.5 | 18.1 | 18.2 | 17.5 | 16 | 16.5 | 10.9 | 10.1 | 10.4 | 10.9 | 10.3 |
| 105 | Mali | 4.2 | 4.2 | 4.1 | 4.7 | 4.3 | 43.3 | 37.5 | 32.6 | 38.9 | 38.6 | 56.7 | 62.5 | 67.4 | 61.1 | 61.4 | 8.2 | 7 | 5.7 | 7.8 | 6.8 |
| 106 | Malta | 8.6 | 8.4 | 8.3 | 8.8 | 8.8 | 67.9 | 69.3 | 67.5 | 68.5 | 68.5 | 32.1 | 30.7 | 32.5 | 31.5 | 31.5 | 11.7 | 11.9 | 11.8 | 13.2 | 12.8 |
| 107 | Marshall Islands | 9.9 | 9.7 | 9.5 | 9.8 | 9.8 | 70.5 | 66.4 | 65.2 | 65 | 64.7 | 29.5 | 33.6 | 34.8 | 35 | 35.3 | 10.7 | 10.9 | 10.8 | 9.6 | 9.6 |
| 108 | Mauritania | 3.4 | 3.6 | 3.6 | 3.7 | 3.6 | 74.5 | 71.1 | 71.9 | 73.5 | 72.4 | 25.5 | 28.9 | 28.1 | 26.5 | 27.6 | 10.2 | 10.1 | 10.5 | 11 | 10.3 |
| 109 | Mauritius | 3 | 3.2 | 3.1 | 3.3 | 3.4 | 61.2 | 62.6 | 62 | 58.7 | 59.5 | 38.8 | 37.4 | 38 | 41.3 | 40.5 | 6.8 | 7 | 7.2 | 6.6 | 7.6 |
| 110 | Mexico | 5.5 | 5.6 | 5.7 | 5.7 | 6.1 | 45.3 | 46.6 | 46.9 | 45.7 | 44.3 | 54.7 | 53.4 | 53.1 | 54.3 | 55.7 | 15 | 16.8 | 17.2 | 16.6 | 16.7 |

| | Member State | External resources for health as % of total expenditure on health | | | | | Social security expenditure on health as % of general government expenditure on health | | | | | Out-of-pocket expenditure as % of private expenditure on health | | | | | Private prepaid plans as % of private expenditure on health | | | | |
|---|---|---|---|---|---|---|---|---|---|---|---|---|---|---|---|---|---|---|---|---|---|
| | | 1997 | 1998 | 1999 | 2000 | 2001 | 1997 | 1998 | 1999 | 2000 | 2001 | 1997 | 1998 | 1999 | 2000 | 2001 | 1997 | 1998 | 1999 | 2000 | 2001 |
| 56 | Equatorial Guinea | 23.6 | 29.2 | 14.9 | 17.2 | 10.6 | 0 | 0 | 0 | 0 | 0 | 95.1 | 95.1 | 89.3 | 70.5 | 52.3 | 0 | 0 | 0 | 0 | 0 |
| 57 | Eritrea | 48.1 | 41.5 | 49.8 | 51.1 | 52.3 | 0 | 0 | 0 | 0 | 0 | 100 | 100 | 100 | 100 | 100 | 0 | 0 | 0 | 0 | 0 |
| 58 | Estonia | 1.7 | 1.5 | 3.5 | 0.9 | 0 | 84.6 | 77.1 | 82 | 85.9 | 86 | 97.9 | 96.6 | 71.3 | 84.9 | 84.7 | 0 | 0 | 4.1 | 4.1 | 4.8 |
| 59 | Ethiopia | 9.3 | 23.5 | 27.6 | 29.6 | 34.3 | 0.7 | 0.7 | 0.8 | 1 | 0.8 | 86.2 | 85.7 | 85.4 | 84.6 | 84.7 | 0 | 0 | 0 | 0 | 0 |
| 60 | Fiji | 4.2 | 7.7 | 11.1 | 10.9 | 10.1 | 0 | 0 | 0 | 0 | 0 | 100 | 100 | 100 | 100 | 100 | 0 | 0 | 0 | 0 | 0 |
| 61 | Finland | 0 | 0 | 0 | 0 | 0 | 18.7 | 19.4 | 19.8 | 20.5 | 20.8 | 82.4 | 81.9 | 82.2 | 81.9 | 82.7 | 11 | 11.1 | 10.8 | 10.5 | 8.3 |
| 62 | France | 0 | 0 | 0 | 0 | 0 | 96.8 | 96.8 | 96.7 | 96.7 | 96.5 | 43.5 | 43.1 | 43 | 43.1 | 42.6 | 52.2 | 52.6 | 52.6 | 52.6 | 53.1 |
| 63 | Gabon | 3.7 | 4 | 4.6 | 1.3 | 1.8 | 0 | 0 | 0 | 0 | 0 | 100 | 100 | 100 | 100 | 100 | 0 | 0 | 0 | 0 | 0 |
| 64 | Gambia | 29.4 | 25 | 28.2 | 26.1 | 26.6 | 0 | 0 | 0 | 0 | 0 | 89.2 | 86.3 | 88.6 | 88.9 | 90 | 0 | 0 | 0 | 0 | 0 |
| 65 | Georgia | 5.4 | 7.1 | 7.3 | 3.1 | 5.1 | 54.3 | 39.3 | 54.4 | 47.9 | 41.5 | 99.7 | 99.5 | 99.5 | 99.7 | 99.7 | 0.3 | 0.5 | 0.5 | 0.3 | 0.3 |
| 66 | Germany | 0 | 0 | 0 | 0 | 0 | 90.7 | 91.4 | 91.5 | 91.6 | 91.8 | 43.9 | 44.5 | 43.2 | 42.2 | 42.4 | 32 | 31.7 | 32.5 | 33.3 | 33.5 |
| 67 | Ghana | 6.8 | 8.2 | 8.6 | 13.2 | 23.2 | 0 | 0 | 0 | 0 | 0 | 100 | 100 | 100 | 100 | 100 | 0 | 0 | 0 | 0 | 0 |
| 68 | Greece | 0 | 0 | 0 | 0 | 0 | 26.9 | 37.5 | 35.4 | 31.9 | 35 | 72.1 | 71 | 69.5 | 74.5 | 73.9 | 4.3 | 4.2 | 4.1 | 4.4 | 4.4 |
| 69 | Grenada | 1 | 0.9 | 0 | 0 | 0 | 0 | 0 | 0 | 0 | 0 | 100 | 100 | 100 | 100 | 100 | 0 | 0 | 0 | 0 | 0 |
| 70 | Guatemala | 3.2 | 5.4 | 5.3 | 4.6 | 1.4 | 49 | 55.3 | 54.8 | 57.1 | 54.1 | 92.2 | 93.2 | 85.6 | 86.2 | 85.7 | 3.8 | 4.5 | 5.4 | 5.2 | 5.3 |
| 71 | Guinea | 14 | 14 | 14.3 | 19.1 | 20.5 | 0 | 0 | 0 | 0 | 0 | 100 | 100 | 100 | 100 | 100 | 0 | 0 | 0 | 0 | 0 |
| 72 | Guinea-Bissau | 22 | 29.4 | 30 | 39.8 | 38.6 | 0.2 | 0.2 | 0.2 | 0.1 | 0.1 | 100 | 100 | 100 | 100 | 100 | 0 | 0 | 0 | 0 | 0 |
| 73 | Guyana | 4.7 | 3.6 | 4 | 3.1 | 2.2 | 0 | 0 | 0 | 0 | 0 | 100 | 100 | 100 | 100 | 100 | 0 | 0 | 0 | 0 | 0 |
| 74 | Haiti | 36.5 | 36.6 | 38.3 | 39.2 | 42.9 | 0 | 0 | 0 | 0 | 0 | 43.2 | 40.2 | 43.3 | 43.3 | 45.3 | n/a | n/a | n/a | n/a | n/a |
| 75 | Honduras | 12.1 | 10.4 | 10.1 | 8.7 | 7.5 | 16.7 | 15.4 | 16.6 | 16.5 | 17.3 | 89.3 | 89 | 89.1 | 88.9 | 88.9 | 7.5 | 7.5 | 7.5 | 7.6 | 7.5 |
| 76 | Hungary | 0 | 0 | 0 | 0 | 0 | 82.8 | 83.4 | 83.8 | 83.9 | 83.2 | n/a | 84.9 | 86.3 | 87 | 85.5 | n/a | 0.2 | 0.5 | 0.8 | 1.3 |
| 77 | Iceland | 0 | 0 | 0 | 0 | 0 | 31.5 | 29.8 | 27.7 | 29.6 | 28.1 | 100 | 100 | 100 | 100 | 100 | 0 | 0 | 0 | 0 | 0 |
| 78 | India | 2.3 | 2.4 | 2.2 | 2.2 | 0.4 | n/a | n/a | n/a | n/a | n/a | 100 | 100 | 100 | 100 | 100 | n/a | n/a | n/a | n/a | n/a |
| 79 | Indonesia | 2.9 | 6.4 | 9.5 | 8.3 | 6.5 | 14.1 | 9 | 7.3 | 7.5 | 7.5 | 95.7 | 93.3 | 89.6 | 91.8 | 91.8 | 4.3 | 6.7 | 10.4 | 8.2 | 8.2 |
| 80 | Iran, Islamic Republic of | 0 | 0 | 0 | 0.1 | 0.1 | 38.8 | 40.8 | 41 | 40.6 | 40.8 | 94.5 | 93.7 | 94.4 | 94.8 | 94.2 | 2.5 | 3 | 2.5 | 2.3 | 2.6 |
| 81 | Iraq | 0 | 0 | 0.1 | 0 | 0.1 | 0 | 0 | 0 | 0 | 0 | 100 | 100 | 100 | 100 | 100 | 0 | 0 | 0 | 0 | 0 |
| 82 | Ireland | 0 | 0 | 0 | 0 | 0 | 1.1 | 1.1 | 1.1 | 1.2 | 1 | 53.1 | 45.6 | 51.4 | 50.5 | 55.2 | 34.1 | 38.1 | 29.3 | 28.4 | 28.4 |
| 83 | Israel | 0 | 0 | 0.3 | 0.4 | 0.1 | 33.1 | 34.3 | 34.9 | 36.4 | 37.1 | 100 | 100 | 100 | 100 | 100 | 0 | 0 | 0 | 0 | 0 |
| 84 | Italy | 0 | 0 | 0 | 0 | 0 | 0.4 | 0.1 | 0.1 | 0.1 | 0.3 | 86.7 | 86.9 | 85.6 | 84.9 | 82.1 | 3.6 | 3.3 | 3.4 | 3.3 | 3.6 |
| 85 | Jamaica | 2.3 | 2.5 | 2.5 | 2 | 3 | 0 | 0 | 0 | 0 | 0 | 69.4 | 66.7 | 70.3 | 65.6 | 73.4 | 25 | 27.2 | 24.3 | 29.5 | 22.5 |
| 86 | Japan | 0 | 0 | 0 | 0 | 0 | 87.1 | 84.5 | 84 | 83.5 | 83.6 | 74.8 | 78.2 | 77.8 | 74.5 | 74.9 | 2.5 | 2.6 | 2.6 | 2.8 | 1.4 |
| 87 | Jordan | 1.5 | 4.1 | 3.5 | 4.5 | 4.4 | 0.7 | 0.6 | 0.8 | 0.8 | 0.7 | 78.5 | 77.9 | 75.8 | 74.1 | 73.9 | 5.8 | 5.9 | 5.7 | 5.6 | 7.4 |
| 88 | Kazakhstan | 0.5 | 0.4 | 3.5 | 4 | 3.5 | 0 | 0 | 0 | 0 | 0 | 100 | 100 | 100 | 100 | 100 | 0 | 0 | 0 | 0 | 0 |
| 89 | Kenya | 7.3 | 7.9 | 9.6 | 9.7 | 9.8 | 0 | 0 | 0 | 0 | 0 | 70 | 70.7 | 68.5 | 69.6 | 67.6 | 7.3 | 6.6 | 9.1 | 8.7 | 9.5 |
| 90 | Kiribati | n/a | n/a | n/a | 2.2 | 4.4 | 0 | 0 | 0 | 0 | 0 | 100 | 100 | 100 | 100 | 100 | 0 | 0 | 0 | 0 | 0 |
| 91 | Kuwait | 0 | 0 | 0 | 0 | 0 | 0 | 0 | 0 | 0 | 0 | 100 | 100 | 100 | 100 | 100 | 0 | 0 | 0 | 0 | 0 |
| 92 | Kyrgyzstan | 6 | 7.4 | 12.8 | 17 | 13 | 0.6 | 4.4 | 8.4 | 10.1 | 10.3 | 100 | 100 | 100 | 100 | 100 | 0 | 0 | 0 | 0 | 0 |
| 93 | Lao People's Democratic Republic | 15.8 | 20.4 | 19.5 | 19.7 | 21.1 | n/a | n/a | n/a | n/a | n/a | 80.1 | 80 | 80 | 80 | 80 | n/a | n/a | n/a | n/a | n/a |
| 94 | Latvia | 0 | 0.8 | 0.8 | 0.7 | 0.7 | 49.9 | 49.3 | 50 | 57 | 52.1 | 100 | 100 | 100 | 100 | 99.7 | 0 | 0 | 0 | 0 | 0.3 |
| 95 | Lebanon | 0.6 | 1.9 | 0.7 | 0.2 | 0.2 | 42.3 | 45.6 | 47.7 | 43 | 50.6 | 80.9 | 81 | 81.8 | 81.1 | 81.2 | 16.7 | 16.7 | 15.8 | 16.4 | 16.5 |
| 96 | Lesotho | 5.3 | 3.9 | 3.2 | 4.7 | 6 | 0 | 0 | 0 | 0 | 0 | 100 | 100 | 100 | 100 | 100 | 0 | 0 | 0 | 0 | 0 |
| 97 | Liberia | 59.4 | 65.5 | 66.2 | 61.9 | 57.2 | 0 | 0 | 0 | 0 | 0 | 86.2 | 87.7 | 88.4 | 84 | 84.2 | 0 | 0 | 0 | 0 | 0 |
| 98 | Libyan Arab Jamahiriya | 0 | 0 | 0 | 0 | 0 | 0 | 0 | 0 | 0 | 0 | 100 | 100 | 100 | 100 | 100 | 0 | 0 | 0 | 0 | 0 |
| 99 | Lithuania | 0 | 0 | 1.1 | 1.4 | 1 | 82.7 | 89.9 | 92.2 | 90.7 | 88.3 | 91.9 | 92 | 91.5 | 92.1 | 91.7 | 0 | 0 | 0 | 0 | 0 |
| 100 | Luxembourg | 0 | 0 | 0 | 0 | 0 | 86 | 82.7 | 77 | 82.9 | 77.6 | 81.9 | 82.4 | 73.9 | 73.2 | 74.6 | 18.1 | 17.6 | 13.4 | 13.8 | 14.6 |
| 101 | Madagascar | 35.8 | 28.6 | 36.3 | 38.1 | 36.8 | 0 | 0 | 0 | 0 | 0 | 73.2 | 89.2 | 89.7 | 87.7 | 85 | 26.8 | 10.8 | 10.3 | 12.3 | 15 |
| 102 | Malawi | 22.8 | 20.4 | 22.9 | 32.3 | 26.5 | 0 | 0 | 0 | 0 | 0 | 40.3 | 40.4 | 41.3 | 39.7 | 43.7 | 1.4 | 1.8 | 1.5 | 1.7 | 1.6 |
| 103 | Malaysia | 0.9 | 1.1 | 1 | 0.8 | 0 | 0.8 | 0.9 | 1 | 0.9 | 1.1 | 100 | 94.2 | 93.9 | 93.4 | 92.8 | n/a | 5.8 | 6.1 | 6.6 | 7.2 |
| 104 | Maldives | 4.2 | 3.6 | 2.6 | 2.2 | 1.9 | 0 | 0 | 0 | 0 | 0 | 100 | 100 | 100 | 100 | 100 | 0 | 0 | 0 | 0 | 0 |
| 105 | Mali | 32 | 24.2 | 18.8 | 24.2 | 20.8 | 0 | 0 | 0 | 0 | 0 | 77.5 | 77.6 | 75.6 | 73.5 | 72.4 | 12.4 | 13.2 | 15.3 | 17.8 | 18.7 |
| 106 | Malta | 0 | 0 | 0 | 0 | 0 | 64.5 | 68.9 | 68 | 59.9 | 58.7 | 100 | 100 | 100 | 100 | 100 | 0 | 0 | 0 | 0 | 0 |
| 107 | Marshall Islands | 13.7 | 13.5 | 38.2 | 36.5 | 25.4 | 0 | 0 | 0 | 0 | 0 | 100 | 100 | 100 | 100 | 100 | 0 | 0 | 0 | 0 | 0 |
| 108 | Mauritania | 24.8 | 19.7 | 21.5 | 24.4 | 23.2 | 0 | 0 | 0 | 0 | 0 | 100 | 100 | 100 | 100 | 100 | 0 | 0 | 0 | 0 | 0 |
| 109 | Mauritius | 1.6 | 1.4 | 1.2 | 1.1 | 1.6 | 5.2 | 6.1 | 6.5 | 7.8 | 8.1 | 100 | 100 | 100 | 100 | 100 | 0 | 0 | 0 | 0 | 0 |
| 110 | Mexico | 0.2 | 0.8 | 0.7 | 0.6 | 0.5 | 68.5 | 68.1 | 69.2 | 67.7 | 66.5 | 92.5 | 92.5 | 92.4 | 92.3 | 92.4 | 3.9 | 3.9 | 4.1 | 4.7 | 4.9 |

## Annex Table 5 Selected national health accounts indicators: measured levels of expenditure on health, 1997–2001

Figures computed by WHO to assure comparability;[a] they are not necessarily the official statistics of Member States, which may use alternative rigorous methods.

| | Member State | Total expenditure on health as % of GDP | | | | | General government expenditure on health as % of total expenditure on health | | | | | Private expenditure on health as % of total expenditure on health | | | | | General government expenditure on health as % of total government expenditure | | | | |
|---|---|---|---|---|---|---|---|---|---|---|---|---|---|---|---|---|---|---|---|---|---|
| | | 1997 | 1998 | 1999 | 2000 | 2001 | 1997 | 1998 | 1999 | 2000 | 2001 | 1997 | 1998 | 1999 | 2000 | 2001 | 1997 | 1998 | 1999 | 2000 | 2001 |
| 111 | Micronesia, Federated States of | 8.3 | 8 | 7.9 | 7.9 | 7.8 | 73.7 | 72.6 | 71.8 | 71.8 | 72 | 26.3 | 27.4 | 28.2 | 28.2 | 28 | 9.8 | 7.9 | 7.9 | 8.5 | 8.5 |
| 112 | Monaco | 7 | 7.2 | 7.4 | 7.4 | 7.6 | 54.7 | 53.6 | 52.7 | 54.5 | 56.1 | 45.3 | 46.4 | 47.3 | 45.5 | 43.9 | 15.9 | 16.1 | 16.3 | 16.8 | 17.7 |
| 113 | Mongolia | 5 | 6.2 | 6.1 | 6.3 | 6.4 | 62.7 | 65.4 | 66.5 | 70.3 | 72.3 | 37.3 | 34.6 | 33.5 | 29.7 | 27.7 | 9.1 | 9 | 9.8 | 10.5 | 10.5 |
| 114 | Morocco | 4.3 | 4.4 | 4.4 | 4.7 | 5.1 | 26 | 28.3 | 29.1 | 34 | 39.3 | 74 | 71.7 | 70.9 | 66 | 60.7 | 3.7 | 4 | 3.9 | 4.7 | 5.3 |
| 115 | Mozambique | 5 | 4.9 | 5 | 5.7 | 5.9 | 60.5 | 62 | 64 | 66.6 | 67.4 | 39.5 | 38 | 36 | 33.4 | 32.6 | 15.1 | 15.5 | 16.5 | 18.2 | 18.9 |
| 116 | Myanmar | 2.1 | 2 | 2 | 2 | 2.1 | 14.3 | 10.6 | 11.7 | 17.1 | 17.8 | 85.7 | 89.4 | 88.3 | 82.9 | 82.2 | 2.7 | 2.5 | 3 | 5 | 5.7 |
| 117 | Namibia | 6.8 | 6.8 | 7 | 6.9 | 7 | 72.8 | 72.2 | 73.3 | 68.9 | 67.8 | 27.2 | 27.8 | 26.7 | 31.1 | 32.2 | 13.1 | 13 | 13.1 | 12.4 | 12.4 |
| 118 | Nauru | 7.6 | 7.9 | 7.7 | 7.7 | 7.5 | 89.1 | 89 | 89.1 | 88.9 | 88.7 | 10.9 | 11 | 10.9 | 11.1 | 11.3 | 9.1 | 9.1 | 9.2 | 9.2 | 9.1 |
| 119 | Nepal | 5.4 | 5.5 | 5.3 | 5.2 | 5.2 | 31.3 | 33.3 | 29.8 | 30.1 | 29.7 | 68.7 | 66.7 | 70.2 | 69.9 | 70.3 | 9.3 | 9.9 | 9 | 9 | 8.1 |
| 120 | Netherlands | 8.2 | 8.6 | 8.7 | 8.6 | 8.9 | 67.8 | 64.4 | 63.3 | 63.4 | 63.3 | 32.2 | 35.6 | 36.7 | 36.6 | 36.7 | 11.5 | 11.7 | 11.7 | 12.1 | 12.2 |
| 121 | New Zealand | 7.5 | 7.9 | 8 | 8 | 8.3 | 77.3 | 77 | 77.9 | 78 | 76.8 | 22.7 | 23 | 22.1 | 22 | 23.2 | 12.7 | 13.5 | 14.1 | 14.5 | 14.8 |
| 122 | Nicaragua | 6.2 | 6 | 5.8 | 7.1 | 7.8 | 53.8 | 60.3 | 54 | 52.5 | 48.5 | 46.2 | 39.7 | 46 | 47.5 | 51.5 | 18.7 | 20.2 | 13.8 | 17 | 17.9 |
| 123 | Niger | 3.4 | 3.3 | 3.2 | 3.6 | 3.7 | 41.7 | 43 | 43.6 | 43.1 | 39.1 | 58.3 | 57 | 56.4 | 56.9 | 60.9 | 8.9 | 8.3 | 7.8 | 8.6 | 7.7 |
| 124 | Nigeria | 2.8 | 3.1 | 3 | 3 | 3.4 | 11.7 | 15.4 | 16 | 14.1 | 23.2 | 88.3 | 84.6 | 84 | 85.9 | 76.8 | 2.1 | 2.3 | 1.7 | 1.7 | 1.9 |
| 125 | Niue | 7.6 | 7.4 | 7.9 | 8 | 7.7 | 97.1 | 97 | 97 | 97 | 97 | 2.9 | 3 | 3 | 3 | 3 | 13 | 13.9 | 15.3 | 15.4 | 14.8 |
| 126 | Norway | 7.8 | 8.5 | 8.5 | 7.6 | 8 | 84.3 | 84.7 | 85.2 | 85.2 | 85.5 | 15.7 | 15.3 | 14.8 | 14.8 | 14.5 | 14 | 14.5 | 15.1 | 14.9 | 15.2 |
| 127 | Oman | 3.4 | 3.8 | 3.5 | 3 | 3 | 81.9 | 82.3 | 82.2 | 81.1 | 80.7 | 18.1 | 17.7 | 17.8 | 18.9 | 19.3 | 7.4 | 7.6 | 7.7 | 7 | 6.5 |
| 128 | Pakistan | 3.8 | 3.9 | 4 | 4.1 | 3.9 | 27.2 | 29.1 | 25.6 | 24.5 | 24.4 | 72.8 | 70.9 | 74.4 | 75.5 | 75.6 | 3.8 | 4.2 | 3.7 | 3.3 | 3.5 |
| 129 | Palau | 8.5 | 8.9 | 9 | 9 | 9.2 | 91.6 | 92.9 | 91.4 | 91.7 | 92 | 8.4 | 7.1 | 8.6 | 8.3 | 8 | 10.7 | 11.3 | 11.3 | 11.3 | 11.6 |
| 130 | Panama | 7.4 | 7.4 | 7.6 | 7.6 | 7 | 68.3 | 70.2 | 69.9 | 69.2 | 69 | 31.7 | 29.8 | 30.1 | 30.8 | 31 | 18.7 | 18.5 | 18.5 | 18.4 | 18.4 |
| 131 | Papua New Guinea | 3.2 | 3.8 | 4.2 | 4.3 | 4.4 | 89 | 90.9 | 89.9 | 89.7 | 89 | 11 | 9.1 | 10.1 | 10.3 | 11 | 9.6 | 12.3 | 13.3 | 12.9 | 13 |
| 132 | Paraguay | 7.6 | 7.3 | 7.9 | 7.9 | 8 | 32.8 | 37.4 | 39.4 | 38.3 | 38.3 | 67.2 | 62.6 | 60.6 | 61.7 | 61.7 | 13.6 | 14.9 | 17.4 | 16.8 | 16.9 |
| 133 | Peru | 4.4 | 4.6 | 4.4 | 4.7 | 4.7 | 51.4 | 54.8 | 55.9 | 55.4 | 55 | 48.6 | 45.2 | 44.1 | 44.6 | 45 | 11.6 | 12.9 | 13 | 12.7 | 12.1 |
| 134 | Philippines | 3.6 | 3.5 | 3.5 | 3.4 | 3.3 | 43.4 | 43.4 | 44.8 | 48.2 | 45.2 | 56.6 | 56.6 | 55.2 | 51.8 | 54.8 | 6.7 | 6.6 | 6.5 | 7.1 | 6.2 |
| 135 | Poland | 6.1 | 6.4 | 6.2 | 5.8 | 6.1 | 72 | 65.4 | 71.1 | 70 | 71.9 | 28 | 34.6 | 28.9 | 30 | 28.1 | 9.5 | 9.4 | 10.6 | 10.2 | 10.9 |
| 136 | Portugal | 8.6 | 8.6 | 8.7 | 9.1 | 9.2 | 64.8 | 65.5 | 67.6 | 68.5 | 69 | 35.2 | 34.5 | 32.4 | 31.5 | 31 | 12.4 | 12.8 | 13 | 13.7 | 13.7 |
| 137 | Qatar | 3.9 | 4.5 | 3.8 | 2.8 | 3.1 | 76.8 | 76.9 | 76 | 74.2 | 73.5 | 23.2 | 23.1 | 24 | 25.8 | 26.5 | 7 | 7.6 | 7.5 | 6.7 | 6.5 |
| 138 | Republic of Korea | 5 | 5.1 | 5.6 | 5.9 | 6 | 41 | 46.2 | 43.1 | 44.4 | 44.4 | 59 | 53.8 | 56.9 | 55.6 | 55.6 | 9 | 9.3 | 9.7 | 10.7 | 9.5 |
| 139 | Republic of Moldova | 8.6 | 7.2 | 5.7 | 5.9 | 5.7 | 70.7 | 60.3 | 50.5 | 49.8 | 49.7 | 29.3 | 39.7 | 49.5 | 50.2 | 50.3 | 12.2 | 10.1 | 8.3 | 8.5 | 9.4 |
| 140 | Romania | 5 | 6.6 | 6.8 | 6.6 | 6.5 | 66.7 | 74.2 | 77.8 | 78.9 | 79.2 | 33.3 | 25.8 | 22.2 | 21.1 | 20.8 | 9.9 | 13.7 | 14.1 | 14.2 | 15.9 |
| 141 | Russian Federation | 5.8 | 5.8 | 5.3 | 5.4 | 5.4 | 72.9 | 68.9 | 64.7 | 69.9 | 68.2 | 27.1 | 31.1 | 35.3 | 30.1 | 31.8 | 9.3 | 9.8 | 9.4 | 10.8 | 10.7 |
| 142 | Rwanda | 5 | 5 | 5.5 | 5.6 | 5.5 | 48.8 | 51.3 | 54 | 52.9 | 55.5 | 51.2 | 48.7 | 46 | 47.1 | 44.5 | 12.5 | 13.8 | 13.5 | 14.8 | 14.2 |
| 143 | Saint Kitts and Nevis | 4.8 | 4.8 | 4.7 | 4.7 | 4.8 | 66.3 | 66.7 | 66.2 | 66.3 | 66.3 | 33.7 | 33.3 | 33.8 | 33.7 | 33.7 | 10.9 | 11 | 10.6 | 10.6 | 10.9 |
| 144 | Saint Lucia | 4.2 | 4.3 | 4.1 | 4.2 | 4.5 | 62.3 | 65.6 | 65.3 | 65.2 | 64.6 | 37.7 | 34.4 | 34.7 | 34.8 | 35.4 | 9 | 8.8 | 8.3 | 8.2 | 8 |
| 145 | Saint Vincent and the Grenadines | 6.1 | 5.9 | 6 | 6 | 6.1 | 63.8 | 62.5 | 62.7 | 65.1 | 63.5 | 36.2 | 37.5 | 37.3 | 34.9 | 36.5 | 9.2 | 8.7 | 9.1 | 9.3 | 9.3 |
| 146 | Samoa | 5.4 | 5.8 | 6.2 | 5.8 | 5.8 | 73.6 | 73.5 | 74.1 | 76.9 | 82.2 | 26.4 | 26.5 | 25.9 | 23.1 | 17.8 | 11.5 | 13.1 | 12.9 | 14.7 | 15.7 |
| 147 | San Marino | 5.9 | 6.1 | 6.3 | 6.7 | 6.8 | 75.1 | 75.4 | 75.8 | 77.1 | 78 | 24.9 | 24.6 | 24.2 | 22.9 | 22 | 11 | 12 | 12.4 | 13.4 | 13.8 |
| 148 | Sao Tome and Principe | 3 | 2.9 | 2.3 | 2.4 | 2.3 | 66.7 | 67.9 | 67.9 | 67.8 | 67.7 | 33.3 | 32.1 | 32.1 | 32.2 | 32.3 | 2.9 | 3.6 | 3.6 | 3.6 | 3.5 |
| 149 | Saudi Arabia | 5.3 | 5.2 | 4.5 | 4.4 | 4.6 | 77.3 | 76.3 | 73.7 | 74.4 | 74.6 | 22.7 | 23.7 | 26.3 | 25.6 | 25.4 | 11.4 | 11.5 | 11 | 9.9 | 10 |
| 150 | Senegal | 5.1 | 4.9 | 4.7 | 4.6 | 4.8 | 54.8 | 57.5 | 56.1 | 56.6 | 58.8 | 45.2 | 42.5 | 43.9 | 43.4 | 41.2 | 14.4 | 15 | 13 | 13.6 | 12.9 |
| 151 | Serbia and Montenegro | 11 | 9.9 | 9.2 | 7.6 | 8.2 | 74 | 71.3 | 70.9 | 77.6 | 79.2 | 26 | 28.7 | 29.1 | 22.4 | 20.8 | 21.1 | 17.5 | 15.9 | 14.7 | 15 |
| 152 | Seychelles | 6.7 | 6.4 | 6.2 | 5.9 | 6 | 72.3 | 69.4 | 68.8 | 66.5 | 68.2 | 27.7 | 30.6 | 31.2 | 33.5 | 31.8 | 8.1 | 7.5 | 7.4 | 6.7 | 7 |
| 153 | Sierra Leone | 3.3 | 3 | 3.7 | 4.3 | 4.3 | 46.8 | 44.2 | 53.8 | 60.4 | 61 | 53.2 | 55.8 | 46.2 | 39.6 | 39 | 8.9 | 9.4 | 9.4 | 9.3 | 9.4 |
| 154 | Singapore | 3.7 | 4.2 | 4 | 3.6 | 3.9 | 39 | 41.6 | 38.3 | 35.2 | 33.5 | 61 | 58.4 | 61.7 | 64.8 | 66.5 | 8.4 | 8.7 | 8.2 | 6.7 | 5.9 |
| 155 | Slovakia | 5.9 | 5.8 | 5.8 | 5.7 | 5.7 | 91.7 | 91.6 | 89.6 | 89.4 | 89.3 | 8.3 | 8.4 | 10.4 | 10.6 | 10.7 | 8.5 | 8.8 | 9.2 | 8.2 | 8.9 |
| 156 | Slovenia | 7.8 | 8.3 | 8.2 | 8 | 8.4 | 79.2 | 75.7 | 75.5 | 76 | 74.9 | 20.8 | 24.3 | 24.5 | 24 | 25.1 | 14.3 | 14.3 | 14 | 14.5 | 14.6 |
| 157 | Solomon Islands | 3.7 | 4.5 | 4.9 | 4.9 | 5 | 92 | 93 | 93.4 | 93.4 | 93.5 | 8 | 7 | 6.6 | 6.6 | 6.5 | 11.4 | 11.4 | 11.1 | 11.4 | 11.5 |
| 158 | Somalia | 2.6 | 2.7 | 2.7 | 2.6 | 2.6 | 45.5 | 46.1 | 45 | 44.8 | 44.6 | 54.5 | 53.9 | 55 | 55.2 | 55.4 | 4.4 | 4.4 | 4.2 | 4.2 | 4.2 |
| 159 | South Africa | 9 | 8.7 | 8.8 | 8.7 | 8.6 | 46.1 | 42.4 | 42.6 | 41.8 | 41.4 | 53.9 | 57.6 | 57.4 | 58.2 | 58.6 | 12.4 | 11.3 | 11.1 | 11.2 | 10.9 |
| 160 | Spain | 7.5 | 7.5 | 7.5 | 7.5 | 7.5 | 72.5 | 72.2 | 72.1 | 71.7 | 71.4 | 27.5 | 27.8 | 27.9 | 28.3 | 28.6 | 13 | 13.1 | 13.4 | 13.4 | 13.6 |
| 161 | Sri Lanka | 3.2 | 3.4 | 3.5 | 3.6 | 3.6 | 49.5 | 51.3 | 49 | 49.2 | 48.9 | 50.5 | 48.7 | 51 | 50.8 | 51.1 | 6 | 5.8 | 5.7 | 6.1 | 6.1 |
| 162 | Sudan | 3.5 | 3.7 | 3.7 | 3.9 | 3.5 | 19.6 | 24.4 | 22.9 | 28.7 | 18.7 | 80.4 | 75.6 | 77.1 | 71.3 | 81.3 | 9.1 | 12 | 9.5 | 9.3 | 4.6 |
| 163 | Suriname | 9.5 | 9.9 | 9.8 | 9.9 | 9.4 | 52.4 | 61.7 | 59.6 | 63.3 | 60.2 | 47.6 | 38.3 | 40.4 | 36.7 | 39.8 | 17.1 | 18.2 | 17.6 | 18.9 | 17 |
| 164 | Swaziland | 3.1 | 3.2 | 3.3 | 3.4 | 3.3 | 71.6 | 70.8 | 67.7 | 69.9 | 68.5 | 28.4 | 29.2 | 32.3 | 30.1 | 31.5 | 7.9 | 7.7 | 7 | 7.8 | 7.5 |
| 165 | Sweden | 8.2 | 8.3 | 8.4 | 8.4 | 8.7 | 85.8 | 85.8 | 85.7 | 85 | 85.2 | 14.2 | 14.2 | 14.3 | 15 | 14.8 | 11.2 | 11.8 | 12 | 12.4 | 13 |

| | Member State | External resources for health as % of total expenditure on health | | | | | Social security expenditure on health as % of general government expenditure on health | | | | | Out-of-pocket expenditure as % of private expenditure on health | | | | | Private prepaid plans as % of private expenditure on health | | | | |
|---|---|---|---|---|---|---|---|---|---|---|---|---|---|---|---|---|---|---|---|---|---|
| | | 1997 | 1998 | 1999 | 2000 | 2001 | 1997 | 1998 | 1999 | 2000 | 2001 | 1997 | 1998 | 1999 | 2000 | 2001 | 1997 | 1998 | 1999 | 2000 | 2001 |
| 111 | Micronesia, Federated States of | n/a | n/a | 22.5 | 22.1 | 16.2 | 0 | 0 | 0 | 0 | 0 | 35.7 | 35.7 | 35.7 | 35.7 | 35.7 | 0 | 0 | 0 | 0 | 0 |
| 112 | Monaco | 0 | 0 | 0 | 0 | 0 | 94.3 | 94.6 | 94.9 | 95.2 | 95.7 | 100 | 100 | 100 | 100 | 100 | 0 | 0 | 0 | 0 | 0 |
| 113 | Mongolia | 4.2 | 9 | 18.9 | 17.2 | 15.4 | 36.8 | 39.9 | 39.3 | 40.2 | 40.3 | 73.3 | 74.5 | 74.1 | 73.9 | 73.4 | 0 | 0 | 0 | 0 | 0 |
| 114 | Morocco | 2.6 | 2.2 | 1.5 | 1.7 | 1.4 | 9.8 | 9 | 9 | 7.6 | 5.8 | 74.3 | 74.4 | 74.3 | 74.3 | 74.1 | 22.8 | 22.5 | 22.7 | 22.6 | 22.7 |
| 115 | Mozambique | 53.1 | 44.2 | 40.3 | 38.2 | 36.9 | 0 | 0 | 0 | 0 | 0 | 42.8 | 40.5 | 39.2 | 39.3 | 39.3 | 0.6 | 0.5 | 0.6 | 0.5 | 0.5 |
| 116 | Myanmar | 0.4 | 0.4 | 0.3 | 0.4 | 0.2 | 3.6 | 3 | 2.1 | 2 | 1.8 | 99.6 | 99.7 | 99.8 | 99.6 | 99.6 | 0 | 0 | 0 | 0 | 0 |
| 117 | Namibia | 2.6 | 2.5 | 2.5 | 3.8 | 3.8 | 1.5 | 1.4 | 1.2 | 1.8 | 1.9 | 22 | 21.9 | 21.2 | 18.2 | 17.9 | 74.6 | 74.6 | 74.6 | 77.3 | 77.9 |
| 118 | Nauru | n/a | n/a | n/a | n/a | n/a | 0 | 0 | 0 | 0 | 0 | 100 | 100 | 100 | 100 | 100 | 0 | 0 | 0 | 0 | 0 |
| 119 | Nepal | 10.6 | 9.9 | 10.2 | 8.3 | 9.4 | 0 | 0 | 0 | 0 | 0 | 94.2 | 94.1 | 94.2 | 93.8 | 93.3 | 0 | 0 | 0 | 0 | 0 |
| 120 | Netherlands | 0 | 0 | 0 | 0 | 0 | 93.6 | 93.3 | 93.2 | 93.6 | 93.8 | 23.8 | 24.7 | 25 | 24.5 | 24.1 | 59.1 | 43.5 | 42.7 | 41.6 | 42.4 |
| 121 | New Zealand | 0 | 0 | 0 | 0 | 0 | 0 | 0 | 0 | 0 | 0 | 68.8 | 70.8 | 70.1 | 69.9 | 72 | 29.8 | 27.7 | 28.1 | 28.5 | 26.5 |
| 122 | Nicaragua | 10.8 | 11.1 | 10 | 7.7 | 7.7 | 24.3 | 23 | 31.5 | 27 | 31.3 | 97.1 | 96.9 | 93.9 | 91.9 | 93.1 | 0.9 | 1.7 | 0.7 | 2.7 | 4 |
| 123 | Niger | 13.7 | 17.7 | 9.2 | 20.9 | 16.9 | 0 | 0 | 0 | 0 | 0 | 84.5 | 83.4 | 82.7 | 83.4 | 85.4 | 3.4 | 2.9 | 3.2 | 3.2 | 2.9 |
| 124 | Nigeria | 1.3 | 1.2 | 3.8 | 7.2 | 7.1 | 0 | 0 | 0 | 0 | 0 | 100 | 100 | 100 | 100 | 100 | 0 | 0 | 0 | 0 | 0 |
| 125 | Niue | n/a | n/a | n/a | n/a | n/a | 0 | 0 | 0 | 0 | 0 | 100 | 100 | 100 | 100 | 100 | 0 | 0 | 0 | 0 | 0 |
| 126 | Norway | 0 | 0 | 0 | 0 | 0 | 0 | 0 | 0 | 0 | 0 | 96.6 | 96.6 | 96.6 | 96.7 | 96.8 | 0 | 0 | 0 | 0 | 0 |
| 127 | Oman | 0 | 0 | 0 | 0.1 | 0 | 0 | 0 | 0 | 0 | 0 | 46.4 | 51.1 | 47.5 | 41.7 | 42.9 | 0 | 0 | 0 | 0 | 0 |
| 128 | Pakistan | 2.7 | 2.2 | 2 | 3.8 | 1.9 | 43.9 | 41.6 | 44.9 | 39.6 | 43.3 | 100 | 100 | 100 | 100 | 100 | 0 | 0 | 0 | 0 | 0 |
| 129 | Palau | 12.5 | 13.5 | 11.9 | 11.4 | 11.8 | 0 | 0 | 0 | 0 | 0 | 100 | 100 | 100 | 100 | 100 | 0 | 0 | 0 | 0 | 0 |
| 130 | Panama | 1.4 | 1.3 | 1.3 | 1.2 | 0.6 | 60.6 | 66.2 | 58.9 | 57.2 | 57.9 | 82.7 | 82 | 81.8 | 81.3 | 81.2 | 17.2 | 18 | 18.2 | 18.7 | 18.7 |
| 131 | Papua New Guinea | 26.8 | 29 | 18.5 | 22.1 | 21.2 | 0 | 0 | 0 | 0 | 0 | 88.7 | 86.4 | 83.4 | 83.9 | 83.3 | 2 | 4.8 | 9.4 | 9.3 | 9.4 |
| 132 | Paraguay | 1.6 | 1.9 | 2 | 2 | 2 | 47.8 | 44.9 | 46.7 | 48.3 | 48.2 | 68.4 | 76.3 | 72.9 | 72.7 | 71.6 | 31.6 | 23.7 | 27.1 | 27.3 | 28.4 |
| 133 | Peru | 2.3 | 2.4 | 2 | 1.4 | 1.7 | 43 | 43.1 | 48.3 | 47.2 | 51.9 | 82.8 | 81.7 | 80 | 81.7 | 81.7 | 15.3 | 16.5 | 18 | 16 | 16.1 |
| 134 | Philippines | 2 | 2.8 | 3.7 | 3.5 | 3.5 | 11.8 | 8.8 | 11.4 | 14.7 | 17.2 | 82.9 | 82.6 | 79.5 | 79.2 | 78.2 | 15.6 | 15.9 | 18.6 | 18.6 | 19.8 |
| 135 | Poland | 0 | 0 | 0 | 0 | 0 | 0 | 0 | 83.4 | 82.4 | 76.7 | 92.7 | 92.8 | 92.3 | 92.4 | 92.4 | 7.3 | 7.2 | 7.7 | 7.6 | 7.6 |
| 136 | Portugal | 0 | 0 | 0 | 0 | 0 | 6.7 | 7.7 | 7.1 | 6.7 | 6.8 | 55.5 | 57.7 | 60.6 | 59.4 | 58.5 | 4.3 | 4.3 | 4.3 | 4.3 | 4.3 |
| 137 | Qatar | 0 | 0 | 0 | 0 | 0 | 0 | 0 | 0 | 0 | 0 | 25.3 | 24.7 | 26.8 | 31.9 | 33.7 | 0 | 0 | 0 | 0 | 0 |
| 138 | Republic of Korea | 0 | 0 | 0 | 0 | 0 | 71.9 | 74.5 | 75.2 | 77.3 | 77.2 | 78.2 | 77.4 | 75.7 | 74.2 | 74.3 | 11.3 | 12.9 | 13.6 | 15.6 | 17.2 |
| 139 | Republic of Moldova | 0.4 | 1 | 3.8 | 6.9 | 7.5 | 0 | 0 | 0 | 0 | 0 | 100 | 100 | 100 | 100 | 100 | n/a | n/a | n/a | n/a | n/a |
| 140 | Romania | 1 | 2.1 | 3 | 2 | 1 | 87.1 | 87 | 87 | 88.6 | 88.3 | 79.4 | 78.8 | 86.7 | 89.2 | 92.1 | 20.6 | 21.2 | 13.3 | 10.8 | 7.9 |
| 141 | Russian Federation | 0.4 | 1.2 | 3.8 | 3.1 | 3.1 | 33.8 | 36.3 | 36.9 | 24.5 | 21.8 | 77.7 | 80.5 | 84.8 | 85.2 | 84.4 | 6.7 | 5.6 | 4.6 | 4.6 | 4.5 |
| 142 | Rwanda | 30.1 | 25.6 | 26.5 | 33.2 | 24.7 | 0.6 | 0.6 | 0.6 | 0.6 | 0.6 | 66.2 | 67 | 64.6 | 61.3 | 66.1 | 0.3 | 0.3 | 0.3 | 0.3 | 0.3 |
| 143 | Saint Kitts and Nevis | 7.2 | 6.8 | 6.7 | 6.2 | 5.6 | 0 | 0 | 0 | 0 | 0 | 100 | 100 | 100 | 100 | 100 | n/a | n/a | n/a | n/a | n/a |
| 144 | Saint Lucia | 0.6 | 0.6 | 0.5 | 0.5 | 0.6 | 35.2 | 17.7 | 14.6 | 24 | 25.5 | 100 | 100 | 100 | 100 | 100 | n/a | n/a | n/a | n/a | n/a |
| 145 | Saint Vincent and the Grenadines | 1.8 | 1.7 | 1.6 | 1.6 | 0.3 | 0 | 0 | 0 | 0 | 0 | 100 | 100 | 100 | 100 | 100 | n/a | n/a | n/a | n/a | n/a |
| 146 | Samoa | 6.1 | 15.8 | 13.8 | 19.1 | 15.6 | 0.6 | 0.6 | 0.3 | 0.3 | 0.2 | 78.1 | 79.4 | 80.1 | 81.7 | 87.5 | 0 | 0 | 0 | 0 | 0 |
| 147 | San Marino | 0 | 0 | 0 | 0 | 0 | 54.8 | 55.7 | 54.9 | 52.7 | 51.7 | 100 | 100 | 100 | 100 | 100 | n/a | n/a | n/a | n/a | n/a |
| 148 | Sao Tome and Principe | 45.3 | 48.6 | 64.1 | 57.8 | 56.4 | 0 | 0 | 0 | 0 | 0 | 100 | 100 | 100 | 100 | 100 | 0 | 0 | 0 | 0 | 0 |
| 149 | Saudi Arabia | 0 | 0 | 0 | 0 | 0 | 0 | 0 | 0 | 0 | 0 | 42.2 | 44.3 | 42.2 | 38.9 | 38 | 33.4 | 32.1 | 33.4 | 35.4 | 36.8 |
| 150 | Senegal | 11.7 | 11.1 | 12.4 | 14.1 | 20.2 | 0 | 0 | 0 | 0 | 0 | 91.3 | 90.6 | 91.2 | 91.3 | 91.6 | 8.7 | 9.4 | 8.8 | 8.7 | 8.4 |
| 151 | Serbia and Montenegro | 0 | 0.1 | 0.3 | 2.2 | 1.4 | 92.7 | 92 | 92.6 | 92.4 | 89.4 | 100 | 100 | 100 | 100 | 100 | 0 | 0 | 0 | 0 | 0 |
| 152 | Seychelles | 13.7 | 12.9 | 12.4 | 11.8 | 11.9 | 0 | 0 | 0 | 0 | 0 | 77.8 | 75.3 | 75 | 74.6 | 75 | 0 | 0 | 0 | 0 | 0 |
| 153 | Sierra Leone | 19.3 | 18.8 | 22.2 | 25.4 | 25.1 | 0 | 0 | 0 | 0 | 0 | 100 | 100 | 100 | 100 | 100 | 0 | 0 | 0 | 0 | 0 |
| 154 | Singapore | 0 | 0 | 0 | 0 | 0 | 20.2 | 17.6 | 19 | 23.3 | 24.5 | 97.5 | 97.3 | 97.4 | 97.2 | 97 | 0 | 0 | 0 | 0 | 0 |
| 155 | Slovakia | 0 | 0 | 0 | 0 | 0 | 96.7 | 96.6 | 94.2 | 94.4 | 95.1 | 100 | 100 | 100 | 100 | 100 | 0 | 0 | 0 | 0 | 0 |
| 156 | Slovenia | 0 | 0 | 0 | 0 | 0 | 87.8 | 87.9 | 87.5 | 87.5 | 77.5 | 48.8 | 44.4 | 39.3 | 38.6 | 41.7 | 51.2 | 55.6 | 60.7 | 61.4 | 58.3 |
| 157 | Solomon Islands | 7 | 7.7 | 7.1 | 16.5 | 15.9 | 0 | 0 | 0 | 0 | 0 | 47 | 45.8 | 47.1 | 48.3 | 49.2 | 0 | 0 | 0 | 0 | 0 |
| 158 | Somalia | 4.3 | 5.3 | 6.1 | 9 | 9.3 | 0 | 0 | 0 | 0 | 0 | 100 | 100 | 100 | 100 | 100 | 0 | 0 | 0 | 0 | 0 |
| 159 | South Africa | 0.2 | 0.2 | 0.1 | 0.4 | 0.4 | 0 | 0 | 0 | 0 | 0 | 19.7 | 21.9 | 21.7 | 21.8 | 22.1 | 78.3 | 76.4 | 76.7 | 76.6 | 72.2 |
| 160 | Spain | 0 | 0 | 0 | 0 | 0 | 13.4 | 11.8 | 9.4 | 9.6 | 9.2 | 83.9 | 83.6 | 83.3 | 83.1 | 82.8 | 12.8 | 13.1 | 13.5 | 13.7 | 14.1 |
| 161 | Sri Lanka | 3.2 | 2.8 | 2.7 | 2.7 | 3.1 | 0 | 0 | 0 | 0 | 0 | 95 | 94.9 | 95.1 | 95 | 95 | 1 | 1 | 1 | 1.1 | 1.1 |
| 162 | Sudan | 1.4 | 2.4 | 4.1 | 2.4 | 2.7 | 0 | 0 | 0 | 0 | 0 | 99.4 | 99.3 | 99.4 | 99.3 | 99.3 | 0 | 0 | 0 | 0 | 0 |
| 163 | Suriname | 9 | 9.5 | 17.6 | 9.8 | 12.4 | 32.2 | 34.9 | 33.3 | 28.1 | 22.8 | 30.5 | 33.7 | 32.7 | 39.9 | 57 | 1.7 | 1.4 | 1.3 | 1 | 0.7 |
| 164 | Swaziland | 9.3 | 1.5 | 5.1 | 0.9 | 7.9 | 0 | 0 | 0 | 0 | 0 | 100 | 100 | 100 | 100 | 100 | 0 | 0 | 0 | 0 | 0 |
| 165 | Sweden | 0 | 0 | 0 | 0 | 0 | 0 | 0 | 0 | 0 | 0 | 100 | 100 | 100 | 100 | 100 | 0 | 0 | 0 | 0 | 0 |

**Annex Table 5 Selected national health accounts indicators: measured levels of expenditure on health, 1997–2001**

Figures computed by WHO to assure comparability;[a] they are not necessarily the official statistics of Member States, which may use alternative rigorous methods.

| | Member State | Total expenditure on health as % of GDP | | | | | General government expenditure on health as % of total expenditure on health | | | | | Private expenditure on health as % of total expenditure on health | | | | | General government expenditure on health as % of total government expenditure | | | | |
|---|---|---|---|---|---|---|---|---|---|---|---|---|---|---|---|---|---|---|---|---|---|
| | | 1997 | 1998 | 1999 | 2000 | 2001 | 1997 | 1998 | 1999 | 2000 | 2001 | 1997 | 1998 | 1999 | 2000 | 2001 | 1997 | 1998 | 1999 | 2000 | 2001 |
| 166 | Switzerland | 10.4 | 10.6 | 10.7 | 10.7 | 11 | 55.2 | 54.9 | 55.3 | 55.6 | 57.1 | 44.8 | 45.1 | 44.7 | 44.4 | 42.9 | 15.3 | 15.4 | 11.9 | 12.5 | 13.2 |
| 167 | Syrian Arab Republic | 5.5 | 5.6 | 5.8 | 5.4 | 5.4 | 37.4 | 38.4 | 39 | 40.8 | 43.9 | 62.6 | 61.6 | 61 | 59.2 | 56.1 | 7.2 | 7.1 | 7.2 | 7.3 | 7 |
| 168 | Tajikistan | 3.2 | 3.6 | 3.4 | 3.3 | 3.3 | 39 | 32.4 | 30.6 | 28.2 | 28.9 | 61 | 67.6 | 69.4 | 71.8 | 71.1 | 7.4 | 7.4 | 6.3 | 6.5 | 6.5 |
| 169 | Thailand | 3.7 | 3.9 | 3.7 | 3.6 | 3.7 | 57.2 | 61.2 | 57.6 | 56.8 | 57.1 | 42.8 | 38.8 | 42.4 | 43.2 | 42.9 | 10.2 | 13.3 | 11.6 | 11.6 | 11.6 |
| 170 | The former Yugoslav Republic of Macedonia | 6.1 | 7.6 | 6.4 | 6 | 6.8 | 83.9 | 87.1 | 85.4 | 84.5 | 84.9 | 16.1 | 12.9 | 14.6 | 15.5 | 15.1 | 14.5 | 19 | 16.3 | 15.6 | 17.4 |
| 171 | Timor-Leste | 9.4 | 6.4 | 9.6 | 7.4 | 9.8 | 90.5 | 85.4 | 88.6 | 74 | 59.5 | 9.5 | 14.6 | 11.4 | 26 | 40.5 | 9 | 5.8 | 9 | 5.8 | 9 |
| 172 | Togo | 3 | 3.5 | 4 | 3 | 2.8 | 50.2 | 59.6 | 62.8 | 48.7 | 48.6 | 49.8 | 40.4 | 37.2 | 51.3 | 51.4 | 8.3 | 9.7 | 12.8 | 7.9 | 9.3 |
| 173 | Tonga | 5.5 | 5.5 | 5.4 | 5.3 | 5.5 | 59.8 | 61.2 | 60.7 | 60.5 | 61.6 | 40.2 | 38.8 | 39.3 | 39.5 | 38.4 | 7.8 | 9.6 | 12.7 | 11.6 | 10.9 |
| 174 | Trinidad and Tobago | 4.5 | 4.8 | 4.5 | 3.9 | 4 | 43 | 46.5 | 46.5 | 45.9 | 43.3 | 57 | 53.5 | 53.5 | 54.1 | 56.7 | 6.6 | 6.7 | 6.7 | 6.7 | 6.4 |
| 175 | Tunisia | 6.4 | 6.3 | 6.3 | 6.2 | 6.4 | 77.7 | 76.7 | 75.9 | 74.3 | 75.7 | 22.3 | 23.3 | 24.1 | 25.7 | 24.3 | 15.5 | 15 | 14.9 | 14.2 | 15.1 |
| 176 | Turkey | 4.2 | 4.8 | 4.9 | 5 | 5 | 71.6 | 71.9 | 71.1 | 71.1 | 71 | 28.4 | 28.1 | 28.9 | 28.9 | 29 | 10.8 | 11.5 | 9.1 | 9 | 9.1 |
| 177 | Turkmenistan | 4.7 | 5 | 5 | 4 | 4.1 | 75.6 | 70.3 | 68 | 74.5 | 73.3 | 24.4 | 29.7 | 32 | 25.5 | 26.7 | 12 | 14.4 | 17.5 | 11.5 | 18.2 |
| 178 | Tuvalu | 5.3 | 5.2 | 5.4 | 5.5 | 5.4 | 59.1 | 59.3 | 57.3 | 53.5 | 53.4 | 40.9 | 40.7 | 42.7 | 46.5 | 46.6 | 5.4 | 3.7 | 3.6 | 3.3 | 2.9 |
| 179 | Uganda | 3.9 | 4 | 4.1 | 5.6 | 5.9 | 29.1 | 38 | 40.9 | 56.1 | 57.5 | 70.9 | 62 | 59.1 | 43.9 | 42.5 | 6.5 | 8.1 | 8.4 | 16.4 | 16.4 |
| 180 | Ukraine | 5.4 | 5 | 4.3 | 4.2 | 4.3 | 75 | 71.7 | 68.3 | 68.2 | 67.8 | 25 | 28.3 | 31.7 | 31.8 | 32.2 | 9.3 | 8 | 8.3 | 7.6 | 7.6 |
| 181 | United Arab Emirates | 3.6 | 4 | 3.7 | 3.5 | 3.5 | 76.7 | 77 | 75.8 | 75.9 | 75.8 | 23.3 | 23 | 24.2 | 24.1 | 24.2 | 28.9 | 28.8 | 27.9 | 31.5 | 32.3 |
| 182 | United Kingdom | 6.8 | 6.9 | 7.2 | 7.3 | 7.6 | 80.1 | 80.2 | 80.5 | 80.9 | 82.2 | 19.9 | 19.8 | 19.5 | 19.1 | 17.8 | 13.4 | 13.9 | 14.8 | 15 | 15.4 |
| 183 | United Republic of Tanzania | 4.1 | 4.4 | 4.3 | 4.4 | 4.4 | 45.9 | 47.1 | 43.4 | 47.1 | 46.7 | 54.1 | 52.9 | 56.6 | 52.9 | 53.3 | 14.4 | 13.1 | 12.4 | 12.1 | 12.1 |
| 184 | United States of America | 13 | 13 | 13 | 13.1 | 13.9 | 45.3 | 44.5 | 44.2 | 44.2 | 44.4 | 54.7 | 55.5 | 55.8 | 55.8 | 55.6 | 16.8 | 16.9 | 16.9 | 17.2 | 17.6 |
| 185 | Uruguay | 10 | 10.2 | 10.7 | 10.9 | 10.9 | 40.8 | 41 | 48.2 | 46.6 | 46.3 | 59.2 | 59 | 51.8 | 53.4 | 53.7 | 12.1 | 12.5 | 14.9 | 14.9 | 14.9 |
| 186 | Uzbekistan | 4.2 | 3.9 | 3.6 | 3.7 | 3.6 | 72.7 | 75.1 | 74 | 74.9 | 74.5 | 27.3 | 24.9 | 26 | 25.1 | 25.5 | 9.3 | 8.8 | 8.6 | 9.6 | 9.2 |
| 187 | Vanuatu | 3.4 | 3.5 | 3.7 | 3.8 | 3.8 | 65.5 | 65.4 | 63.6 | 60.9 | 59.2 | 34.5 | 34.6 | 36.4 | 39.1 | 40.8 | 10.2 | 8.7 | 10.3 | 10.1 | 9.7 |
| 188 | Venezuela, Bolivarian Republic of | 5.4 | 5.4 | 5.6 | 5.9 | 6 | 57.1 | 54.4 | 53.9 | 57.1 | 62.1 | 42.9 | 45.6 | 46.1 | 42.9 | 37.9 | 12.5 | 12.4 | 13.6 | 13.8 | 14.7 |
| 189 | Viet Nam | 4.4 | 4.9 | 4.9 | 5.2 | 5.1 | 31.5 | 32.7 | 32.7 | 28.5 | 28.5 | 68.5 | 67.3 | 67.3 | 71.5 | 71.5 | 5.6 | 7.1 | 6.7 | 6.1 | 6.1 |
| 190 | Yemen | 3.8 | 4.4 | 4 | 4 | 4.5 | 30.4 | 39.5 | 32.5 | 34.6 | 34.1 | 69.6 | 60.5 | 67.5 | 65.4 | 65.9 | 3.5 | 4.8 | 4.8 | 3.9 | 4 |
| 191 | Zambia | 6 | 6 | 5.7 | 5.5 | 5.7 | 55.1 | 56.9 | 54.8 | 52.5 | 53.1 | 44.9 | 43.1 | 45.2 | 47.5 | 46.9 | 13.1 | 12.5 | 13.7 | 13.6 | 13.5 |
| 192 | Zimbabwe | 9.3 | 11.4 | 7.9 | 7.4 | 6.2 | 59.1 | 55.9 | 48.9 | 50.7 | 45.3 | 40.9 | 44.1 | 51.1 | 49.3 | 54.7 | 15.4 | 12.2 | 10 | 7.1 | 8 |

[a] See explanatory notes for sources and methods.

n/a Used when the information accessed indicates that a cell should have an entry but no estimates could be made.

0 Used when no evidence of the schemes to which the cell relates exist. Some estimates yielding a ratio inferior to 0.04% are shown as 0.

| | Member State | External resources for health as % of total expenditure on health | | | | | Social security expenditure on health as % of general government expenditure on health | | | | | Out-of-pocket expenditure as % of private expenditure on health | | | | | Private prepaid plans as % of private expenditure on health | | | | |
|---|---|---|---|---|---|---|---|---|---|---|---|---|---|---|---|---|---|---|---|---|---|
| | | 1997 | 1998 | 1999 | 2000 | 2001 | 1997 | 1998 | 1999 | 2000 | 2001 | 1997 | 1998 | 1999 | 2000 | 2001 | 1997 | 1998 | 1999 | 2000 | 2001 |
| 166 | Switzerland | 0 | 0 | 0 | 0 | 0 | 71.6 | 72.3 | 72.1 | 72.6 | 70.4 | 72 | 72.6 | 74.5 | 74.1 | 73.9 | 25.7 | 25.2 | 23.3 | 23.6 | 23.8 |
| 167 | Syrian Arab Republic | 0.3 | 0.2 | 0.1 | 0.1 | 0.3 | 0 | 0 | 0 | 0 | 0 | 100 | 100 | 100 | 100 | 100 | 0 | 0 | 0 | 0 | 0 |
| 168 | Tajikistan | 5.6 | 6.2 | 3.1 | 7.6 | 7.4 | 0 | 0 | 0 | 0 | 0 | 100 | 100 | 100 | 100 | 100 | 0 | 0 | 0 | 0 | 0 |
| 169 | Thailand | 0.3 | 0.4 | 0.5 | 0.5 | 0.1 | 30.2 | 25.8 | 26.9 | 27 | 26.8 | 86.2 | 84.9 | 84.9 | 85 | 85 | 8.6 | 9.6 | 9.6 | 9.6 | 9.6 |
| 170 | The former Yugoslav Republic of Macedonia | 2.6 | 2.6 | 2.6 | 3.1 | 3.5 | 96.3 | 96.8 | 94.8 | 91.9 | 87.5 | 100 | 100 | 100 | 100 | 100 | 0 | 0 | 0 | 0 | 0 |
| 171 | Timor-Leste | 41.8 | 66.7 | 87.2 | 64.6 | 53.8 | 0.9 | 1.2 | n/a | n/a | n/a | 93 | 88.6 | 75.8 | 43.1 | 20.8 | 0 | 0 | 0 | 0 | 0 |
| 172 | Togo | 8.1 | 9.8 | 5.3 | 31.2 | 8.1 | 0 | 0 | 0 | 0 | 0 | 100 | 100 | 100 | 100 | 100 | n/a | n/a | n/a | n/a | n/a |
| 173 | Tonga | 6.3 | 5.9 | 8.8 | 10.2 | 20.7 | 0 | 0 | 0 | 0 | 0 | 100 | 100 | 100 | 100 | 100 | 0 | 0 | 0 | 0 | 0 |
| 174 | Trinidad and Tobago | 5.2 | 4.6 | 4.4 | 4.2 | 3.8 | 0 | 0 | 0 | 0 | 0 | 86.9 | 87.1 | 86.4 | 85.7 | 86.5 | 6.2 | 6.2 | 6.7 | 7.6 | 7.1 |
| 175 | Tunisia | 0.6 | 0.6 | 0.6 | 0.6 | 0.6 | 45.3 | 52.7 | 54.9 | 57.3 | 53.4 | 77.2 | 76 | 77.1 | 78 | 77.6 | 22.8 | 24 | 22.9 | 22 | 22.4 |
| 176 | Turkey | 0.4 | 0.4 | 0.1 | 0.1 | 0 | 38.8 | 43.8 | 28.4 | 28.4 | 28.6 | 99.6 | 99.6 | 99.8 | 99.9 | 98.8 | 0.2 | 0.2 | 0.2 | 0.1 | 1.2 |
| 177 | Turkmenistan | 2.1 | 2.6 | 1.4 | 0.9 | 0.6 | 8.4 | 16.2 | 23.5 | 26.4 | 26.8 | 71.4 | 76.6 | 78.1 | 72.6 | 73.7 | 28.6 | 23.4 | 21.9 | 27.4 | 26.3 |
| 178 | Tuvalu | 6.9 | 7.1 | 6.4 | 6.4 | 29.4 | 0 | 0 | 0 | 0 | 0 | 100 | 100 | 100 | 100 | 100 | 0 | 0 | 0 | 0 | 0 |
| 179 | Uganda | 24.4 | 41.7 | 22.9 | 41.2 | 24.8 | 0 | 0 | 0 | 0 | 0 | 54 | 54 | 55.4 | 55.6 | 53.4 | 0.5 | 0.5 | 0.5 | 0.5 | 0.5 |
| 180 | Ukraine | 0.6 | 0.4 | 0.3 | 0.7 | 0.7 | 0 | 0 | 0 | 0 | 0 | 100 | 100 | 100 | 100 | 100 | 0 | 0 | 0 | 0 | 0 |
| 181 | United Arab Emirates | 0 | 0 | 0 | 0 | 0 | 0 | 0 | 0 | 0 | 0 | 69.4 | 69.5 | 67 | 66 | 65.6 | 16.4 | 16.9 | 19 | 19.1 | 19.1 |
| 182 | United Kingdom | 0 | 0 | 0 | 0 | 0 | 0 | 0 | 0 | 0 | 0 | 53.5 | 55.1 | 54.7 | 55 | 55.3 | 17 | 17.2 | 16.7 | 16.7 | 17.2 |
| 183 | United Republic of Tanzania | 16 | 22 | 35.3 | 30 | 29.5 | 0 | 0 | 0 | 0 | 0 | 87 | 87.5 | 83.5 | 83 | 83.1 | 0 | 0 | 4.5 | 4.4 | 4.4 |
| 184 | United States of America | 0 | 0 | 0 | 0 | 0 | 32.1 | 33.3 | 33.3 | 33.9 | 32.9 | 27.6 | 28 | 27.6 | 27.2 | 26.5 | 61.2 | 61 | 61.7 | 62.8 | 64.1 |
| 185 | Uruguay | 0.6 | 0.6 | 0.1 | 0.5 | 0.8 | 45.6 | 46.8 | 37.6 | 34.7 | 35.8 | 33.5 | 32.9 | 33.2 | 31.2 | 30.4 | 66.5 | 67.1 | 66.8 | 68.8 | 69.6 |
| 186 | Uzbekistan | 1 | 1.3 | 1.5 | 0.9 | 1.7 | 0 | 0 | 0 | 0 | 0 | 100 | 100 | 100 | 100 | 100 | 0 | 0 | 0 | 0 | 0 |
| 187 | Vanuatu | 20 | 30.4 | 28.7 | 28.5 | 8.4 | 0 | 0 | 0 | 0 | 0 | 100 | 100 | 100 | 100 | 100 | 0 | 0 | 0 | 0 | 0 |
| 188 | Venezuela, Bolivarian Republic of | 1.3 | 1.2 | 1 | 0.4 | 0.1 | 20.9 | 18.6 | 25 | 24.7 | 20.2 | 78.6 | 77.9 | 79.9 | 73.8 | 95.4 | 4.6 | 4.8 | 4.4 | 4 | 4.6 |
| 189 | Viet Nam | 5.6 | 2.8 | 3.4 | 2.7 | 2.6 | 13 | 11.5 | 9.5 | 10.9 | 10.9 | 93.5 | 89.7 | 86.5 | 87.7 | 87.6 | 0 | 3.4 | 3.7 | 4.2 | 4.2 |
| 190 | Yemen | 6.2 | 5.2 | 5.1 | 4.1 | 3.7 | 0 | 0 | 0 | 0 | 0 | 87.4 | 87.9 | 88.2 | 87.8 | 88.7 | 0 | 0 | 0 | 0 | 0 |
| 191 | Zambia | 23.5 | 26.1 | 40.1 | 33.5 | 48.7 | 0 | 0 | 0 | 0 | 0 | 70.9 | 74.1 | 70.7 | 71.1 | 71.8 | 0 | 0 | 0 | 0 | 0 |
| 192 | Zimbabwe | 2.3 | 17.2 | 13 | 12.5 | 7.8 | 0 | 0 | 0 | 0 | 0 | 67 | 75.2 | 44.9 | 48 | 52.2 | 21 | 16.4 | 39.6 | 39.2 | 34.8 |

## Annex Table 6 Selected national health accounts indicators: measured levels of per capita expenditure on health, 1997–2001

Figures computed by WHO to assure comparability;[a] they are not necessarily the official statistics of Member States, which may use alternative rigorous methods.

| | Member State | Per capita total expenditure on health at average exchange rate (US$) | | | | | Per capita total expenditure on health at international dollar rate | | | | | Per capita government expenditure on health at average exchange rate (US$) | | | | | Per capita government expenditure on health at international dollar rate | | | | |
|---|---|---|---|---|---|---|---|---|---|---|---|---|---|---|---|---|---|---|---|---|---|
| | | 1997 | 1998 | 1999 | 2000 | 2001 | 1997 | 1998 | 1999 | 2000 | 2001 | 1997 | 1998 | 1999 | 2000 | 2001 | 1997 | 1998 | 1999 | 2000 | 2001 |
| 1 | Afghanistan | n/a | n/a | n/a | 9 | 8 | 34 | 35 | 38 | 40 | 34 | n/a | n/a | n/a | 5 | 4 | 17 | 19 | 20 | 22 | 18 |
| 2 | Albania | 28 | 34 | 43 | 46 | 48 | 108 | 108 | 125 | 144 | 150 | 17 | 21 | 27 | 30 | 31 | 66 | 67 | 78 | 92 | 97 |
| 3 | Algeria | 57 | 59 | 59 | 68 | 73 | 122 | 133 | 138 | 151 | 169 | 41 | 42 | 41 | 48 | 55 | 87 | 94 | 96 | 106 | 127 |
| 4 | Andorra | 1328 | 1670 | 1285 | 1200 | 1233 | 1601 | 2021 | 1610 | 1723 | 1821 | 950 | 1313 | 920 | 841 | 875 | 1145 | 1589 | 1152 | 1208 | 1292 |
| 5 | Angola | 26 | 19 | 17 | 26 | 31 | 56 | 51 | 48 | 55 | 70 | 12 | 8 | 7 | 14 | 19 | 25 | 20 | 21 | 30 | 44 |
| 6 | Antigua and Barbuda | 448 | 464 | 485 | 509 | 531 | 484 | 496 | 526 | 581 | 614 | 278 | 290 | 297 | 305 | 323 | 300 | 310 | 322 | 348 | 374 |
| 7 | Argentina | 668 | 680 | 700 | 683 | 679 | 1014 | 1065 | 1140 | 1099 | 1130 | 371 | 376 | 394 | 377 | 363 | 563 | 588 | 641 | 607 | 604 |
| 8 | Armenia | 36 | 42 | 46 | 49 | 54 | 171 | 190 | 224 | 246 | 273 | 13 | 16 | 19 | 20 | 22 | 60 | 70 | 92 | 99 | 112 |
| 9 | Australia | 1909 | 1709 | 1870 | 1808 | 1741 | 1978 | 2093 | 2230 | 2363 | 2532 | 1293 | 1165 | 1293 | 1246 | 1182 | 1341 | 1427 | 1542 | 1629 | 1718 |
| 10 | Austria | 2027 | 2100 | 2086 | 1873 | 1866 | 1881 | 1972 | 2070 | 2236 | 2259 | 1438 | 1500 | 1461 | 1305 | 1293 | 1334 | 1409 | 1450 | 1559 | 1566 |
| 11 | Azerbaijan | 11 | 13 | 11 | 11 | 11 | 44 | 50 | 46 | 46 | 48 | 8 | 9 | 8 | 8 | 8 | 32 | 37 | 32 | 31 | 32 |
| 12 | Bahamas | 701 | 754 | 807 | 863 | 864 | 829 | 922 | 1057 | 1117 | 1220 | 390 | 434 | 463 | 490 | 492 | 461 | 531 | 606 | 635 | 695 |
| 13 | Bahrain | 484 | 480 | 479 | 484 | 500 | 702 | 715 | 670 | 568 | 664 | 341 | 335 | 332 | 334 | 345 | 495 | 498 | 464 | 393 | 458 |
| 14 | Bangladesh | 10 | 10 | 11 | 13 | 12 | 40 | 41 | 47 | 56 | 58 | 3 | 4 | 4 | 6 | 5 | 13 | 15 | 17 | 26 | 26 |
| 15 | Barbados | 495 | 531 | 569 | 603 | 613 | 775 | 783 | 839 | 881 | 940 | 323 | 348 | 374 | 397 | 406 | 505 | 514 | 551 | 581 | 623 |
| 16 | Belarus | 82 | 67 | 63 | 56 | 68 | 375 | 391 | 415 | 424 | 464 | 71 | 58 | 54 | 48 | 59 | 327 | 337 | 355 | 362 | 402 |
| 17 | Belgium | 2016 | 2059 | 2095 | 1916 | 1983 | 1988 | 1969 | 2105 | 2272 | 2481 | 1441 | 1481 | 1512 | 1382 | 1421 | 1422 | 1417 | 1519 | 1639 | 1778 |
| 18 | Belize | 130 | 133 | 149 | 156 | 167 | 228 | 236 | 257 | 257 | 278 | 66 | 69 | 72 | 75 | 75 | 116 | 122 | 125 | 123 | 125 |
| 19 | Benin | 14 | 15 | 15 | 15 | 16 | 28 | 29 | 31 | 35 | 39 | 5 | 5 | 6 | 7 | 8 | 9 | 11 | 12 | 15 | 18 |
| 20 | Bhutan | 8 | 8 | 8 | 9 | 9 | 48 | 52 | 52 | 61 | 64 | 7 | 7 | 7 | 8 | 8 | 43 | 47 | 47 | 55 | 58 |
| 21 | Bolivia | 48 | 53 | 53 | 52 | 49 | 104 | 114 | 120 | 122 | 125 | 31 | 35 | 35 | 35 | 33 | 66 | 75 | 79 | 81 | 83 |
| 22 | Bosnia and Herzegovina | 69 | 89 | 94 | 87 | 85 | 192 | 237 | 241 | 259 | 268 | 36 | 36 | 37 | 34 | 31 | 100 | 95 | 95 | 103 | 99 |
| 23 | Botswana | 169 | 158 | 164 | 173 | 190 | 260 | 260 | 294 | 309 | 381 | 100 | 95 | 100 | 107 | 126 | 153 | 155 | 178 | 192 | 252 |
| 24 | Brazil | 362 | 348 | 246 | 265 | 222 | 528 | 526 | 560 | 556 | 573 | 157 | 153 | 105 | 108 | 92 | 229 | 231 | 240 | 227 | 238 |
| 25 | Brunei Darussalam | 429 | 463 | 484 | 479 | 453 | 525 | 570 | 607 | 617 | 638 | 340 | 376 | 384 | 383 | 359 | 416 | 464 | 482 | 493 | 507 |
| 26 | Bulgaria | 58 | 60 | 80 | 75 | 81 | 227 | 200 | 272 | 283 | 303 | 48 | 47 | 67 | 62 | 67 | 188 | 159 | 227 | 233 | 248 |
| 27 | Burkina Faso | 7 | 8 | 8 | 6 | 6 | 25 | 26 | 30 | 29 | 27 | 5 | 5 | 5 | 4 | 3 | 17 | 17 | 20 | 18 | 16 |
| 28 | Burundi | 5 | 5 | 4 | 4 | 4 | 15 | 17 | 16 | 18 | 19 | 2 | 3 | 2 | 2 | 2 | 8 | 9 | 9 | 10 | 11 |
| 29 | Cambodia | 30 | 26 | 28 | 30 | 30 | 146 | 146 | 152 | 174 | 184 | 3 | 3 | 3 | 4 | 4 | 15 | 15 | 15 | 25 | 27 |
| 30 | Cameroon | 23 | 23 | 19 | 19 | 20 | 45 | 38 | 36 | 39 | 42 | 5 | 4 | 4 | 7 | 8 | 9 | 7 | 8 | 13 | 16 |
| 31 | Canada | 1864 | 1835 | 1949 | 2102 | 2163 | 2187 | 2288 | 2433 | 2580 | 2792 | 1305 | 1297 | 1372 | 1490 | 1533 | 1532 | 1617 | 1713 | 1828 | 1978 |
| 32 | Cape Verde | 46 | 52 | 54 | 54 | 57 | 108 | 123 | 128 | 153 | 165 | 35 | 41 | 43 | 45 | 47 | 82 | 97 | 102 | 127 | 138 |
| 33 | Central African Republic | 10 | 12 | 12 | 12 | 12 | 41 | 47 | 50 | 55 | 58 | 4 | 5 | 6 | 6 | 6 | 16 | 21 | 24 | 27 | 30 |
| 34 | Chad | 6 | 5 | 5 | 5 | 5 | 17 | 14 | 16 | 19 | 17 | 5 | 4 | 4 | 4 | 4 | 13 | 10 | 12 | 15 | 13 |
| 35 | Chile | 371 | 369 | 331 | 336 | 303 | 643 | 699 | 686 | 681 | 792 | 140 | 146 | 135 | 143 | 133 | 243 | 277 | 280 | 290 | 348 |
| 36 | China | 33 | 36 | 40 | 45 | 49 | 135 | 155 | 176 | 200 | 224 | 13 | 14 | 15 | 17 | 18 | 54 | 60 | 67 | 73 | 83 |
| 37 | Colombia | 205 | 140 | 133 | 108 | 105 | 497 | 373 | 395 | 350 | 356 | 98 | 84 | 82 | 73 | 69 | 237 | 225 | 245 | 236 | 234 |
| 38 | Comoros | 10 | 10 | 10 | 9 | 9 | 28 | 27 | 27 | 26 | 29 | 6 | 6 | 6 | 5 | 6 | 17 | 16 | 16 | 16 | 17 |
| 39 | Congo | 23 | 19 | 19 | 18 | 18 | 33 | 34 | 28 | 20 | 22 | 16 | 14 | 13 | 13 | 12 | 23 | 26 | 20 | 15 | 14 |
| 40 | Cook Islands | 258 | 216 | 214 | 196 | 198 | 430 | 452 | 442 | 444 | 598 | 188 | 155 | 139 | 126 | 134 | 312 | 325 | 288 | 286 | 404 |
| 41 | Costa Rica | 236 | 254 | 268 | 280 | 293 | 445 | 477 | 496 | 533 | 562 | 167 | 171 | 184 | 192 | 201 | 315 | 323 | 339 | 365 | 385 |
| 42 | Côte d'Ivoire | 48 | 54 | 51 | 42 | 41 | 107 | 117 | 119 | 123 | 127 | 9 | 10 | 10 | 6 | 7 | 20 | 22 | 24 | 19 | 20 |
| 43 | Croatia | 373 | 429 | 402 | 388 | 394 | 569 | 637 | 651 | 715 | 726 | 300 | 351 | 332 | 323 | 322 | 458 | 521 | 538 | 595 | 593 |
| 44 | Cuba | 137 | 143 | 163 | 175 | 185 | 166 | 170 | 188 | 193 | 229 | 114 | 121 | 139 | 150 | 160 | 139 | 144 | 161 | 166 | 198 |
| 45 | Cyprus | 909 | 991 | 862 | 909 | 932 | 938 | 948 | 917 | 905 | 941 | 457 | 516 | 436 | 443 | 445 | 472 | 493 | 464 | 441 | 449 |
| 46 | Czech Republic | 364 | 392 | 380 | 358 | 407 | 930 | 944 | 972 | 1031 | 1129 | 334 | 360 | 347 | 327 | 372 | 853 | 867 | 889 | 942 | 1031 |
| 47 | Democratic People's Republic of Korea | 10 | 16 | 19 | 21 | 22 | 27 | 47 | 54 | 41 | 44 | 7 | 12 | 14 | 15 | 16 | 19 | 36 | 40 | 30 | 32 |
| 48 | Democratic Republic of the Congo | 4 | 4 | 8 | 10 | 5 | 13 | 12 | 11 | 11 | 12 | 2 | 2 | 4 | 5 | 2 | 6 | 5 | 5 | 5 | 5 |
| 49 | Denmark | 2629 | 2725 | 2769 | 2474 | 2545 | 2099 | 2238 | 2344 | 2398 | 2503 | 2163 | 2234 | 2276 | 2042 | 2097 | 1727 | 1835 | 1927 | 1979 | 2063 |
| 50 | Djibouti | 60 | 59 | 58 | 58 | 58 | 90 | 89 | 88 | 89 | 90 | 35 | 34 | 34 | 34 | 34 | 52 | 52 | 51 | 52 | 53 |
| 51 | Dominica | 190 | 193 | 214 | 200 | 203 | 274 | 278 | 305 | 291 | 312 | 143 | 144 | 159 | 143 | 145 | 205 | 208 | 227 | 208 | 222 |
| 52 | Dominican Republic | 111 | 114 | 121 | 145 | 153 | 262 | 279 | 298 | 345 | 353 | 35 | 36 | 39 | 51 | 55 | 84 | 88 | 96 | 122 | 127 |
| 53 | Ecuador | 88 | 85 | 50 | 52 | 76 | 168 | 167 | 131 | 149 | 177 | 47 | 43 | 28 | 29 | 38 | 89 | 84 | 73 | 82 | 89 |
| 54 | Egypt | 47 | 48 | 52 | 52 | 46 | 121 | 125 | 134 | 139 | 153 | 21 | 22 | 24 | 24 | 22 | 56 | 57 | 62 | 64 | 75 |
| 55 | El Salvador | 153 | 165 | 163 | 169 | 174 | 332 | 347 | 348 | 364 | 376 | 59 | 70 | 71 | 76 | 81 | 128 | 148 | 151 | 164 | 175 |

| | Member State | Per capita total expenditure on health at average exchange rate (US$) | | | | | Per capita total expenditure on health at international dollar rate | | | | | Per capita government expenditure on health at average exchange rate (US$) | | | | | Per capita government expenditure on health at international dollar rate | | | | |
|---|---|---|---|---|---|---|---|---|---|---|---|---|---|---|---|---|---|---|---|---|---|
| | | 1997 | 1998 | 1999 | 2000 | 2001 | 1997 | 1998 | 1999 | 2000 | 2001 | 1997 | 1998 | 1999 | 2000 | 2001 | 1997 | 1998 | 1999 | 2000 | 2001 |
| 56 | Equatorial Guinea | 36 | 44 | 42 | 56 | 76 | 58 | 99 | 73 | 65 | 106 | 23 | 27 | 26 | 35 | 46 | 36 | 61 | 45 | 40 | 64 |
| 57 | Eritrea | 9 | 10 | 11 | 9 | 10 | 25 | 29 | 31 | 32 | 36 | 6 | 7 | 7 | 6 | 6 | 17 | 19 | 21 | 22 | 23 |
| 58 | Estonia | 182 | 223 | 244 | 222 | 226 | 430 | 494 | 548 | 551 | 562 | 158 | 193 | 196 | 170 | 176 | 373 | 427 | 440 | 423 | 438 |
| 59 | Ethiopia | 4 | 4 | 3 | 3 | 3 | 12 | 11 | 11 | 11 | 14 | 1 | 1 | 1 | 1 | 1 | 5 | 4 | 4 | 4 | 6 |
| 60 | Fiji | 106 | 82 | 85 | 80 | 79 | 187 | 189 | 184 | 213 | 224 | 71 | 54 | 56 | 52 | 53 | 125 | 124 | 120 | 139 | 150 |
| 61 | Finland | 1737 | 1734 | 1713 | 1550 | 1631 | 1543 | 1528 | 1614 | 1696 | 1845 | 1322 | 1323 | 1290 | 1164 | 1233 | 1174 | 1165 | 1215 | 1274 | 1395 |
| 62 | France | 2261 | 2307 | 2285 | 2067 | 2109 | 2028 | 2079 | 2204 | 2382 | 2567 | 1723 | 1754 | 1738 | 1568 | 1603 | 1546 | 1581 | 1676 | 1806 | 1951 |
| 63 | Gabon | 131 | 137 | 131 | 130 | 127 | 178 | 228 | 204 | 176 | 197 | 86 | 91 | 85 | 65 | 61 | 116 | 152 | 132 | 88 | 94 |
| 64 | Gambia | 22 | 24 | 23 | 20 | 19 | 62 | 74 | 73 | 73 | 78 | 10 | 10 | 11 | 9 | 9 | 29 | 32 | 34 | 34 | 39 |
| 65 | Georgia | 19 | 16 | 13 | 20 | 22 | 71 | 60 | 65 | 95 | 108 | 8 | 7 | 5 | 7 | 8 | 28 | 27 | 25 | 32 | 41 |
| 66 | Germany | 2753 | 2773 | 2731 | 2408 | 2412 | 2458 | 2515 | 2621 | 2766 | 2820 | 2073 | 2075 | 2043 | 1807 | 1807 | 1851 | 1882 | 1961 | 2075 | 2113 |
| 67 | Ghana | 15 | 17 | 17 | 11 | 12 | 44 | 49 | 49 | 52 | 60 | 7 | 9 | 9 | 6 | 7 | 21 | 26 | 27 | 29 | 36 |
| 68 | Greece | 1092 | 1087 | 1149 | 1015 | 1001 | 1326 | 1407 | 1523 | 1553 | 1522 | 577 | 566 | 614 | 570 | 560 | 701 | 732 | 813 | 872 | 852 |
| 69 | Grenada | 179 | 205 | 225 | 245 | 262 | 298 | 331 | 372 | 416 | 445 | 118 | 135 | 157 | 171 | 188 | 197 | 218 | 259 | 291 | 320 |
| 70 | Guatemala | 64 | 78 | 78 | 79 | 86 | 140 | 167 | 186 | 190 | 199 | 24 | 37 | 38 | 38 | 41 | 52 | 79 | 90 | 90 | 96 |
| 71 | Guinea | 18 | 15 | 16 | 13 | 13 | 54 | 52 | 58 | 57 | 61 | 10 | 8 | 9 | 7 | 7 | 31 | 27 | 32 | 30 | 33 |
| 72 | Guinea-Bissau | 12 | 9 | 10 | 10 | 8 | 44 | 31 | 36 | 41 | 37 | 5 | 4 | 5 | 5 | 5 | 19 | 14 | 18 | 23 | 20 |
| 73 | Guyana | 48 | 48 | 44 | 48 | 50 | 176 | 182 | 184 | 196 | 215 | 40 | 40 | 37 | 40 | 40 | 147 | 152 | 154 | 162 | 171 |
| 74 | Haiti | 20 | 23 | 24 | 22 | 22 | 51 | 54 | 53 | 56 | 56 | 10 | 11 | 12 | 11 | 12 | 26 | 27 | 27 | 28 | 30 |
| 75 | Honduras | 42 | 48 | 48 | 54 | 59 | 126 | 134 | 130 | 145 | 153 | 22 | 26 | 25 | 29 | 31 | 67 | 72 | 67 | 78 | 81 |
| 76 | Hungary | 309 | 315 | 320 | 305 | 345 | 684 | 731 | 771 | 813 | 914 | 251 | 251 | 250 | 231 | 258 | 556 | 581 | 602 | 614 | 686 |
| 77 | Iceland | 2190 | 2509 | 2877 | 2759 | 2441 | 2003 | 2226 | 2563 | 2607 | 2643 | 1820 | 2084 | 2417 | 2309 | 2025 | 1665 | 1848 | 2154 | 2182 | 2192 |
| 78 | India | 23 | 22 | 23 | 23 | 24 | 64 | 65 | 71 | 74 | 80 | 4 | 4 | 4 | 4 | 4 | 10 | 12 | 13 | 13 | 14 |
| 79 | Indonesia | 26 | 11 | 17 | 20 | 16 | 82 | 72 | 76 | 85 | 77 | 6 | 3 | 5 | 5 | 4 | 19 | 20 | 21 | 20 | 19 |
| 80 | Iran, Islamic Republic of | 149 | 172 | 243 | 310 | 350 | 326 | 342 | 382 | 390 | 422 | 67 | 76 | 102 | 129 | 152 | 147 | 150 | 160 | 162 | 183 |
| 81 | Iraq | 146 | 170 | 199 | 214 | 225 | 63 | 70 | 80 | 91 | 97 | 48 | 54 | 62 | 67 | 72 | 21 | 22 | 25 | 28 | 31 |
| 82 | Ireland | 1404 | 1451 | 1591 | 1586 | 1714 | 1417 | 1439 | 1625 | 1797 | 1935 | 1047 | 1110 | 1159 | 1162 | 1303 | 1057 | 1101 | 1183 | 1317 | 1470 |
| 83 | Israel | 1551 | 1505 | 1492 | 1612 | 1641 | 1656 | 1674 | 1725 | 1748 | 1839 | 1148 | 1084 | 1059 | 1124 | 1135 | 1226 | 1206 | 1224 | 1219 | 1272 |
| 84 | Italy | 1570 | 1606 | 1605 | 1518 | 1584 | 1682 | 1786 | 1876 | 2047 | 2204 | 1133 | 1154 | 1155 | 1114 | 1193 | 1214 | 1283 | 1351 | 1502 | 1660 |
| 85 | Jamaica | 177 | 179 | 169 | 173 | 191 | 227 | 226 | 215 | 224 | 253 | 100 | 107 | 86 | 82 | 80 | 128 | 135 | 110 | 105 | 106 |
| 86 | Japan | 2337 | 2216 | 2634 | 2890 | 2627 | 1734 | 1730 | 1852 | 2002 | 2131 | 1803 | 1715 | 2056 | 2245 | 2046 | 1338 | 1339 | 1445 | 1555 | 1660 |
| 87 | Jordan | 129 | 135 | 143 | 154 | 163 | 323 | 324 | 350 | 383 | 412 | 70 | 77 | 73 | 72 | 76 | 176 | 185 | 178 | 178 | 194 |
| 88 | Kazakhstan | 44 | 48 | 37 | 39 | 44 | 150 | 163 | 174 | 186 | 204 | 32 | 34 | 24 | 24 | 27 | 109 | 114 | 110 | 117 | 123 |
| 89 | Kenya | 29 | 33 | 28 | 30 | 29 | 110 | 116 | 111 | 124 | 114 | 6 | 8 | 5 | 7 | 6 | 24 | 28 | 21 | 30 | 24 |
| 90 | Kiribati | 53 | 47 | 49 | 45 | 40 | 141 | 141 | 144 | 148 | 143 | 53 | 46 | 48 | 44 | 40 | 139 | 140 | 143 | 146 | 141 |
| 91 | Kuwait | 596 | 562 | 536 | 553 | 537 | 638 | 750 | 617 | 540 | 612 | 474 | 443 | 422 | 435 | 423 | 507 | 591 | 486 | 425 | 482 |
| 92 | Kyrgyzstan | 21 | 19 | 13 | 12 | 12 | 130 | 131 | 119 | 108 | 108 | 10 | 10 | 6 | 6 | 6 | 63 | 65 | 58 | 52 | 53 |
| 93 | Lao People's Democratic Republic | 10 | 6 | 8 | 9 | 10 | 39 | 33 | 43 | 45 | 51 | 6 | 3 | 4 | 5 | 6 | 24 | 16 | 21 | 24 | 29 |
| 94 | Latvia | 157 | 171 | 190 | 191 | 210 | 385 | 412 | 439 | 446 | 509 | 89 | 104 | 113 | 107 | 110 | 219 | 250 | 262 | 249 | 267 |
| 95 | Lebanon | 532 | 594 | 587 | 607 | 500 | 642 | 701 | 719 | 794 | 673 | 165 | 162 | 157 | 178 | 141 | 200 | 191 | 192 | 232 | 189 |
| 96 | Lesotho | 31 | 30 | 31 | 29 | 23 | 94 | 98 | 105 | 109 | 101 | 24 | 23 | 25 | 24 | 18 | 71 | 77 | 85 | 88 | 80 |
| 97 | Liberia | 1 | 1 | 2 | 2 | 1 | 91 | 99 | 110 | 114 | 127 | 1 | 1 | 1 | 1 | 1 | 63 | 73 | 84 | 87 | 97 |
| 98 | Libyan Arab Jamahiriya | 250 | 249 | 177 | 175 | 143 | 274 | 301 | 282 | 233 | 239 | 120 | 124 | 87 | 90 | 80 | 131 | 149 | 138 | 120 | 134 |
| 99 | Lithuania | 165 | 197 | 190 | 200 | 206 | 401 | 454 | 431 | 454 | 478 | 126 | 148 | 140 | 141 | 146 | 306 | 341 | 317 | 321 | 337 |
| 100 | Luxembourg | 2492 | 2612 | 2756 | 2411 | 2600 | 2239 | 2405 | 2631 | 2659 | 2905 | 2272 | 2373 | 2463 | 2152 | 2336 | 2041 | 2185 | 2352 | 2374 | 2611 |
| 101 | Madagascar | 4 | 7 | 6 | 6 | 6 | 16 | 24 | 23 | 23 | 20 | 3 | 4 | 4 | 4 | 4 | 12 | 15 | 13 | 15 | 13 |
| 102 | Malawi | 21 | 15 | 14 | 12 | 13 | 41 | 41 | 42 | 42 | 39 | 8 | 5 | 5 | 4 | 4 | 15 | 14 | 16 | 15 | 14 |
| 103 | Malaysia | 129 | 99 | 109 | 129 | 143 | 237 | 237 | 257 | 297 | 345 | 69 | 51 | 58 | 69 | 77 | 127 | 122 | 136 | 158 | 185 |
| 104 | Maldives | 83 | 85 | 95 | 104 | 98 | 180 | 190 | 219 | 272 | 263 | 68 | 70 | 78 | 87 | 82 | 147 | 155 | 181 | 228 | 220 |
| 105 | Mali | 10 | 11 | 10 | 10 | 11 | 25 | 25 | 25 | 32 | 30 | 5 | 4 | 3 | 4 | 4 | 11 | 9 | 8 | 13 | 12 |
| 106 | Malta | 738 | 784 | 760 | 807 | 808 | 739 | 759 | 782 | 804 | 813 | 501 | 543 | 513 | 553 | 554 | 502 | 526 | 528 | 551 | 557 |
| 107 | Marshall Islands | 186 | 187 | 182 | 188 | 190 | 332 | 331 | 327 | 340 | 343 | 131 | 124 | 118 | 122 | 123 | 234 | 220 | 213 | 221 | 222 |
| 108 | Mauritania | 15 | 14 | 13 | 13 | 12 | 38 | 40 | 43 | 45 | 45 | 11 | 10 | 9 | 9 | 9 | 28 | 29 | 31 | 33 | 33 |
| 109 | Mauritius | 109 | 114 | 113 | 127 | 128 | 227 | 256 | 259 | 288 | 323 | 67 | 72 | 70 | 74 | 76 | 139 | 160 | 160 | 169 | 192 |
| 110 | Mexico | 231 | 244 | 277 | 327 | 370 | 418 | 446 | 471 | 501 | 544 | 105 | 114 | 130 | 150 | 164 | 190 | 208 | 221 | 229 | 241 |

### Annex Table 6 Selected national health accounts indicators: measured levels of per capita expenditure on health, 1997–2001

Figures computed by WHO to assure comparability;[a] they are not necessarily the official statistics of Member States, which may use alternative rigorous methods.

| | Member State | Per capita total expenditure on health at average exchange rate (US$) | | | | | Per capita total expenditure on health at international dollar rate | | | | | Per capita government expenditure on health at average exchange rate (US$) | | | | | Per capita government expenditure on health at international dollar rate | | | | |
|---|---|---|---|---|---|---|---|---|---|---|---|---|---|---|---|---|---|---|---|---|---|
| | | 1997 | 1998 | 1999 | 2000 | 2001 | 1997 | 1998 | 1999 | 2000 | 2001 | 1997 | 1998 | 1999 | 2000 | 2001 | 1997 | 1998 | 1999 | 2000 | 2001 |
| 111 | Micronesia, Federated States of | 170 | 167 | 169 | 169 | 172 | 315 | 304 | 302 | 296 | 319 | 125 | 121 | 121 | 121 | 124 | 232 | 221 | 217 | 212 | 230 |
| 112 | Monaco | 1689 | 1783 | 1812 | 1610 | 1653 | 1516 | 1608 | 1751 | 1863 | 2016 | 924 | 956 | 955 | 878 | 927 | 829 | 862 | 923 | 1016 | 1131 |
| 113 | Mongolia | 22 | 24 | 21 | 23 | 25 | 84 | 106 | 110 | 118 | 122 | 14 | 16 | 14 | 16 | 18 | 52 | 69 | 73 | 83 | 88 |
| 114 | Morocco | 52 | 56 | 54 | 54 | 59 | 147 | 160 | 159 | 171 | 199 | 13 | 16 | 16 | 18 | 23 | 38 | 45 | 46 | 58 | 78 |
| 115 | Mozambique | 10 | 11 | 11 | 12 | 11 | 29 | 32 | 35 | 40 | 47 | 6 | 7 | 7 | 8 | 8 | 18 | 20 | 23 | 27 | 32 |
| 116 | Myanmar | 81 | 109 | 147 | 162 | 197 | 21 | 21 | 22 | 23 | 26 | 12 | 12 | 17 | 28 | 35 | 3 | 2 | 3 | 4 | 5 |
| 117 | Namibia | 141 | 128 | 127 | 126 | 114 | 305 | 307 | 323 | 330 | 342 | 103 | 92 | 93 | 87 | 77 | 222 | 221 | 236 | 228 | 232 |
| 118 | Nauru | 719 | 640 | 705 | 643 | 588 | 981 | 987 | 941 | 921 | 1015 | 640 | 570 | 628 | 571 | 521 | 874 | 878 | 839 | 819 | 900 |
| 119 | Nepal | 12 | 11 | 12 | 12 | 12 | 58 | 60 | 59 | 61 | 63 | 4 | 4 | 3 | 4 | 3 | 18 | 20 | 18 | 18 | 19 |
| 120 | Netherlands | 1968 | 2151 | 2191 | 2012 | 2138 | 1951 | 2164 | 2305 | 2358 | 2612 | 1335 | 1385 | 1386 | 1275 | 1354 | 1323 | 1393 | 1458 | 1495 | 1654 |
| 121 | New Zealand | 1301 | 1125 | 1169 | 1054 | 1073 | 1357 | 1440 | 1534 | 1611 | 1724 | 1005 | 867 | 911 | 822 | 823 | 1049 | 1109 | 1195 | 1257 | 1323 |
| 122 | Nicaragua | 45 | 44 | 44 | 55 | 60 | 117 | 110 | 113 | 147 | 158 | 24 | 27 | 24 | 29 | 29 | 63 | 66 | 61 | 77 | 77 |
| 123 | Niger | 6 | 7 | 6 | 6 | 6 | 21 | 22 | 22 | 21 | 22 | 3 | 3 | 3 | 2 | 2 | 9 | 9 | 9 | 9 | 9 |
| 124 | Nigeria | 35 | 37 | 10 | 12 | 15 | 23 | 26 | 26 | 26 | 31 | 4 | 6 | 2 | 2 | 3 | 3 | 4 | 4 | 4 | 7 |
| 125 | Niue | 344 | 330 | 335 | 290 | 289 | 945 | 910 | 990 | 1068 | 1041 | 334 | 321 | 325 | 281 | 280 | 917 | 883 | 961 | 1036 | 1010 |
| 126 | Norway | 2797 | 2867 | 3025 | 2817 | 2981 | 2193 | 2438 | 2550 | 2755 | 2920 | 2357 | 2428 | 2576 | 2400 | 2550 | 1848 | 2065 | 2172 | 2347 | 2497 |
| 127 | Oman | 229 | 219 | 221 | 230 | 225 | 348 | 392 | 357 | 316 | 343 | 187 | 180 | 182 | 187 | 181 | 285 | 322 | 294 | 256 | 277 |
| 128 | Pakistan | 19 | 19 | 18 | 18 | 16 | 73 | 77 | 80 | 85 | 85 | 5 | 6 | 5 | 4 | 4 | 20 | 22 | 20 | 21 | 21 |
| 129 | Palau | 498 | 502 | 447 | 454 | 426 | 695 | 789 | 823 | 835 | 886 | 456 | 466 | 408 | 416 | 392 | 636 | 733 | 753 | 766 | 816 |
| 130 | Panama | 231 | 244 | 252 | 260 | 258 | 398 | 411 | 434 | 452 | 458 | 158 | 171 | 176 | 180 | 178 | 272 | 289 | 303 | 313 | 316 |
| 131 | Papua New Guinea | 32 | 29 | 28 | 27 | 24 | 107 | 121 | 144 | 145 | 144 | 28 | 26 | 25 | 24 | 21 | 95 | 110 | 129 | 130 | 128 |
| 132 | Paraguay | 143 | 121 | 115 | 112 | 97 | 320 | 305 | 326 | 323 | 332 | 47 | 45 | 45 | 43 | 37 | 105 | 114 | 129 | 124 | 127 |
| 133 | Peru | 106 | 105 | 99 | 97 | 97 | 207 | 216 | 231 | 228 | 231 | 54 | 57 | 55 | 54 | 53 | 107 | 118 | 129 | 126 | 127 |
| 134 | Philippines | 41 | 31 | 36 | 34 | 30 | 168 | 162 | 165 | 169 | 169 | 18 | 14 | 16 | 16 | 14 | 73 | 70 | 74 | 81 | 77 |
| 135 | Poland | 228 | 264 | 249 | 245 | 289 | 461 | 543 | 558 | 572 | 629 | 164 | 173 | 177 | 171 | 208 | 332 | 355 | 397 | 400 | 452 |
| 136 | Portugal | 903 | 956 | 986 | 938 | 982 | 1339 | 1370 | 1457 | 1512 | 1618 | 586 | 626 | 666 | 642 | 677 | 868 | 898 | 985 | 1036 | 1116 |
| 137 | Qatar | 813 | 819 | 824 | 860 | 885 | 842 | 1006 | 874 | 720 | 782 | 624 | 630 | 626 | 638 | 650 | 647 | 773 | 665 | 534 | 574 |
| 138 | Republic of Korea | 520 | 352 | 484 | 577 | 532 | 657 | 628 | 762 | 893 | 948 | 213 | 163 | 209 | 256 | 236 | 270 | 290 | 329 | 396 | 421 |
| 139 | Republic of Moldova | 38 | 28 | 16 | 18 | 20 | 159 | 125 | 99 | 106 | 112 | 27 | 17 | 8 | 9 | 10 | 112 | 76 | 50 | 53 | 56 |
| 140 | Romania | 79 | 124 | 108 | 109 | 117 | 320 | 409 | 424 | 428 | 460 | 53 | 92 | 84 | 86 | 93 | 214 | 303 | 330 | 338 | 365 |
| 141 | Russian Federation | 167 | 112 | 71 | 95 | 115 | 390 | 382 | 378 | 420 | 454 | 122 | 77 | 46 | 66 | 78 | 284 | 263 | 245 | 293 | 310 |
| 142 | Rwanda | 16 | 15 | 14 | 13 | 11 | 39 | 39 | 41 | 43 | 44 | 8 | 8 | 8 | 7 | 6 | 19 | 20 | 22 | 23 | 24 |
| 143 | Saint Kitts and Nevis | 304 | 323 | 335 | 364 | 393 | 464 | 495 | 507 | 535 | 576 | 202 | 216 | 222 | 241 | 260 | 307 | 330 | 336 | 355 | 382 |
| 144 | Saint Lucia | 169 | 187 | 192 | 195 | 199 | 240 | 257 | 254 | 263 | 272 | 105 | 123 | 125 | 127 | 129 | 150 | 169 | 166 | 171 | 176 |
| 145 | Saint Vincent and the Grenadines | 155 | 161 | 170 | 170 | 178 | 295 | 302 | 324 | 341 | 358 | 99 | 101 | 106 | 111 | 113 | 188 | 189 | 203 | 222 | 227 |
| 146 | Samoa | 79 | 76 | 84 | 80 | 74 | 167 | 185 | 210 | 219 | 199 | 58 | 56 | 62 | 61 | 61 | 123 | 136 | 156 | 168 | 164 |
| 147 | San Marino | 1188 | 1252 | 1286 | 1196 | 1222 | 1275 | 1391 | 1511 | 1610 | 1711 | 892 | 944 | 974 | 922 | 953 | 957 | 1049 | 1145 | 1240 | 1334 |
| 148 | Sao Tome and Principe | 10 | 8 | 8 | 7 | 7 | 26 | 25 | 21 | 22 | 22 | 6 | 6 | 5 | 5 | 5 | 17 | 17 | 14 | 15 | 15 |
| 149 | Saudi Arabia | 432 | 368 | 340 | 376 | 375 | 680 | 680 | 583 | 565 | 591 | 334 | 281 | 251 | 280 | 280 | 526 | 519 | 430 | 421 | 441 |
| 150 | Senegal | 25 | 25 | 24 | 22 | 22 | 53 | 53 | 56 | 58 | 63 | 14 | 14 | 14 | 12 | 13 | 29 | 30 | 31 | 33 | 37 |
| 151 | Serbia and Montenegro | 198 | 149 | 185 | 89 | 103 | 621 | 542 | 601 | 528 | 616 | 147 | 106 | 131 | 69 | 82 | 460 | 386 | 426 | 409 | 488 |
| 152 | Seychelles | 490 | 500 | 491 | 444 | 450 | 732 | 752 | 746 | 733 | 770 | 355 | 347 | 338 | 295 | 307 | 529 | 522 | 513 | 487 | 525 |
| 153 | Sierra Leone | 7 | 5 | 6 | 6 | 7 | 23 | 21 | 23 | 25 | 26 | 3 | 2 | 3 | 4 | 4 | 11 | 9 | 13 | 15 | 16 |
| 154 | Singapore | 936 | 902 | 851 | 826 | 816 | 834 | 926 | 947 | 925 | 993 | 365 | 375 | 327 | 291 | 274 | 325 | 385 | 363 | 326 | 333 |
| 155 | Slovakia | 230 | 235 | 218 | 208 | 216 | 608 | 636 | 664 | 642 | 681 | 211 | 215 | 196 | 186 | 192 | 558 | 583 | 595 | 574 | 608 |
| 156 | Slovenia | 712 | 813 | 829 | 765 | 821 | 1097 | 1223 | 1299 | 1421 | 1545 | 564 | 616 | 626 | 582 | 615 | 868 | 927 | 981 | 1080 | 1157 |
| 157 | Solomon Islands | 45 | 40 | 42 | 39 | 40 | 100 | 106 | 113 | 141 | 133 | 41 | 37 | 39 | 37 | 37 | 92 | 99 | 106 | 132 | 124 |
| 158 | Somalia | 5 | 6 | 7 | 6 | 6 | 19 | 18 | 18 | 15 | 15 | 2 | 3 | 3 | 3 | 3 | 9 | 8 | 8 | 7 | 7 |
| 159 | South Africa | 315 | 270 | 264 | 253 | 222 | 622 | 604 | 623 | 633 | 652 | 145 | 114 | 113 | 106 | 92 | 287 | 256 | 265 | 265 | 270 |
| 160 | Spain | 1067 | 1115 | 1140 | 1048 | 1088 | 1273 | 1347 | 1428 | 1505 | 1607 | 773 | 805 | 822 | 751 | 778 | 922 | 973 | 1030 | 1078 | 1148 |
| 161 | Sri Lanka | 27 | 29 | 30 | 32 | 30 | 91 | 102 | 112 | 121 | 122 | 13 | 15 | 15 | 16 | 15 | 45 | 52 | 55 | 60 | 60 |
| 162 | Sudan | 13 | 14 | 12 | 14 | 14 | 31 | 39 | 38 | 41 | 39 | 2 | 3 | 3 | 4 | 3 | 6 | 9 | 9 | 12 | 7 |
| 163 | Suriname | 207 | 194 | 104 | 186 | 153 | 371 | 404 | 402 | 407 | 398 | 108 | 120 | 62 | 118 | 92 | 194 | 249 | 239 | 258 | 240 |
| 164 | Swaziland | 45 | 43 | 43 | 45 | 41 | 137 | 146 | 152 | 163 | 167 | 32 | 30 | 29 | 31 | 28 | 98 | 103 | 103 | 114 | 115 |
| 165 | Sweden | 2300 | 2336 | 2395 | 2268 | 2150 | 1855 | 1903 | 2053 | 2195 | 2270 | 1975 | 2005 | 2053 | 1929 | 1832 | 1592 | 1633 | 1760 | 1866 | 1935 |

| | Member State | Per capita total expenditure on health at average exchange rate (US$) | | | | | Per capita total expenditure on health at international dollar rate | | | | | Per capita government expenditure on health at average exchange rate (US$) | | | | | Per capita government expenditure on health at international dollar rate | | | | |
|---|---|---|---|---|---|---|---|---|---|---|---|---|---|---|---|---|---|---|---|---|---|
| | | 1997 | 1998 | 1999 | 2000 | 2001 | 1997 | 1998 | 1999 | 2000 | 2001 | 1997 | 1998 | 1999 | 2000 | 2001 | 1997 | 1998 | 1999 | 2000 | 2001 |
| 166 | Switzerland | 3759 | 3909 | 3875 | 3574 | 3779 | 2841 | 2952 | 3080 | 3160 | 3322 | 2073 | 2145 | 2144 | 1988 | 2159 | 1567 | 1619 | 1704 | 1758 | 1897 |
| 167 | Syrian Arab Republic | 59 | 60 | 63 | 64 | 65 | 427 | 452 | 473 | 439 | 427 | 22 | 23 | 25 | 26 | 29 | 160 | 174 | 184 | 179 | 188 |
| 168 | Tajikistan | 6 | 8 | 6 | 5 | 6 | 38 | 36 | 36 | 38 | 43 | 2 | 3 | 2 | 2 | 2 | 15 | 12 | 11 | 11 | 12 |
| 169 | Thailand | 95 | 73 | 75 | 73 | 69 | 247 | 234 | 233 | 241 | 254 | 54 | 45 | 43 | 41 | 39 | 141 | 143 | 134 | 137 | 145 |
| 170 | The former Yugoslav Republic of Macedonia | 114 | 135 | 117 | 106 | 115 | 263 | 340 | 303 | 302 | 331 | 96 | 118 | 100 | 90 | 98 | 221 | 296 | 259 | 255 | 281 |
| 171 | Timor-Leste | 46 | 32 | 30 | 28 | 42 | n/a | n/a | n/a | n/a | n/a | 41 | 27 | 27 | 20 | 25 | n/a | n/a | n/a | n/a | n/a |
| 172 | Togo | 11 | 12 | 13 | 8 | 8 | 40 | 51 | 55 | 45 | 45 | 5 | 7 | 8 | 4 | 4 | 20 | 30 | 34 | 22 | 22 |
| 173 | Tonga | 97 | 87 | 87 | 81 | 73 | 192 | 194 | 203 | 209 | 223 | 58 | 53 | 53 | 49 | 45 | 115 | 119 | 123 | 126 | 138 |
| 174 | Trinidad and Tobago | 203 | 229 | 238 | 248 | 279 | 332 | 378 | 379 | 360 | 388 | 87 | 106 | 111 | 114 | 121 | 143 | 175 | 176 | 165 | 168 |
| 175 | Tunisia | 132 | 133 | 139 | 126 | 134 | 360 | 367 | 398 | 417 | 463 | 102 | 102 | 106 | 94 | 101 | 280 | 282 | 302 | 310 | 350 |
| 176 | Turkey | 125 | 149 | 137 | 148 | 109 | 272 | 301 | 291 | 311 | 294 | 90 | 107 | 98 | 105 | 77 | 195 | 217 | 207 | 222 | 209 |
| 177 | Turkmenistan | 28 | 34 | 42 | 42 | 57 | 170 | 195 | 226 | 222 | 245 | 21 | 24 | 29 | 31 | 42 | 129 | 137 | 153 | 166 | 180 |
| 178 | Tuvalu | 71 | 68 | 75 | 74 | 66 | 495 | 558 | 566 | 553 | 673 | 42 | 41 | 43 | 39 | 35 | 293 | 330 | 324 | 296 | 359 |
| 179 | Uganda | 12 | 11 | 11 | 14 | 14 | 32 | 32 | 37 | 52 | 57 | 3 | 4 | 5 | 8 | 8 | 9 | 12 | 15 | 29 | 33 |
| 180 | Ukraine | 53 | 42 | 27 | 27 | 33 | 179 | 166 | 145 | 156 | 176 | 40 | 30 | 19 | 18 | 22 | 134 | 119 | 99 | 107 | 120 |
| 181 | United Arab Emirates | 703 | 724 | 729 | 821 | 849 | 727 | 754 | 710 | 781 | 921 | 539 | 557 | 552 | 623 | 643 | 558 | 580 | 538 | 593 | 698 |
| 182 | United Kingdom | 1563 | 1683 | 1792 | 1783 | 1835 | 1516 | 1573 | 1704 | 1827 | 1989 | 1253 | 1349 | 1442 | 1444 | 1508 | 1214 | 1261 | 1371 | 1479 | 1634 |
| 183 | United Republic of Tanzania | 10 | 11 | 11 | 11 | 12 | 21 | 23 | 23 | 25 | 26 | 4 | 5 | 5 | 5 | 5 | 9 | 11 | 10 | 12 | 12 |
| 184 | United States of America | 3939 | 4095 | 4287 | 4540 | 4887 | 3939 | 4095 | 4287 | 4540 | 4887 | 1784 | 1824 | 1895 | 2005 | 2168 | 1784 | 1824 | 1895 | 2005 | 2168 |
| 185 | Uruguay | 662 | 696 | 675 | 653 | 603 | 894 | 965 | 988 | 986 | 971 | 270 | 286 | 326 | 304 | 279 | 364 | 396 | 477 | 459 | 450 |
| 186 | Uzbekistan | 27 | 24 | 25 | 21 | 17 | 89 | 85 | 82 | 88 | 91 | 19 | 18 | 19 | 15 | 12 | 65 | 64 | 60 | 66 | 68 |
| 187 | Vanuatu | 47 | 43 | 44 | 44 | 42 | 102 | 105 | 109 | 109 | 107 | 31 | 28 | 28 | 27 | 25 | 67 | 69 | 70 | 66 | 63 |
| 188 | Venezuela, Bolivarian Republic of | 210 | 221 | 244 | 296 | 307 | 338 | 333 | 324 | 353 | 386 | 120 | 120 | 132 | 169 | 191 | 193 | 181 | 175 | 201 | 240 |
| 189 | Viet Nam | 16 | 18 | 18 | 21 | 21 | 92 | 108 | 113 | 128 | 134 | 5 | 6 | 6 | 6 | 6 | 29 | 35 | 37 | 36 | 38 |
| 190 | Yemen | 16 | 16 | 17 | 19 | 20 | 52 | 63 | 58 | 59 | 69 | 5 | 6 | 5 | 7 | 7 | 16 | 25 | 19 | 21 | 24 |
| 191 | Zambia | 24 | 20 | 19 | 18 | 19 | 51 | 48 | 47 | 47 | 52 | 13 | 12 | 11 | 10 | 10 | 28 | 28 | 26 | 25 | 27 |
| 192 | Zimbabwe | 66 | 59 | 35 | 42 | 45 | 221 | 275 | 192 | 182 | 142 | 39 | 33 | 17 | 22 | 20 | 131 | 154 | 94 | 92 | 64 |

a See explanatory notes for sources and methods.

n/a Used when the information accessed indicates that a cell should have an entry but no estimates could be made.

**Annex Table 7 Millennium Development Goals: selected health indicators in all WHO Member States, 2000 (unless specified)**

Figures computed by WHO to assure comparability;[a] they are not necessarily the official statistics of Member States, which may use alternative rigorous methods

| | Member State | Children under five years of age underweight for age (%) | Children under five years of age underweight for age Year | Under-five mortality rate (per 1000 live births) | Infant mortality rate (per 1000 live births) | One-year-olds immunized against measles (%) (2001) | Maternal mortality ratio (per 100 000 live births) | Births attended by skilled health personnel (%) |
|---|---|---|---|---|---|---|---|---|
| 1 | Afghanistan | 49.3 | 1997 | 257 | 189 | 46 | 1900 | n/a |
| 2 | Albania | 14.3 | 2000 | 27 | 23 | 95 | 55 | 99.1 |
| 3 | Algeria | 6 | 2000 | 51 | 42 | 83 | 140 | 92 |
| 4 | Andorra | n/a | n/a | 5 | 4 | 90 | n/a | n/a |
| 5 | Angola | 30.5 | 2001 | 262 | 153 | 72 | 1700 | 22.5 |
| 6 | Antigua and Barbuda | n/a | n/a | 21 | 16 | 97 | n/a | 100 |
| 7 | Argentina | 5.4 | 1995-96 | 19 | 17 | 94 | 70 | 97.5 |
| 8 | Armenia | 2.6 | 2000-01 | 37 | 31 | 93 | 55 | 96.9 |
| 9 | Australia | 0 | 1995-96 | 6 | 5 | 93 | 6 | 100 |
| 10 | Austria | n/a | n/a | 6 | 5 | 79 | 5 | n/a |
| 11 | Azerbaijan | 16.8 | 2000 | 75 | 61 | 99 | 94 | 87.5 |
| 12 | Bahamas | n/a | n/a | 18 | 15 | 92 | 60 | 99 |
| 13 | Bahrain | 8.7 | 1995 | 13 | 10 | 98 | 33 | 98.4 |
| 14 | Bangladesh | 47.7 | 1999-00 | 82 | 63 | 76 | 380 | 12.1 |
| 15 | Barbados | 5.9 | 1981 | 19 | 17 | 92 | 95 | 91 |
| 16 | Belarus | n/a | n/a | 14 | 10 | 99 | 36 | n/a |
| 17 | Belgium | n/a | n/a | 6 | 5 | 75 | 10 | n/a |
| 18 | Belize | 6.2 | 1992 | 41 | 33 | 93 | 140 | 76.9 |
| 19 | Benin | 22.9 | 2001 | 161 | 96 | 65 | 850 | 59.8 |
| 20 | Bhutan | 18.7 | 1999 | 98 | 75 | 78 | 420 | 15 |
| 21 | Bolivia | 9.5 | 1998 | 80 | 63 | 79 | 420 | 59.3 |
| 22 | Bosnia and Herzegovina | 4.1 | 2000 | 18 | 15 | 92 | 31 | 99.5 |
| 23 | Botswana | 12.5 | 2000 | 93 | 60 | 90 | 100 | 98.5 |
| 24 | Brazil | 5.7 | 1996 | 41 | 37 | 95 | 260 | 87.6 |
| 25 | Brunei Darussalam | n/a | n/a | 14 | 11 | 99 | 37 | 99 |
| 26 | Bulgaria | n/a | n/a | 16 | 14 | 90 | 32 | n/a |
| 27 | Burkina Faso | 34.3 | 1998-99 | 225 | 117 | 46 | 1000 | 31 |
| 28 | Burundi | 45.1 | 2000 | 190 | 116 | 75 | 1000 | 24.9 |
| 29 | Cambodia | 45.2 | 2000 | 134 | 106 | 59 | 450 | 31.8 |
| 30 | Cameroon | 22.2 | 1998 | 155 | 91 | 62 | 730 | 56.1 |
| 31 | Canada | n/a | n/a | 6 | 5 | 96 | 5 | 98 |
| 32 | Cape Verde | 13.5 | 1994 | 40 | 32 | 72 | 150 | 53.2 |
| 33 | Central African Republic | 24.3 | 2000 | 179 | 120 | 35 | 1100 | 44 |
| 34 | Chad | 28 | 2000 | 193 | 112 | 36 | 1100 | 16.2 |
| 35 | Chile | 0.8 | 1999 | 16 | 14 | 99 | 30 | 100 |
| 36 | China | 10 | 2000 | 37 | 31 | 79 | 56 | 89.3 |
| 37 | Colombia | 6.7 | 2000 | 24 | 22 | 90 | 130 | 86.4 |
| 38 | Comoros | 25.4 | 2000 | 82 | 65 | 70 | 480 | 61.8 |
| 39 | Congo | 23.9 | 1987 | 106 | 68 | 35 | 510 | n/a |
| 40 | Cook Islands | n/a | n/a | 23 | 18 | 84 | n/a | 100 |
| 41 | Costa Rica | 5.1 | 1996 | 11 | 10 | 82 | 25 | 98.2 |
| 42 | Côte d'Ivoire | 21.2 | 1998-99 | 167 | 113 | 61 | 690 | 46.9 |
| 43 | Croatia | 0.6 | 1995-96 | 8 | 7 | 94 | 10 | n/a |
| 44 | Cuba | 3.9 | 2000 | 9 | 7 | 99 | 33 | 100 |
| 45 | Cyprus | n/a | n/a | 8 | 7 | 86 | 47 | n/a |
| 46 | Czech Republic | 1 | 1991 | 5 | 4 | 97 | 9 | n/a |
| 47 | Democratic People's Republic of Korea | 27.9 | 2000 | 55 | 43 | n/a | 67 | n/a |
| 48 | Democratic Republic of the Congo | 31 | 2001 | 212 | 127 | 37 | 990 | 69.7 |
| 49 | Denmark | n/a | n/a | 6 | 5 | 94 | 7 | n/a |
| 50 | Djibouti | 18.2 | 1996 | 150 | 94 | 49 | 730 | n/a |
| 51 | Dominica | n/a | n/a | 14 | 11 | 99 | n/a | 100 |
| 52 | Dominican Republic | 4.6 | 2000 | 37 | 31 | 98 | 150 | 95.5 |
| 53 | Ecuador | 14.3 | 1998 | 36 | 26 | 99 | 130 | 68.7 |
| 54 | Egypt | 10.7 | 1998 | 45 | 38 | 97 | 84 | 60.9 |
| 55 | El Salvador | 9.5 | 1998 | 37 | 28 | 82 | 150 | 58 |

| | HIV prevalence among 15–49-year-olds (%) | Malaria mortality rate (per 100 000) | Tuberculosis prevalence (per 100 000) | Tuberculosis mortality rate (per 100 000) | Tuberculosis cases | | Population using solid fuels (%) | Population with sustainable access to an improved water source (%) | | Population with access to improved sanitation (%) | |
|---|---|---|---|---|---|---|---|---|---|---|---|
| | | | | | Detected under DOTS (2001) | Cured under DOTS | | Urban | Rural | Urban | Rural |
| 1 | <0.1 | 10 | 708 | 96 | 15 | 86 | >95 | 19 | 11 | 25 | 8 |
| 2 | <0.1 | 0 | 30 | 3 | 20 | n/a | 76 | 99 | 95 | 99 | 85 |
| 3 | 0.1 | 23 | 48 | 2 | 100 | 87 | <5 | 94 | 82 | 99 | 81 |
| 4 | 0.7 | 0 | 20 | 1 | 34 | 50 | <5 | 100 | 100 | 100 | 100 |
| 5 | 1.6 | 383 | 577 | 64 | ... | ... | >95 | 34 | 40 | 70 | 30 |
| 6 | 0.7 | 0 | 9 | 1 | 52 | 100 | <5 | 95 | 89 | 98 | 94 |
| 7 | 0.7 | 0 | 68 | 2 | 39 | 55 | <5 | 85 | 30 | 89 | 48 |
| 8 | 0.1 | 0 | 94 | 6 | 22 | 87 | 66 | n/a | n/a | n/a | n/a |
| 9 | 0.1 | 0 | 6 | 0 | 14 | 74 | <5 | 100 | 100 | 100 | 100 |
| 10 | 0.2 | 0 | 9 | 1 | 46 | 73 | <5 | 100 | 100 | 100 | 100 |
| 11 | <0.1 | 0 | 112 | 10 | 0 | 91 | 37 | 93 | 58 | 90 | 70 |
| 12 | 3.7 | 0 | 50 | 3 | ... | ... | <5 | 98 | 86 | 100 | 100 |
| 13 | 0.3 | 0 | 38 | 2 | 59 | 73 | <5 | 100[b] | n/a | 100[b] | n/a |
| 14 | <0.1 | 9 | 479 | 56 | 26 | 83 | >95 | 99 | 97 | 71 | 41 |
| 15 | 1.4 | 0 | 20 | 0 | 30 | n/a | 57 | 100 | 100 | 100 | 100 |
| 16 | 0.4 | 0 | 114 | 8 | ... | ... | 11 | 100 | 100 | n/a | n/a |
| 17 | 0.2 | 0 | 15 | 1 | 75 | n/a | <5 | n/a | n/a | n/a | n/a |
| 18 | 1.9 | 0 | 72 | 14 | n/a | 78 | <5 | 100 | 82 | 71 | 25 |
| 19 | 2.3 | 190 | 122 | 10 | ... | ... | 89 | 74 | 55 | 46 | 6 |
| 20 | <0.1 | 12 | 223 | 19 | 26 | 90 | <5 | 86 | 60 | 65 | 70 |
| 21 | <0.1 | 0 | 322 | 36 | 81 | 79 | 61 | 95 | 64 | 86 | 42 |
| 22 | <0.1 | 0 | 76 | 6 | 71 | 94 | 74 | n/a | n/a | n/a | n/a |
| 23 | 37.5 | 8 | 288 | 28 | 75 | 77 | 65 | 100 | 90 | 88 | 43 |
| 24 | 0.6 | 0 | 103 | 9 | 8 | 73 | 27 | 95 | 53 | 84 | 43 |
| 25 | <0.1 | 0 | 39 | 3 | 100 | 63 | 70 | n/a | n/a | n/a | n/a |
| 26 | <0.1 | 0 | 67 | 4 | 15 | n/a | 31 | 100 | 100 | 100 | 100 |
| 27 | 4.2 | 223 | 269 | 30 | 15 | 60 | >95 | 66 | 37 | 39 | 27 |
| 28 | 6.4 | 149 | 445 | 50 | 39 | 80 | >95 | 91 | 77 | 68 | 90 |
| 29 | 2.8 | 24 | 743 | 91 | 41 | 91 | >95 | 54 | 26 | 56 | 10 |
| 30 | 7.4 | 116 | 232 | 25 | ... | ... | 77 | 78 | 39 | 92 | 66 |
| 31 | 0.3 | 0 | 5 | 1 | 56 | 80 | <5 | 100 | 99 | 100 | 99 |
| 32 | <0.1 | 20 | 402 | 44 | 40 | n/a | <5 | 64 | 89 | 95 | 32 |
| 33 | 12.8 | 132 | 461 | 51 | 8 | 57 | >95 | 89 | 57 | 38 | 16 |
| 34 | 4.9 | 232 | 370 | 41 | ... | ... | 95 | 31 | 26 | 81 | 13 |
| 35 | 0.3 | 0 | 23 | 4 | 97 | 82 | 15 | 99 | 58 | 96 | 97 |
| 36 | <0.1 | 0 | 250 | 21 | 29 | 95 | 80 | 93.7 | 66.1 | 68.5 | 25.8 |
| 37 | 0.4 | 1 | 62 | 6 | ... | ... | 36 | 99 | 70 | 96 | 56 |
| 38 | 0.1 | 65 | 125 | 9 | ... | ... | <5 | 98 | 95 | 98 | 98 |
| 39 | 5.5 | 54 | 322 | 36 | 10 | 69 | 67 | 71 | 17 | 14 | n/a |
| 40 | <0.1 | 0 | 56 | 6 | 67 | n/a | <5 | 100 | 100 | 100 | 100 |
| 41 | 0.6 | 0 | 16 | 2 | 89 | 76 | 58 | 99 | 92 | 89 | 97 |
| 42 | 9.7 | 118 | 520 | 57 | 10 | n/a | 93 | 92 | 72 | 71 | 35 |
| 43 | <0.1 | 0 | 73 | 4 | n/a | n/a | 16 | n/a | n/a | n/a | n/a |
| 44 | <0.1 | 0 | 16 | 1 | 85 | 93 | 42 | 95 | 77 | 99 | 95 |
| 45 | 0.3 | 0 | 8 | 1 | ... | ... | 24 | 100 | 100 | 100 | 100 |
| 46 | <0.1 | 0 | 13 | 1 | 59 | 70 | <5 | n/a | n/a | n/a | n/a |
| 47 | 0.1 | 0 | 346 | 31 | n/a | 91 | 68 | 100 | 100 | 99 | 100 |
| 48 | 4.3 | 452 | 511 | 57 | n/a | 78 | >95 | 89 | 26 | 54 | 6 |
| 49 | 0.2 | 0 | 12 | 1 | ... | ... | <5 | 100 | 100 | n/a | n/a |
| 50 | 5.1 | 114 | 534 | 61 | 65 | 62 | 6 | 100 | 100 | 99 | 50 |
| 51 | 0.3 | 0 | 26 | 5 | ... | ... | <5 | 100 | 90 | 86 | 75 |
| 52 | 1.8 | 0 | 149 | 19 | 7 | 79 | 48 | 90 | 78 | 70 | 60 |
| 53 | 0.3 | 1 | 239 | 32 | 5 | n/a | 28 | 90 | 75 | 92 | 74 |
| 54 | <0.1 | 8 | 42 | 4 | 39 | 87 | 23 | 99 | 96 | 100 | 96 |
| 55 | 0.6 | 0 | 91 | 10 | 58 | 80 | 65 | 91 | 64 | 89 | 76 |

### Annex Table 7 Millennium Development Goals: selected health indicators in all WHO Member States, 2000 (unless specified)

Figures computed by WHO to assure comparability;[a] they are not necessarily the official statistics of Member States, which may use alternative rigorous methods

| | Member State | Children under five years of age underweight for age (%) | Year | Under-five mortality rate (per 1000 live births) | Infant mortality rate (per 1000 live births) | One-year-olds immunized against measles (%) (2001) | Maternal mortality ratio (per 100 000 live births) | Births attended by skilled health personnel (%) |
|---|---|---|---|---|---|---|---|---|
| 56 | Equatorial Guinea | n/a | n/a | 156 | 97 | 51 | 880 | n/a |
| 57 | Eritrea | 43.7 | 1995-96 | 112 | 65 | 84 | 630 | 20.6 |
| 58 | Estonia | n/a | n/a | 11 | 9 | 95 | 38 | n/a |
| 59 | Ethiopia | 47.2 | 2000 | 179 | 114 | 52 | 850 | 9.7 |
| 60 | Fiji | 7.9 | 1993 | 28 | 22 | 90 | 75 | n/a |
| 61 | Finland | n/a | n/a | 4 | 4 | 96 | 5 | n/a |
| 62 | France | n/a | n/a | 6 | 5 | 84 | 17 | n/a |
| 63 | Gabon | 11.9 | 2000-01 | 91 | 64 | 55 | 420 | 85.5 |
| 64 | Gambia | 17 | 2000 | 128 | 81 | 90 | 540 | 51 |
| 65 | Georgia | 3.1 | 1999 | 23 | 21 | 73 | 32 | 96.4 |
| 66 | Germany | n/a | n/a | 5 | 4 | 89 | 9 | n/a |
| 67 | Ghana | 24.9 | 1998-99 | 105 | 62 | 81 | 540 | 44.3 |
| 68 | Greece | n/a | n/a | 7 | 6 | 88 | 10 | n/a |
| 69 | Grenada | n/a | n/a | 23 | 17 | 96 | n/a | 100 |
| 70 | Guatemala | 24.2 | 1998-99 | 56 | 45 | 91 | 240 | 40.6 |
| 71 | Guinea | 23.2 | 1999 | 163 | 94 | 52 | 740 | 34.8 |
| 72 | Guinea-Bissau | 25 | 2000 | 215 | 128 | 48 | 1100 | 34.7 |
| 73 | Guyana | 13.6 | 2000 | 58 | 45 | 92 | 170 | 95 |
| 74 | Haiti | 17.3 | 2000 | 136 | 92 | 53 | 680 | 24.2 |
| 75 | Honduras | 16.6 | 2001 | 44 | 35 | 95 | 110 | 62 |
| 76 | Hungary | 2.2 | 1980-88 | 11 | 9 | 99 | 11 | n/a |
| 77 | Iceland | n/a | n/a | 3 | 3 | 88 | 0 | n/a |
| 78 | India | 46.7 | 1998-99 | 96 | 77 | 56 | 540 | 42.3 |
| 79 | Indonesia | 27.3 | 2002 | 50 | 39 | 76 | 230 | 55.8 |
| 80 | Iran, Islamic Republic of | 10.9 | 1998 | 45 | 36 | 96 | 76 | n/a |
| 81 | Iraq | 15.9 | 2000 | 118 | 93 | 90 | 250 | n/a |
| 82 | Ireland | n/a | n/a | 7 | 6 | 73 | 4 | n/a |
| 83 | Israel | n/a | n/a | 7 | 5 | 94 | 13 | n/a |
| 84 | Italy | 1.5 | 1975-77 | 6 | 5 | 70 | 5 | n/a |
| 85 | Jamaica | 3.8 | 1999 | 16 | 13 | 85 | 87 | 94.6 |
| 86 | Japan | 3.7 | 1978-81 | 5 | 3 | 98 | 10 | 100 |
| 87 | Jordan | 5.1 | 1997 | 28 | 25 | 99 | 41 | 96.7 |
| 88 | Kazakhstan | 4.2 | 1999 | 36 | 33 | 96 | 210 | 99.1 |
| 89 | Kenya | 21.2 | 2000 | 113 | 79 | 78 | 1000 | 44.3 |
| 90 | Kiribati | 12.9 | 1985 | 77 | 54 | 76 | n/a | 85 |
| 91 | Kuwait | 10.5 | 1994-95 | 11 | 9 | 99 | 12 | 98.2 |
| 92 | Kyrgyzstan | 11 | 1997 | 63 | 52 | 99 | 110 | 98.1 |
| 93 | Lao People's Democratic Republic | 40 | 2000 | 143 | 107 | 50 | 650 | 21.4 |
| 94 | Latvia | n/a | n/a | 14 | 12 | 98 | 61 | 100 |
| 95 | Lebanon | 3 | 1996 | 34 | 27 | 94 | 150 | 88 |
| 96 | Lesotho | 17.9 | 2000 | 149 | 94 | 70 | 550 | 59.7 |
| 97 | Liberia | 26.5 | 1999-00 | 232 | 136 | 78 | 760 | n/a |
| 98 | Libyan Arab Jamahiriya | 4.7 | 1995 | 20 | 16 | 93 | 97 | 94.4 |
| 99 | Lithuania | n/a | n/a | 11 | 9 | 97 | 19 | n/a |
| 100 | Luxembourg | n/a | n/a | 5 | 4 | 91 | 28 | n/a |
| 101 | Madagascar | 40 | 1997 | 139 | 89 | 55 | 550 | 47.3 |
| 102 | Malawi | 25.4 | 2000 | 197 | 117 | 82 | 1800 | 55.6 |
| 103 | Malaysia | 20.1 | 1995 | 10 | 8 | 92 | 41 | 96.2 |
| 104 | Maldives | 45 | 1997-98 | 50 | 37 | 99 | 110 | n/a |
| 105 | Mali | 33.2 | 2001 | 233 | 131 | 37 | 1200 | 23.7 |
| 106 | Malta | n/a | n/a | 7 | 6 | 65 | n/a | n/a |
| 107 | Marshall Islands | n/a | n/a | 44 | 32 | 89 | n/a | 94.9 |
| 108 | Mauritania | 31.8 | 2000-01 | 173 | 105 | 58 | 1000 | 40 |
| 109 | Mauritius | 14.9 | 1995 | 18 | 16 | 90 | 37 | n/a |
| 110 | Mexico | 7.5 | 1998-99 | 29 | 25 | 95 | 83 | 85.7 |

| | HIV prevalence among 15–49-year-olds (%) | Malaria mortality rate (per 100 000) | Tuberculosis prevalence (per 100 000) | Tuberculosis mortality rate (per 100 000) | Tuberculosis cases | | Population using solid fuels (%) | Population with sustainable access to an improved water source (%) | | Population with access to improved sanitation (%) | |
|---|---|---|---|---|---|---|---|---|---|---|---|
| | | | | | Detected under DOTS (2001) | Cured under DOTS | | Urban | Rural | Urban | Rural |
| 56 | 9.2 | 165 | 350 | 40 | … | … | 83 | 45 | 42 | 60 | 46 |
| 57 | 2.9 | 68 | 361 | 44 | 15 | 76 | >95 | 63 | 42 | 66 | 1 |
| 58 | 1.0 | 0 | 61 | 8 | 67 | 70 | 34 | n/a | n/a | 93 | n/a |
| 59 | 5.0 | 80 | 440 | 52 | 42 | 80 | >95 | 81 | 12 | 33 | 7 |
| 60 | <0.1 | 0 | 49 | 6 | 59 | 86 | <5 | 43 | 51 | 75 | 12 |
| 61 | <0.1 | 0 | 16 | 3 | … | … | <5 | 100 | 100 | 100 | 100 |
| 62 | 0.3 | 0 | 16 | 2 | … | … | <5 | n/a | n/a | n/a | n/a |
| 63 | 5.0 | 74 | 444 | 49 | … | … | 34 | 95 | 47 | 55 | 43 |
| 64 | 1.3 | 58 | 499 | 55 | … | … | >95 | 80 | 53 | 41 | 35 |
| 65 | <0.1 | 0 | 93 | 13 | 48 | 63 | 71 | 90 | 61 | 100 | 99 |
| 66 | 0.1 | 0 | 10 | 1 | 46 | 77 | <5 | n/a | n/a | n/a | n/a |
| 67 | 3.2 | 66 | 381 | 42 | 45 | 50 | 95 | 91 | 62 | 74 | 70 |
| 68 | 0.2 | 0 | 24 | 1 | … | … | <5 | n/a | n/a | n/a | n/a |
| 69 | 1.1 | 0 | 8 | 0 | … | … | <5 | 97 | 93 | 96 | 97 |
| 70 | 1.0 | 1 | 113 | 13 | 39 | 86 | 73 | 98 | 88 | 83 | 79 |
| 71 | 2.5 | 206 | 344 | 38 | … | … | >95 | 72 | 36 | 94 | 41 |
| 72 | 3.4 | 139 | 281 | 33 | … | … | 95 | 79 | 49 | 95 | 44 |
| 73 | 2.7 | 5 | 142 | 7 | 21 | 91 | <5 | 98 | 91 | 97 | 81 |
| 74 | 5.5 | 2 | 444 | 58 | 31 | 73 | 82 | 49[b] | 45[b] | 50[b] | 16[b] |
| 75 | 1.4 | 2 | 120 | 11 | 100 | 89 | 66 | 95 | 81 | 93 | 55 |
| 76 | <0.1 | 0 | 33 | 4 | 35 | 64 | 26 | 100 | 98 | 100 | 98 |
| 77 | 0.2 | 0 | 4 | 1 | 69 | n/a | <5 | n/a | n/a | n/a | n/a |
| 78 | 0.8 | 3 | 431 | 41 | 23 | 84 | 81 | 95 | 79 | 61 | 15 |
| 79 | <0.1 | 4 | 742 | 67 | 21 | 87 | 50 | 90 | 69 | 69 | 46 |
| 80 | <0.1 | 1 | 39 | 4 | 33 | 85 | <5 | 98 | 83 | 86 | 79 |
| 81 | <0.1 | 11 | 216 | 30 | 26 | 92 | <5 | 96 | 48 | 93 | 31 |
| 82 | 0.1 | 0 | 15 | 1 | … | … | <5 | n/a | n/a | n/a | n/a |
| 83 | 0.1 | 0 | 10 | 2 | 63 | n/a | <5 | n/a | n/a | n/a | n/a |
| 84 | 0.4 | 0 | 7 | 1 | 10 | 74 | <5 | n/a | n/a | n/a | n/a |
| 85 | 0.7 | 0 | 9 | 1 | 84 | 46 | 47 | 98 | 85 | 99 | 99 |
| 86 | <0.1 | 0 | 46 | 4 | 28 | 70 | <5 | n/a | n/a | n/a | n/a |
| 87 | <0.1 | 0 | 7 | 1 | 47 | 90 | 10 | 100 | 84 | 100 | 98 |
| 88 | <0.1 | 0 | 153 | 21 | 69 | 79 | 51 | 98 | 82 | 100 | 98 |
| 89 | 12.3 | 67 | 462 | 49 | 47 | 80 | 85 | 88 | 42 | 96 | 82 |
| 90 | <0.1 | 1 | 90 | 7 | n/a | 91 | <5 | 82 | 25 | 54 | 44 |
| 91 | <0.1 | 0 | 28 | 1 | … | … | <5 | n/a | n/a | n/a | n/a |
| 92 | <0.1 | 0 | 156 | 20 | n/a | 82 | >95 | 98 | 66 | 100 | 100 |
| 93 | <0.1 | 22 | 373 | 29 | 40 | 82 | 95 | 61 | 29 | 67 | 19 |
| 94 | 0.4 | 0 | 85 | 13 | 77 | 72 | 19 | n/a | n/a | n/a | n/a |
| 95 | <0.1 | 0 | 17 | 2 | 54 | 92 | <5 | 100 | 100 | 100 | 87 |
| 96 | 29.9 | 65 | 310 | 36 | … | … | 85 | 88 | 74 | 72 | 40 |
| 97 | 4.7 | 164 | 485 | 55 | … | … | 83 | n/a | n/a | n/a | n/a |
| 98 | 0.2 | 0 | 22 | 2 | … | … | <5 | 72 | 68 | 97 | 96 |
| 99 | <0.1 | 0 | 107 | 11 | 30 | 92 | 42 | n/a | n/a | n/a | n/a |
| 100 | 0.2 | 0 | 12 | 1 | 40 | n/a | <5 | n/a | n/a | n/a | n/a |
| 101 | 0.2 | 138 | 471 | 54 | 60 | 70 | >95 | 85 | 31 | 70 | 30 |
| 102 | 16.0 | 212 | 439 | 49 | 40 | 73 | >95 | 95 | 44 | 96 | 70 |
| 103 | 0.4 | 0 | 128 | 15 | … | … | 29 | n/a | 94 | n/a | 98 |
| 104 | <0.1 | 5 | 68 | 5 | 88 | 95 | <5 | 100 | 100 | 100 | 41 |
| 105 | 1.9 | 260 | 661 | 73 | … | … | >95 | 74 | 61 | 93 | 58 |
| 106 | 0.1 | 0 | 7 | 1 | 25 | 100 | <5 | 100 | 100 | 100 | 100 |
| 107 | <0.1 | 2 | 113 | 13 | 76 | 91 | <5 | n/a | n/a | n/a | n/a |
| 108 | 0.4 | 103 | 498 | 55 | … | … | 69 | 34 | 40 | 44 | 19 |
| 109 | 0.1 | 0 | 135 | 1 | 24 | 93 | 75 | 100 | 100 | 100 | 99 |
| 110 | 0.2 | 0 | 49 | 4 | 95 | 76 | 22 | 95 | 69 | 88 | 34 |

**Annex Table 7 Millennium Development Goals: selected health indicators in all WHO Member States, 2000 (unless specified)**

Figures computed by WHO to assure comparability;[a] they are not necessarily the official statistics of Member States, which may use alternative rigorous methods

| | Member State | Children under five years of age underweight for age (%) | Children under five years of age underweight for age Year | Under-five mortality rate (per 1000 live births) | Infant mortality rate (per 1000 live births) | One-year-olds immunized against measles (%) (2001) | Maternal mortality ratio (per 100 000 live births) | Births attended by skilled health personnel (%) |
|---|---|---|---|---|---|---|---|---|
| 111 | Micronesia, Federated States of | n/a | n/a | 60 | 47 | 84 | n/a | 92.8 |
| 112 | Monaco | n/a | n/a | 5 | 4 | 99 | n/a | n/a |
| 113 | Mongolia | 12.7 | 2000 | 79 | 57 | 95 | 110 | 96.6 |
| 114 | Morocco | 9.5 | 1992 | 46 | 38 | 96 | 220 | 39.6 |
| 115 | Mozambique | 26.1 | 1997 | 206 | 146 | 58 | 1000 | 44.2 |
| 116 | Myanmar | 35.3 | 2000 | 108 | 83 | 73 | 360 | 56.4 |
| 117 | Namibia | 24 | 1992 | 85 | 56 | 58 | 300 | 75.7 |
| 118 | Nauru | n/a | n/a | 16 | 11 | 95 | n/a | n/a |
| 119 | Nepal | 48.3 | 2001 | 95 | 72 | 71 | 740 | 11.9 |
| 120 | Netherlands | 0.7 | 1980 | 6 | 5 | 96 | 16 | 99.9 |
| 121 | New Zealand | n/a | n/a | 8 | 6 | 85 | 7 | 100 |
| 122 | Nicaragua | 9.6 | 2001 | 38 | 32 | 99 | 230 | 64.6 |
| 123 | Niger | 40.1 | 2000 | 255 | 122 | 51 | 1600 | 15.7 |
| 124 | Nigeria | 30.7 | 1999 | 183 | 103 | 40 | 800 | 41.6 |
| 125 | Niue | n/a | n/a | 28 | 22 | 99 | n/a | 100 |
| 126 | Norway | n/a | n/a | 5 | 4 | 93 | 10 | n/a |
| 127 | Oman | 17.8 | 1998 | 18 | 15 | 99 | 87 | 91 |
| 128 | Pakistan | 37.4 | 2001-02 | 110 | 86 | 57 | 500 | 20 |
| 129 | Palau | n/a | n/a | 24 | 20 | 91 | n/a | 100 |
| 130 | Panama | 8.1 | 1997 | 25 | 19 | 95 | 160 | 90 |
| 131 | Papua New Guinea | 29.9 | 1982-83 | 99 | 75 | 58 | 300 | 53.2 |
| 132 | Paraguay | 3.7 | 1990 | 33 | 26 | 77 | 170 | 58.1 |
| 133 | Peru | 7.1 | 2000 | 42 | 32 | 97 | 410 | 56.4 |
| 134 | Philippines | 31.8 | 1998 | 40 | 28 | 75 | 200 | 56.4 |
| 135 | Poland | n/a | n/a | 9 | 8 | 97 | 10 | n/a |
| 136 | Portugal | n/a | n/a | 7 | 6 | 87 | 8 | 99.7 |
| 137 | Qatar | 5.5 | 1995 | 15 | 14 | 92 | 7 | n/a |
| 138 | Republic of Korea | n/a | n/a | 7 | 5 | 97 | 20 | 100 |
| 139 | Republic of Moldova | n/a | n/a | 29 | 24 | 81 | 36 | 99.1 |
| 140 | Romania | 5.7 | 1991 | 22 | 19 | 98 | 58 | 97.9 |
| 141 | Russian Federation | n/a | n/a | 19 | 16 | 98 | 65 | n/a |
| 142 | Rwanda | 24.3 | 2000 | 182 | 111 | 69 | 1400 | 30.8 |
| 143 | Saint Kitts and Nevis | n/a | n/a | 22 | 18 | 94 | n/a | 100 |
| 144 | Saint Lucia | 13.8 | 1976 | 14 | 12 | 89 | n/a | 100 |
| 145 | Saint Vincent and the Grenadines | n/a | n/a | 23 | 19 | 98 | n/a | 100 |
| 146 | Samoa | n/a | n/a | 26 | 20 | 92 | n/a | 100 |
| 147 | San Marino | n/a | n/a | 5 | 5 | 74 | n/a | n/a |
| 148 | Sao Tome and Principe | 12.9 | 2000 | 90 | 59 | 75 | n/a | 86 |
| 149 | Saudi Arabia | n/a | n/a | 29 | 24 | 94 | 23 | 91.4 |
| 150 | Senegal | 22.7 | 2000 | 138 | 73 | 48 | 690 | 50.5 |
| 151 | Serbia and Montenegro | n/a | n/a | 15 | 13 | 90 | 9 | n/a |
| 152 | Seychelles | 5.7 | 1987-88 | 14 | 11 | 95 | n/a | n/a |
| 153 | Sierra Leone | 27.2 | 2000 | 316 | 181 | 53 | 2000 | 41.7 |
| 154 | Singapore | 2.9 | 2000 | 4 | 3 | 89 | 15 | 100 |
| 155 | Slovakia | n/a | n/a | 10 | 8 | 99 | 10 | n/a |
| 156 | Slovenia | n/a | n/a | 6 | 5 | 94 | 17 | n/a |
| 157 | Solomon Islands | 21.3 | 1989 | 81 | 65 | 78 | 130 | 85 |
| 158 | Somalia | 25.8 | 2000 | 219 | 130 | 36 | 1100 | 34.2 |
| 159 | South Africa | 9.2 | 1994-95 | 71 | 49 | 72 | 230 | 84.4 |
| 160 | Spain | n/a | n/a | 6 | 4 | 96 | 5 | n/a |
| 161 | Sri Lanka | 32.9 | 1995 | 20 | 16 | 99 | 92 | 94.1 |
| 162 | Sudan | 40.7 | 2000 | 110 | 71 | 67 | 590 | 86.3 |
| 163 | Suriname | 13.2 | 1999-00 | 31 | 24 | 90 | 110 | 84.5 |
| 164 | Swaziland | 10.3 | 2000 | 135 | 86 | 72 | 370 | 55.4 |
| 165 | Sweden | n/a | n/a | 4 | 3 | 94 | 8 | n/a |

| | HIV prevalence among 15–49-year-olds (%) | Malaria mortality rate (per 100 000) | Tuberculosis prevalence (per 100 000) | Tuberculosis mortality rate (per 100 000) | Tuberculosis cases | | Population using solid fuels (%) | Population with sustainable access to an improved water source (%) | | Population with access to improved sanitation (%) | |
|---|---|---|---|---|---|---|---|---|---|---|---|
| | | | | | Detected under DOTS (2001) | Cured under DOTS | | Urban | Rural | Urban | Rural |
| 111 | <0.1 | 1 | 116 | 13 | 17 | 93 | <5 | n/a | n/a | n/a | n/a |
| 112 | 0.5 | 0 | 3 | 0 | … | … | <5 | 100 | 100 | 100 | 100 |
| 113 | <0.1 | 0 | 305 | 38 | 73 | 87 | 67 | 77 | 30 | 46 | 2 |
| 114 | <0.1 | 3 | 104 | 11 | 81 | 89 | 11 | 98 | 56 | 86 | 44 |
| 115 | 11.9 | 263 | 473 | 52 | 68 | 75 | 87 | 81 | 41 | 68 | 26 |
| 116 | 0.9 | 15 | 255 | 33 | 59 | 82 | >95 | 89 | 66 | 84 | 57 |
| 117 | 20.8 | 39 | 411 | 45 | 98 | 53 | 83 | 100 | 67 | 96 | 17 |
| 118 | 0.4 | 0 | 52 | 4 | n/a | 25 | <5 | n/a | n/a | n/a | n/a |
| 119 | 0.3 | 20 | 299 | 27 | 60 | 86 | >95 | 94 | 87 | 73 | 22 |
| 120 | 0.2 | 0 | 7 | 1 | 56 | 76 | <5 | 100 | 100 | 100 | 100 |
| 121 | 0.1 | 0 | 8 | 1 | 37 | 30 | <5 | 100 | n/a | n/a | n/a |
| 122 | 0.2 | 1 | 96 | 10 | 94 | 83 | 72 | 91 | 59 | 95 | 72 |
| 123 | 1.7 | 329 | 330 | 37 | … | … | >95 | 70 | 56 | 79 | 5 |
| 124 | 5.7 | 209 | 491 | 54 | 16 | 79 | 67 | 78 | 49 | 66 | 45 |
| 125 | <0.1 | 0 | 67 | 7 | n/a | n/a | <5 | 100 | 100 | 100 | 100 |
| 126 | <0.1 | 0 | 8 | 1 | 50 | 70 | <5 | 100 | 100 | n/a | n/a |
| 127 | 0.1 | 1 | 13 | 1 | 100 | 93 | <5 | 41 | 30 | 98 | 61 |
| 128 | <0.1 | 9 | 415 | 48 | 6 | 75 | 76 | 95 | 87 | 95 | 43 |
| 129 | <0.1 | 0 | 180 | 13 | … | … | <5 | 100 | 20 | 100 | 100 |
| 130 | 0.6 | 0 | 65 | 6 | 71 | 67 | 37 | 99 | 79 | 99 | 83 |
| 131 | 0.3 | 17 | 648 | 57 | 9 | 63 | >95 | 88 | 32 | 92 | 80 |
| 132 | 0.3 | 0 | 112 | 13 | 5 | 77 | 64 | 93 | 59 | 94 | 93 |
| 133 | 0.4 | 0 | 275 | 26 | 95 | 90 | 40 | 87 | 62 | 79 | 49 |
| 134 | <0.1 | 1 | 582 | 61 | 58 | 88 | 85 | 91 | 79 | 93 | 69 |
| 135 | <0.1 | 0 | 55 | 3 | 3 | 72 | 37 | n/a | n/a | n/a | n/a |
| 136 | 0.5 | 0 | 41 | 4 | 84 | 79 | <5 | n/a | n/a | n/a | n/a |
| 137 | <0.1 | 0 | 69 | 6 | 100 | 66 | <5 | n/a | n/a | n/a | n/a |
| 138 | <0.1 | 0 | 140 | 10 | … | … | <5 | 97 | 71 | 76 | 4 |
| 139 | 0.2 | 0 | 213 | 17 | 37 | 83 | 72 | 97 | 88 | 100 | 98 |
| 140 | <0.1 | 0 | 189 | 10 | 11 | 80 | 45 | 91 | 16 | 86 | 10 |
| 141 | 0.7 | 0 | 170 | 21 | 5 | 68 | 7 | 100 | 96 | n/a | n/a |
| 142 | 7.0 | 186 | 500 | 55 | 32 | 61 | >95 | 60 | 40 | 12 | 8 |
| 143 | 0.3 | 0 | 23 | 4 | n/a | n/a | <5 | n/a | n/a | n/a | n/a |
| 144 | 0.3 | 0 | 30 | 4 | 55 | 100 | <5 | n/a | n/a | n/a | n/a |
| 145 | 1.7 | 0 | 42 | 1 | n/a | 100 | <5 | n/a | n/a | n/a | n/a |
| 146 | <0.1 | 1 | 42 | 5 | 50 | 92 | <5 | 95 | 100 | 95 | 100 |
| 147 | 0.3 | 0 | 7 | 0 | n/a | 0 | <5 | n/a | n/a | n/a | n/a |
| 148 | <0.1 | 57 | 299 | 33 | … | … | <5 | n/a | n/a | n/a | n/a |
| 149 | <0.1 | 4 | 61 | 5 | 40 | 73 | <5 | 100 | 64 | 100 | 100 |
| 150 | 0.8 | 71 | 416 | 46 | 85 | 52 | 79 | 92 | 65 | 94 | 48 |
| 151 | 0.2 | 0 | 65 | 4 | n/a | n/a | 70 | 99 | 97 | 100 | 99 |
| 152 | 0.1 | 3 | 60 | 1 | 77 | 82 | <5 | n/a | n/a | n/a | n/a |
| 153 | 2.0 | 321 | 573 | 63 | 39 | 77 | 92 | 75 | 46 | 88 | 53 |
| 154 | 0.2 | 0 | 28 | 3 | 21 | 85 | <5 | 100 | n/a | 100 | n/a |
| 155 | <0.1 | 0 | 34 | 1 | 38 | 82 | 24 | 100 | 100 | 100 | 100 |
| 156 | <0.1 | 0 | 23 | 1 | 68 | 84 | <5 | 100 | 100 | n/a | n/a |
| 157 | <0.1 | 1 | 111 | 13 | 67 | 81 | <5 | 94 | 65 | 98 | 18 |
| 158 | 0.7 | 82 | 747 | 115 | 32 | 83 | <5 | n/a | n/a | n/a | n/a |
| 159 | 19.6 | 0 | 483 | 46 | 72 | 66 | 28 | 99 | 73 | 93 | 80 |
| 160 | 0.5 | 0 | 33 | 1 | … | … | <5 | n/a | n/a | n/a | n/a |
| 161 | <0.1 | 6 | 97 | 9 | 74 | 77 | 89 | 98 | 70 | 97 | 93 |
| 162 | 3.0 | 70 | 363 | 53 | 35 | 79 | <5 | 86 | 69 | 87 | 48 |
| 163 | 1.3 | 2 | 111 | 13 | … | … | 69 | 93 | 50 | 99 | 75 |
| 164 | 31.2 | 0 | 856 | 92 | … | … | 88 | n/a | n/a | n/a | n/a |
| 165 | <0.1 | 0 | 5 | 1 | 54 | 80 | <5 | 100 | 100 | 100 | 100 |

**Annex Table 7 Millennium Development Goals: selected health indicators in all WHO Member States, 2000 (unless specified)**

Figures computed by WHO to assure comparability;[a] they are not necessarily the official statistics of Member States, which may use alternative rigorous methods

| | Member State | Children under five years of age underweight for age (%) | Year | Under-five mortality rate (per 1000 live births) | Infant mortality rate (per 1000 live births) | One-year-olds immunized against measles (%) (2001) | Maternal mortality ratio (per 100 000 live births) | Births attended by skilled health personnel (%) |
|---|---|---|---|---|---|---|---|---|
| 166 | Switzerland | n/a | n/a | 6 | 5 | 81 | 7 | n/a |
| 167 | Syrian Arab Republic | 6.9 | 2000 | 27 | 24 | 93 | 160 | 76 |
| 168 | Tajikistan | n/a | n/a | 63 | 51 | 86 | 100 | 76.8 |
| 169 | Thailand | 17.6 | 1995 | 31 | 27 | 94 | 44 | 85 |
| 170 | The former Yugoslav Republic of Macedonia | 5.9 | 1999 | 19 | 16 | 92 | 13 | n/a |
| 171 | Timor-Leste | 42.6 | 2003 | 126 | 88 | n/a | n/a | n/a |
| 172 | Togo | 25.1 | 1998 | 141 | 83 | 58 | 570 | 50.5 |
| 173 | Tonga | n/a | n/a | 21 | 17 | 93 | n/a | 92.1 |
| 174 | Trinidad and Tobago | 5.9 | 2000 | 21 | 18 | 91 | 110 | 99 |
| 175 | Tunisia | 4 | 2000 | 30 | 24 | 92 | 120 | 89.9 |
| 176 | Turkey | 8.3 | 1998 | 44 | 36 | 90 | 70 | 80.6 |
| 177 | Turkmenistan | 12 | 2000 | 59 | 51 | 98 | 31 | 97.2 |
| 178 | Tuvalu | n/a | n/a | 65 | 49 | 99 | n/a | 99 |
| 179 | Uganda | 22.8 | 2000-01 | 147 | 89 | 61 | 880 | 37.8 |
| 180 | Ukraine | 3.2 | 2000 | 21 | 16 | 99 | 38 | 99 |
| 181 | United Arab Emirates | n/a | n/a | 10 | 8 | 94 | 54 | 99.2 |
| 182 | United Kingdom | 1.3 | 2001 | 7 | 6 | 85 | 11 | 99 |
| 183 | United Republic of Tanzania | 29.4 | 1999 | 156 | 109 | 83 | 1500 | 35.8 |
| 184 | United States of America | 1.4 | 1988-94 | 9 | 7 | 91 | 14 | 99 |
| 185 | Uruguay | 4.4 | 1992-93 | 16 | 14 | 94 | 20 | 99 |
| 186 | Uzbekistan | 18.8 | 1996 | 36 | 30 | 99 | 24 | 96 |
| 187 | Vanuatu | 19.7 | 1983 | 44 | 35 | 94 | n/a | 89.1 |
| 188 | Venezuela, Bolivarian Republic of | 4.4 | 2000 | 23 | 19 | 98 | 78 | 95 |
| 189 | Viet Nam | 33.8 | 2000 | 39 | 31 | 97 | 130 | 69.6 |
| 190 | Yemen | 46.1 | 1997 | 110 | 86 | 79 | 570 | 22 |
| 191 | Zambia | 25 | 1999 | 185 | 111 | 85 | 750 | 46.5 |
| 192 | Zimbabwe | 13 | 1999 | 108 | 71 | 68 | 1100 | 72.5 |

[a] See explanatory notes for sources and methods.

[b] Estimates from the 1990s.

... Countries not implementing DOTs or not reporting to WHO.

n/a Data not available.

| | HIV prevalence among 15–49-year-olds (%) | Malaria mortality rate (per 100 000) | Tuberculosis prevalence (per 100 000) | Tuberculosis mortality rate (per 100 000) | Tuberculosis cases | | Population using solid fuels (%) | Population with sustainable access to an improved water source (%) | | Population with access to improved sanitation (%) | |
|---|---|---|---|---|---|---|---|---|---|---|---|
| | | | | | Detected under DOTS (2001) | Cured under DOTS | | Urban | Rural | Urban | Rural |
| 166 | 0.5 | 0 | 9 | 1 | … | … | <5 | 100 | 100 | 100 | 100 |
| 167 | <0.1 | 0 | 60 | 5 | 27 | 79 | 19 | 94 | 64 | 98 | 81 |
| 168 | <0.1 | 1 | 163 | 19 | … | … | >95 | 93 | 47 | 97 | 88 |
| 169 | 1.9 | 7 | 225 | 18 | 75 | 69 | 72 | 95 | 81 | 96 | 96 |
| 170 | <0.1 | 0 | 68 | 5 | 51 | 86 | 58 | n/a | n/a | n/a | n/a |
| 171 | <0.1 | 4 | 798 | 101 | n/a | n/a | >95 | n/a | n/a | n/a | n/a |
| 172 | 4.8 | 46 | 661 | 63 | … | … | >95 | 85 | 38 | 69 | 17 |
| 173 | <0.1 | 1 | 43 | 4 | 53 | 93 | <5 | 100 | 100 | n/a | n/a |
| 174 | 2.9 | 0 | 26 | 3 | … | … | <5 | n/a | n/a | n/a | n/a |
| 175 | <0.1 | 0 | 28 | 2 | 73 | 91 | 29 | 92 | 58 | 96 | 62 |
| 176 | <0.1 | 0 | 55 | 6 | … | … | 11 | 81 | 86 | 97 | 70 |
| 177 | <0.1 | 0 | 169 | 13 | 36 | 70 | 50 | n/a | n/a | n/a | n/a |
| 178 | <0.1 | 0 | 67 | 6 | … | … | <5 | 100 | 100 | 100 | 100 |
| 179 | 5.8 | 151 | 544 | 61 | 52 | 63 | >95 | 80 | 47 | 93 | 77 |
| 180 | 1.1 | 0 | 118 | 10 | n/a | n/a | 56 | 100 | 94 | 100 | 98 |
| 181 | 0.1 | 0 | 28 | 2 | 29 | 74 | <5 | n/a | n/a | n/a | n/a |
| 182 | 0.1 | 0 | 12 | 1 | … | … | <5 | 100 | 100 | 100 | 100 |
| 183 | 7.1 | 181 | 439 | 47 | 47 | 79 | >95 | 90 | 57 | 99 | 86 |
| 184 | 0.6 | 0 | 4 | 0 | 90 | 76 | <5 | 100 | 100 | 100 | 100 |
| 185 | 0.3 | 0 | 30 | 2 | 78 | 85 | <5 | 98 | 93 | 95 | 85 |
| 186 | <0.1 | 0 | 140 | 13 | 8 | 81 | 79 | 94 | 79 | 97 | 85 |
| 187 | <0.1 | 2 | 126 | 14 | 60 | 89 | <5 | 63 | 94 | 100 | 100 |
| 188 | 0.1 | 0 | 40 | 3 | 68 | 76 | <5 | 85 | 70 | 71 | 48 |
| 189 | 0.2 | 6 | 264 | 25 | 85 | 92 | >95 | 95 | 72 | 82 | 38 |
| 190 | 0.1 | 8 | 178 | 13 | 47 | 75 | 66 | 74 | 68 | 89 | 21 |
| 191 | 16.8 | 158 | 852 | 89 | … | … | 87 | 88 | 48 | 99 | 64 |
| 192 | 24.8 | 1 | 412 | 50 | 47 | n/a | 67 | 100 | 73 | 71 | 57 |

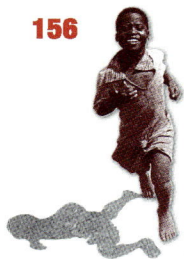

# List of Member States
## by WHO region and
## mortality stratum

To aid in cause-of-death and burden-of-disease analyses, the 192 Member States of the World Health Organization have been divided into five mortality strata on the basis of their levels of mortality in children under five years of age (5q0) and in males 15–59 years old (45q15). This classification was carried out using population estimates for 1999 (using United Nations Population Division data) and estimates of 5q0 and 45q15 based on WHO analyses of mortality rates for 1999.

Quintiles of the distribution of child mortality for both sexes combined (5q0) were used to define some countries as ***very low child mortality*** (1st quintile), some as ***low child mortality*** (2nd and 3rd quintiles) and others as ***high child mortality*** (4th and 5th quintiles). Adult mortality (the risk of death between ages 15 and 60 years, i.e. 45q15) was regressed on 5q0 and the regression line used to divide countries with high child mortality into ***high adult mortality*** (stratum D) and ***very high adult mortality*** (stratum E). Stratum E includes the countries in sub-Saharan Africa where HIV/AIDS has had a very substantial impact.

The adjacent table summarizes the five mortality strata. When these mortality strata are applied to the six WHO regions, they produce 14 subregions, which are used in the Annex Tables to present results. The WHO Member States in each region are grouped by subregion as listed opposite. This classification has no official status and is for analytical purposes only.

The total number of WHO Member States is 192, the latest addition being Timor-Leste, which is classified in the high-mortality developing region of Sear-D. In 2003, the Fifty-sixth World Health Assembly endorsed the reassignment of Cyprus to the European Region from the Eastern Mediterranean Region.

## Definitions of mortality strata used to define subregions

| Mortality stratum | Child mortality | Adult mortality |
|---|---|---|
| A | Very low | Very low |
| B | Low | Low |
| C | Low | High |
| D | High | High |
| E | High | Very high |

# WHO Member States, by region and mortality stratum

| Region and mortality stratum | Description | Broad grouping | Member States |
|---|---|---|---|
| **Africa** | | | |
| Afr-D | Africa with high child and high adult mortality | High-mortality developing | Algeria, Angola, Benin, Burkina Faso, Cameroon, Cape Verde, Chad, Comoros, Equatorial Guinea, Gabon, Gambia, Ghana, Guinea, Guinea-Bissau, Liberia, Madagascar, Mali, Mauritania, Mauritius, Niger, Nigeria, Sao Tome and Principe, Senegal, Seychelles, Sierra Leone, Togo |
| Afr-E | Africa with high child and very high adult mortality | High-mortality developing | Botswana, Burundi, Central African Republic, Congo, Côte d'Ivoire, Democratic Republic of the Congo, Eritrea, Ethiopia, Kenya, Lesotho, Malawi, Mozambique, Namibia, Rwanda, South Africa, Swaziland, Uganda, United Republic of Tanzania, Zambia, Zimbabwe |
| **Americas** | | | |
| Amr-A | Americas with very low child and very low adult mortality | Developed | Canada, Cuba, United States of America |
| Amr-B | Americas with low child and low adult mortality | Low-mortality developing | Antigua and Barbuda, Argentina, Bahamas, Barbados, Belize, Brazil, Chile, Colombia, Costa Rica, Dominica, Dominican Republic, El Salvador, Grenada, Guyana, Honduras, Jamaica, Mexico, Panama, Paraguay, Saint Kitts and Nevis, Saint Lucia, Saint Vincent and the Grenadines, Suriname, Trinidad and Tobago, Uruguay, Venezuela (Bolivarian Republic of) |
| Amr-D | Americas with high child and high adult mortality | High-mortality developing | Bolivia, Ecuador, Guatemala, Haiti, Nicaragua, Peru |
| **South-East Asia** | | | |
| Sear-B | South-East Asia with low child and low adult mortality | Low-mortality developing | Indonesia, Sri Lanka, Thailand |
| Sear-D | South-East Asia with high child and high adult mortality | High-mortality developing | Bangladesh, Bhutan, Democratic People's Republic of Korea, India, Maldives, Myanmar, Nepal, Timor-Leste |
| **Europe** | | | |
| Eur-A | Europe with very low child and very low adult mortality | Developed | Andorra, Austria, Belgium, Croatia, Cyprus, Czech Republic, Denmark, Finland, France, Germany, Greece, Iceland, Ireland, Israel, Italy, Luxembourg, Malta, Monaco, Netherlands, Norway, Portugal, San Marino, Slovenia, Spain, Sweden, Switzerland, United Kingdom |
| Eur-B | Europe with low child and low adult mortality | Developed | Albania, Armenia, Azerbaijan, Bosnia and Herzegovina, Bulgaria, Georgia, Kyrgyzstan, Poland, Romania, Serbia and Montenegro, Slovakia, Tajikistan, The former Yugoslav Republic of Macedonia, Turkey, Turkmenistan, Uzbekistan |
| Eur-C | Europe with low child and high adult mortality | Developed | Belarus, Estonia, Hungary, Kazakhstan, Latvia, Lithuania, Republic of Moldova, Russian Federation, Ukraine |
| **Eastern Mediterranean** | | | |
| Emr-B | Eastern Mediterranean with low child and low adult mortality | Low-mortality developing | Bahrain, Iran (Islamic Republic of), Jordan, Kuwait, Lebanon, Libyan Arab Jamahiriya, Oman, Qatar, Saudi Arabia, Syrian Arab Republic, Tunisia, United Arab Emirates |
| Emr-D | Eastern Mediterranean with high child and high adult mortality | High-mortality developing | Afghanistan, Djibouti, Egypt,[a] Iraq, Morocco, Pakistan, Somalia, Sudan, Yemen |
| **Western Pacific** | | | |
| Wpr-A | Western Pacific with very low child and very low adult mortality | Developed | Australia, Brunei Darussalam, Japan, New Zealand, Singapore |
| Wpr-B | Western Pacific with low child and low adult mortality | Low-mortality developing | Cambodia,[b] China, Cook Islands, Fiji, Kiribati, Lao People's Democratic Republic,[b] Malaysia, Marshall Islands, Micronesia (Federated States of), Mongolia, Nauru, Niue, Palau, Papua New Guinea,[b] Philippines, Republic of Korea, Samoa, Solomon Islands, Tonga, Tuvalu, Vanuatu, Viet Nam |

[a] Following improvements in child mortality over recent years, Egypt meets criteria for inclusion in subregion Emr-B with low child and low adult mortality. Egypt has been included in Emr-D for the presentation of subregional totals for mortality and burden to ensure comparability with previous editions of *The World Health Report* and other WHO publications.

[b] Although Cambodia, the Lao People's Democratic Republic, and Papua New Guinea meet criteria for high child mortality, they have been included in the Wpr-B subregion with other developing countries of the Western Pacific Region for reporting purposes.

# index

## A

## B



## C

# D

# E



# F



# G

# H

## I



## J



## K

# L



# M



# N

# S

# T



# U



# V

# W

waiting lists  35
water source, improved access to  108–109
western Africa, HIV prevalence  3
western Europe, incidence of sexually transmitted infections  4
WHO
    AIDS Medicines and Diagnostics Service  xiv, 24, 26
    collaborative assessment of child mortality levels  94
    Evidence and Information for Policy cluster  93
    guidance on ethical aspects  36, 37
    guidelines  17, 23, 26, 27
    Member States  156
    Multi-Country Survey Study (MCSS)  96
    responsibility for reporting on Millennium Development Goals  102
    Scientific Peer Review Group (SPRG)  97
    stewardship function  22
    support for 3 by 5 strategy  21, 25–27, 32
    working in partnership  xiii–xiv, xv–xvi, 22, 26, 39
William J. Clinton Foundation  xii, 30, 33, 67
women
    access to treatment  37
    discrimination against  84
    disproportionate risk of HIV/AIDS  1, 8–9
    effect of food insecurity  82
    obstacles to adherence  78
    protecting with microbicides  77
    risk of earlier death  5
Women Fighting AIDS in Kenya  46
women-led groups  46
World Bank  xii, xiv, 24, 85, 102
    Multi-Country HIV/AIDS Program  27, 28, 67
    reports  99
World Trade Organization  47
    Agreement on Trade-Related Aspects of Intellectual Property (TRIPS)  33

# Y

years of life lost (YLL)  96
years lost through disability (YLD)  96
young people, prevention programmes  13

# Z

Zambia
    antiretroviral drugs imported from Asia  33
    Chikankata faith-based district hospital  49
    health workers killed by AIDS  64
    HIV testing  5
    home-based care  60
    national commitment to 3 by 5 initiative  35
    teachers killed by AIDS  3
    WHO working in partnership  xiii
zidovudine, resistance  29
Zimbabwe
    adult mortality  6
    census and survey data  5
    HIV testing  5